Essential Paediatrics

Essential Paediatrics

David Hull
BSc, MB, FRCP, DObstRCOG, DCH
Professor of Child Health, University of Nottingham

Derek I. Johnston
MA, MD, FRCP, DCH
Consultant Paediatrician, University Hospital, Nottingham

Illustrated by Geoffrey Lyth BA

THIRD EDITION

CHURCHILL LIVINGSTONE
EDINBURGH, LONDON, MADRID, MELBOURNE, NEW YORK AND TOKYO 1993

CHURCHILL LIVINGSTONE
Medical Division of Longman Group UK Limited

Distributed in the United States of America by
Churchill Livingstone Inc., 650 Avenue of the Americas, New York,
N.Y. 10011, and by associated companies, branches and
representatives throughout the world.

First published 1981
    Reprinted 1981
    Reprinted 1982
    Reprinted 1984
    Reprinted 1986
Second edition 1987
    Reprinted 1988
    Reprinted 1990
Third edition 1993

ISBN 0-443-04782-0

British Library Cataloguing Data

A catalogue record for this book is available from
the British Library.

Produced by Longman Singapore Publishers (Pte) Ltd.
Printed in Singapore

Preface

The main objective of each edition of *Essential Paediatrics* has been to provide medical students with an introduction to paediatrics which is sufficiently comprehensive and yet compatible with the brief time set aside for this purpose in their clinical course. We hope that it will also assist other health professionals who require easy access to the core of paediatric knowledge. Emphasis is given to common disorders, and to appreciating the importance of priority when considering differential diagnosis and management.

The maturation of *Essential Paediatrics* over three editions has had some parallels with the developing child. The anxieties of the gestation and birth are receding into the past, and we have watched its passage through the first decade with the usual blend of parental pride and concern. An extended family of contributors, students and reviewers has continued to counsel us on faults and scope for improvement. This new edition has given us the opportunity to follow this advice, and plan for substantial revision with the incorporation of much fresh material, a new format and greater use of colour. We particularly welcome our new contributors who have already had a much valued impact on the Nottingham teaching programme. This programme, incorporating community and hospital children's services, remains the infrastructure on which the text is based.

No book is an alternative to clinical experience acquired by talking to and examining children, and discussing their problems with parents. We hope that by providing a text that covers most aspects of paediatric practice, readers will feel more confident about approaching sick children and anxious families. It is in the interest of all of us that we generate an enduring enthusiasm for the care of children.

Once again we are indebted to our contributors who have worked so hard to bring sections up to date while retaining relevance and balance. This rebirth has been made possible by the skill of Mrs Kath Walter who has, with her usual proficiency, taken in her stride all the advances and confusion created by word-processing technology.

Nottingham, 1993

D.H.
D.I.J.

Acknowledgement

Many of the colour illustrations in the Dermatology chapter were reproduced by kind permission from Churchill Livingstone's Colour Guide series: Thomas R & Harvey D: Neonatology; Thomas R & Harvey D: Paediatrics; Wilkinson J D, Shaw S, Fenton DS: Dermatology.

Contributors

Peter R. H. Barbor
BA, MB, BChir, FRCP
Consultant Paediatrician, University Hospital, Nottingham

David A. Curnock
MA, MB, BChir, FRCP, DCH, DObstRCOG
Consultant Paediatrician, City Hospital, Nottingham

E. Joan Hiller
BSc, MB, BS, FRCP, DObstRCOG
Consultant Paediatrician, City Hospital, Nottingham

Leela Kapila
MB, BS, FRCS
Consultant Paediatric Surgeon, University and City Hospitals, Nottingham

David H. Mellor
MD, FRCP, DCH
Consultant Paediatric Neurologist, University and City Hospitals, Nottingham

John B. Pearce
MB, BS, MPhil, MRCP, FRCPsych
Professor of Child and Adolescent Psychiatry, University of Nottingham

Constance R. Pullan
MD, FRCP
Consultant Paediatrician (Community Child Health), Nottingham

Nicholas Rutter
BA, MD, FRCP
Reader in Child Health and Honorary Consultant Paediatrician,
University of Nottingham

Terence J. Stephenson
BSc, BM, BCh, MRCP
Senior Lecturer in Child Health and Honorary Consultant Paediatrician,
University of Nottingham

Helen Venning
BMedSci, BM, BS, MRCP
Consultant Paediatrician (Community Child Health), Nottingham

Alan R. Watson
MB, ChB, FRCP
Consultant Paediatric Nephrologist, City Hospital, Nottingham

David Walker
BMedSci, BM, BS, MRCP
Senior Lecturer in Paediatric Oncology and Honorary Consultant Paediatrician,
University of Nottingham

Ian D. Young
MD, MSc, FRCP
Consultant Clinical Geneticist, City Hospital, Nottingham

Contents

Editors' note

For ease of reading, the masculine gender is used throughout this book, except where obviously inappropriate, but the feminine is intended to be equally applicable.

The Ill Child and his Doctor

In paediatric practice it is not possible to make a full diagnosis or draw up an appropriate care programme without some knowledge of the child, his age, size, abilities and personality. Furthermore, a child is part of a family; to understand him one must know something of his family, his parents, their life styles, their family life, their capacity to look after their children and in particular their relationships to our patient and attitudes towards his illness. Families live in communities and as the child grows older and becomes more independent he relates more directly to the community, to his school and his peers. Thus, it is helpful to know the main features of that community and the child's and family's relationship to it. The mode of presentation, the symptoms and even the signs of disease may be influenced by the nature of the child, his family and their surroundings and experiences. Likewise, treatment will depend on the reserves and resources of the family and community.

THE INTERVIEW

First impressions are important. Even very young children are quick to sense an atmosphere and the reactions of their parents to it. As they grow older they become expert at masking their feelings. In uncertain situations they are more likely to demonstrate what they think by actions rather than words. They will look to and reach for those they trust. Children, not unlike adults, warm to those who like and admire them, and they are less suspicious than adults of ulterior motives. A relaxed, friendly beginning to the interview not only eases its passage, but is essential for its success.

Establishing trust

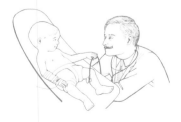

It is a matter of sensitivity and judgement to know how to make the first introductions. In the UK shaking hands is probably right for most parents but not for most children. It is impolite not to know the child's name and what he would like to be called. All Susans do not like to be called 'Suzie'. The sex of the child is not always evident from appearances. Sometimes the dress and hair style may be very misleading and you may wonder why. Even under such circumstances, to call a boy 'she' is a mistake. His mother will not like it and neither will he if he is

The interview

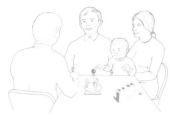

old enough to understand. Never refer to the baby as 'it'. Next ascertain the names and the relationship to the child of the adults who accompany him. Children belong to their parents, parents are responsible for their children so it is the parents' point of view that, in the first instance, you want to know. Not infrequently parents differ in their interpretation of their child's symptoms and signs. Neither parent has a monopoly on objectivity. Sometimes an unaccompanied mother will say, referring to her husband, that 'he disagrees with me and says I fuss too much', or alternatively that 'he told me to bring the child along because he is not right'. Some grandparents are a tremendous support to their children when they start their own families but others tend to be interfering busy bodies. The latter, if they are present at the interview, should be encouraged not to interrupt or enlarge upon the history given by the parents, though their attempts to do so may help in understanding the total situation.

The ability and willingness of children to describe their own symptoms varies widely. If in doubt always ask. It is instructive, for example, to find out why the child thinks he has been brought to see you. The answers are often revealing if not too helpful with the diagnosis. Another very important question, possibly best asked at the end of the interview, is what does the child and what do the parents think is the cause of the child's illness? In particular, what do they fear it might be?

In the main, children are not interested in adult talk so as the interview gets underway the majority of the younger ones will become restless and seek ways of entertaining themselves; but never make the mistake of thinking that they are not listening to what is being said. Toys for every age group should be scattered on the desk, shelves and floor. Play will not only occupy the youngster, it will also give valuable clues to his motor skills, mental abilities, interests and personality. So whilst taking the history watch the child. In particular, watch the way he moves, how he uses his eyes and ears and hands and feet. Does he follow up a challenge? Is he constructive? Is he relaxed? Watch the interplay between the child and his parents, and the child and yourself. It will not only help interpret the history but also give some indication of how best to examine the child later to get the most information. For

Suggested types of toys to have on hand

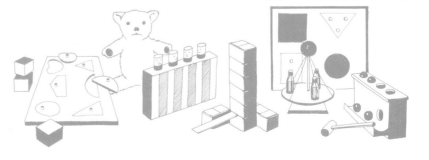

example, if a 4-year-old stays on his mother's knee and demands that the toys be brought to him, he is obviously feeling very threatened or is limited either by his illness or in his abilities. In these circumstances it is probably wisest to make the preliminary examination at least, whilst the child is on his mother's knee. Know something about the toys in the room; for example, at what stage can a child be expected to put a square block in a square hole, or to lift it out to find pictures underneath, or to name what he sees. If he does not do it you have not learnt much – it might be simply because of the situation – but if he does you may have learnt a great deal.

History

Every doctor develops his or her own way of collecting information. It is best to start by noting the main complaint or complaints. If there are a number, then a simple opening problem list helps. Then enlarge and define each problem and enquire about associated problems. An obsessional enquiry about all the bodily functions is not usually necessary, it wastes time and may interrupt the flow of the interview. However for most medical problems, and always for any child admitted to hospital, certain background information is essential.

Firstly, it is important to collect information about the child's own life. Was the pregnancy, labour and birth normal? What was the birth weight? How was he in the first days of life? It may be important to note whether he was breast or bottle fed and when he was weaned. Has he had the common childhood infections? Has he been immunised? Has he been treated in hospital and, if so, when and where and for what?

Secondly, an assessment should be made as to how the child is progressing. Full assessment of motor and language achievement and mental and social responses demands considerable skill and experience. However, for most purposes a simple enquiry about the principal stages of development is all that is required and should be within the competence of anyone presuming to advise parents about the care of their children. Plot on the charts of normal development what his parents say he can do — and they are usually right — and what he is observed to do in clinic. For the older child, ask about progress at school. It is not acceptable to make a note that the child is slow or retarded without

Steps in development?

 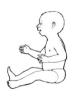 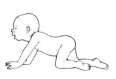

Lifts head clear
of ground

Sits with
support

Sits on
own

Crawling

Stages in development

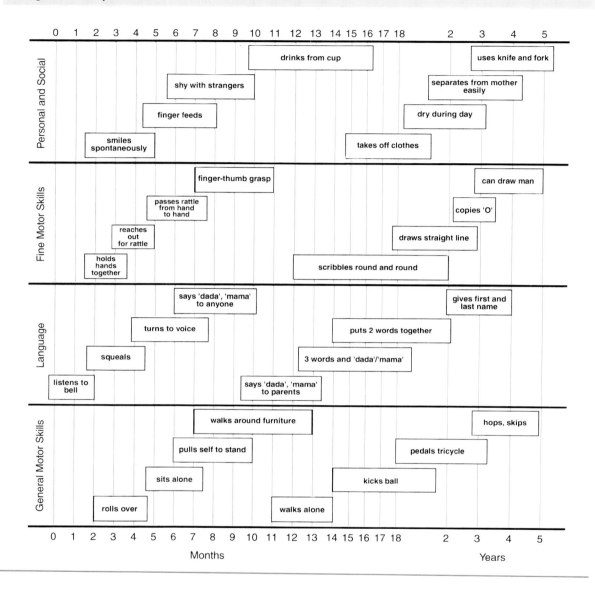

indicating the basis for that conclusion. Indeed, labels of that nature are best avoided altogether. If a child is not speaking at three years of age, write that he has delayed speech, but do not guess at the likely cause, even if, for instance, his mother appears not to understand even your simplest questions.

Always ask about the health of the rest of the family. This is important for a variety of reasons. The first, and perhaps the most obvious, is that the child might have an inherited disorder. Collect the information carefully and record it using accepted symbols and notation (see Ch. 2).

Secondly, if environmental factors are important, then other members of the family may also be affected. This might include anything from respiratory infections to the inhalation of lead. Thirdly, the presence of chronic illness in other members of the family may be the reason why the parents are concerned about the child before you. It may be that the family's stress has helped precipitate the child's problems. The fourth, though not the most important, is probably the most interesting reason. There are often family complaints, headaches, stomach aches, weariness, which determine the family language of disease and colour the way the child and his parents interpret his symptoms and signs. This will be particularly so if there is a strong behavioural component to his problem.

Examination

Examining children can be fun, but it may involve games when you do not want to play, and occasionally it can be singularly frustrating. Children, even the smallest infants, will try and work out your intentions by looking into your eyes. People with kind eyes do not mean to hurt! The parents may be more nervous about what you might do than the child himself, so they need reassurance as well. Some parents attempt to comfort their child by telling him not to worry 'the doctor won't hurt you'. Up until that time it may not have entered his head that you might, so be prepared for the protests. Some mothers may say such things in an attempt to put you off any examination which might be uncomfortable or embarrassing. Always encourage the parents to help you with the examination by holding or distracting the child, unless, of course, the youngster is approaching puberty when his independence is to be respected.

Clinicians have different practices about clothes. Undressing disturbs babies and they do not like it. Older infants hold onto their clothes as a protection, so they may object to their removal. From three years onwards there is usually no problem until puberty. Then the youngster must be handled with all the care and sensitivity you would extend to royalty! So it can be very useful to make observations whilst the child is clothed and undisturbed. Palpation and auscultation can easily be performed through vest and pants. On the other hand, some babies and children will remain undisturbed and, indeed, may expect you to undress them, and you can learn a great deal by the handling involved. It is a form of palpation which the children understand and further palpation afterwards is usually acceptable. But if the child shows uncertainty ask the parents to undress him. Even the most defensive child is usually happy for you to observe him naked from a distance.

Although the collection of the information may be disorderly, its recording in the notes must not be. In most situations it is important to record aspects of the child's size. Weight and length or height must be measured accurately. In certain situations, skull circumference and very occasionally skin fold thicknesses may also be measured. The data is recorded in the notes and on the appropriate charts.

Note the child's general behaviour and awareness. You may wish to make your own evaluation of the child's capabilities and record them with the parents' reports of his achievements.

Next, observe the child. Much of the information you seek may be obtained by careful observation. In general terms, is his appearance at all unusual? If so, try to define why: is it the shape of his head, the mould of his ears, the position of his eyes, his bodily proportions or the posture? Does he look like his parents? Has he got any of the recognised major or minor anomalies?

Then specifically assess his general size, proportions and nutritional state. Note the nature and distribution of any skin lesions or rashes. Then examine the system or systems that are the source of the complaint.

Respiratory disorders are often most easily observed. Avoid percussion or auscultation until you have noted the respiratory rate and the movement of the diaphragm and chest wall with quiet breathing and the effect of a stronger respiratory effort performed on request in an older child, or with a cry in a baby.

Determine whether or not the lung is over-inflated by percussion of the upper edge of the liver.

Listen to the heart

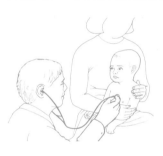

Interpretation of breath sounds and additional noises can be difficult in the very young. Fine crackling noises on inspiration (crepitations) may be heard on careful auscultation in apparently normal babies. If they are persistent and bilateral in a distressed toddler they usually indicate bronchiolitis or, very rarely, left heart failure. Coarse intermittent noises during both inspiration and expiration (rales) usually signify liquid debris in the larger airways. They may be transmitted from the back of the throat. Harsh and more persistent noises superadded on the breath sounds (rhonchi), indicating a more persistent obstruction, are less frequently heard in children. Continuous noises, hardening and extending the breath sounds (bronchial breathing) may be heard in babies over most of the upper back, and usually are transmitted sounds from the main airway. When the airway is partially obstructed the noise becomes harsher and more vibrant and is called a stridor. This term covers a wide range of sounds, some fine and high pitched, some low and coarse. The character depends on the site, the nature of the obstruction and the narrowness of the aperture. Wheezing is heard when the mid airways are narrowed; always check if it is bilateral.

Percuss the liver

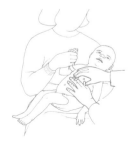

Examination of the cardiovascular system begins by recording the rate, rhythm, strength and character of the peripheral pulses. Palpate and percuss the anterior chest wall to determine the heart size, the site and nature of the apex beat and to detect the presence, if any, of a thrill. Then listen to the first heart sound, then the second, then the sounds in between and then the murmurs between the heart sounds. For each murmur you will wish to know its timing, character, loudness, site and distribution. Check if it is transmitted into the neck.

Always observe the abdomen before you palpate. Look for swellings and movements. Ask if anywhere is tender, and if you can, watch the child's face and not his abdomen whilst you palpate. After general palpation in the four quadrants, systematically determine the position and size of the liver, spleen, kidneys and bladder. If an organ is enlarged, note its position, size, surface and texture, the character of the edge if it

Palpate the fontanelle

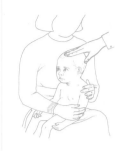

Look at the ear drum

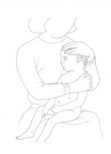

has one, and whether or not it is tender. When examining the back of the chest, look at the spine, particularly the lower end.

Again, examination of the locomotor and nervous systems is more by observation than manipulation. In babies and infants always palpate the anterior fontanelle or head 'soft spot'. It usually closes in the middle of the second year.

Note if it is pulsating: it usually does. You can record the heart rate from it. The fontanelle may be full or flat. Ask yourself the following questions: Can the child see? Can he hear? Does he move his eyes and head well and in all directions? Does he move all limbs, is the movement normal and full? Is the contour and position of each limb normal? Is the power good? When you handle the infant, note the tone on passive movement of the limb. Is there any limitation in the movement at any joint? Are the joints unduly lax and hyperextendable? Again, watch the child's face whilst you move his limbs. Eliciting the reflex responses rarely adds useful information in children but it is as well to keep up the habit for the odd occasion when it does. In the infant the percussing finger can be used as the hammer.

Finally, examine with the light. If necessary, check the eyes and then the ear drums and finally the throat. Never force yourself upon the child. Never force his mouth open against his will: be patient. Ask yourself, is the information you wish to gather as important as all that? Why use a nasty dry stick to depress the tongue when a smooth teaspoon handle will do just as well, and spoons are meant to go into mouths anyway.

Before you finish, should you bother to record the blood pressure? If disease of the kidney or heart is suspected, the answer is yes.

This completes the general examination. During it you may have included specific observations or examinations, for example, to see if the testes are in the scrotum, femoral pulses are present, the hips in joint, the characteristic of unusual lumps, the presence of the signs of puberty, etc.

Once the clinical enquiry is complete the next step is to re-examine the initial list of problems; some may be easily dealt with by appropriate advice, on the other hand new problems may have arisen. Draw up a new list and indicate what steps by way of further enquiry, investigation or treatment you propose to follow, and discuss these with the parents and to the extent that he may understand it, with your patient.

THE PROBLEMS

Every week a practising paediatrician sees a condition, anomaly, or a sign that he has never seen before and in such a situation his actions depend on his basic scientific knowledge. Every month he will treat a condition which is known but rare, then he relies on colleagues who have reported their observations in the medical literature. However, the substance of a doctor's practice is with diseases he has seen before, and his management of these problems will be influenced as much by his own previous experience and by his knowledge of his own patients and their community, as it is by therapies recommended in textbooks. What are these common problems? Obviously, this will vary from place to place and from community to community, and on whether the doctor works in family practice, child health clinic, or district hospital.

Family practice

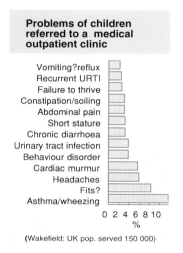

Problems of children referred to a medical outpatient clinic

Vomiting?reflux
Recurrent URTI
Failure to thrive
Constipation/soiling
Abdominal pain
Short stature
Chronic diarrhoea
Urinary tract infection
Behaviour disorder
Cardiac murmur
Headaches
Fits?
Asthma/wheezing

0 2 4 6 8 10
%

(Wakefield: UK pop. served 150 000)

If we assume that each family doctor has about 2500 people in his practice — in the UK the average is a little less — then with a birth rate running at 12.0 births per 1000 population, there will be 30 births in the practice each year and 450 child patients spread between 0 and 15 years of age. Between 15 and 20 per cent of the family doctor's work is with children. Disorders of the respiratory system are by far the commonest, followed by skin conditions, infectious diseases, gastrointestinal disorders, problems with eyes, ears and teeth. Social and administrative problems form the bulk of the remainder. Only 10 per cent of children's disorders are judged to be serious and in need of specific therapy, though it is likely that medicine will be prescribed in over half the cases.

Only occasionally will an individual family doctor have to care for a child with some of the conditions which are often seen in hospital. Thus, on average, a family doctor will see a child presenting with mental retardation, diabetes or epilepsy every five years or so, a child with Down syndrome every 20 years, cystic fibrosis every 40 years and muscular dystrophy every 480 years!

Hospital service

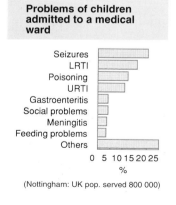

Problems of children admitted to a medical ward

Seizures
LRTI
Poisoning
URTI
Gastroenteritis
Social problems
Meningitis
Feeding problems
Others

0 5 10 15 20 25
%

(Nottingham: UK pop. served 800 000)

Children who fall ill suddenly are usually brought directly to the hospital emergency and accident department. Over half of the children admitted to hospital are brought by their parents directly to hospital. Here the conditions commonly seen are home and road accidents, accidental poisoning, acute respiratory illness, fevers, convulsions and acute bowel upsets.

Patients referred to the Paediatric consultancy service usually have less acute conditions. The commoner problems include recurrent respiratory infections, asthma, failure to thrive, small size, suspected developmental delay, convulsions or suspected convulsions, nocturnal enuresis and constipation. There are usually special clinics for children with chronic illnesses, for example for children with diabetes, leukaemia, neurology, short stature, cystic fibrosis and renal disorders. Children with physical and mental handicaps are assessed in a special developmental assessment unit by a team which includes physiotherapists, occupational therapists, psychologists, teachers, audiometricians as well as doctors from various disciplines.

Child health service

Many family doctors work in group practices in health centres. Working with them in the primary care team are health visitors. In some centres one doctor in the group, with the health visitors, holds regular child health clinics in order to examine routinely every child and provides a preventive health service. In others a special clinical medical officer attends the clinic. Healthy babies are examined routinely at six weeks of age and then at regular intervals afterwards. The predominant problems in the early months are related to feeding, nutrition, bowels and general growth and development. Hearing is assessed at 6 to 9 months of age. The infants are examined for vision abnormalities and the development of squints. The clinics also have responsibilities for the immunisation programme and health education. After the age of five years surveillance is continued by the school health services.

Child health surveillance programme: see Appendix A (p. 338) for details

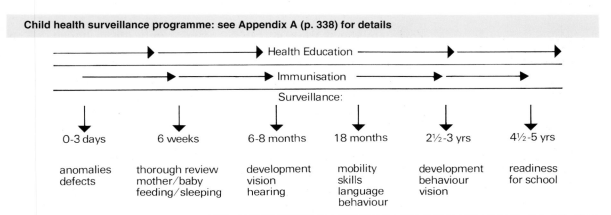

0-3 days	6 weeks	6-8 months	18 months	2½-3 yrs	4½-5 yrs
anomalies defects	thorough review mother/baby feeding/sleeping	development vision hearing	mobility skills language behaviour	development behaviour vision	readiness for school

Social paediatrics

The distribution of health problems differs across the town. Certain inner city areas, deprived by most material and social standards, have a higher incidence of most medical problems and the children who live there are, in general, less physically, mentally and socially able. At a disadvantage from birth, these children 'born to fail', are less able to form secure relationships and thus are themselves less likely to establish a strong family environment for their own children. Breaking this circle of events is one of the major tasks of community paediatric care. It is a challenge that the health service staff share with social workers and teachers.

Association between social factors and child abuse, deaths, and mental retardation (population study from Mansfield area, data drom Dr C Maddock and colleagues)

Social risk factor	Population (%)	Abuse/1000	Inevitable deaths/1000	Possible preventable deaths/1000	Moderate retardation /1000	Severe retardation /1000
0	60	1.8	0.8	1.1	1.4	1.5
1	30	5.8	0.3	2.1	5.5	1.8
2	7	35.1	5.2	3.9	18.2	3.9
3	2	50.9	9.2	18.5	37.0	13.9
4/5	1	135.6	16.9	33.9	84.7	33.9
Total	100	7.1	1.2	2.1	5.0	2.2

Perinatal mortality. Happily, infant and child mortality rates continue to fall. The rates are highest for the very young. Around 30 per cent of neonatal deaths are due to congenital abnormalities incompatible with independent life, and over 40 per cent are very immature and even with artificial respiratory and nutritional support do not survive the first few days after birth. Improvements in general health, antenatal care, and appropriate genetic counselling may accelerate the fall in the perinatal mortality rate.

Post-neonatal mortality. Older infants rarely die in hospital. The majority of children dying between four weeks and one year, post-neonatal infant deaths, die suddenly at home. The 'sudden infant death syndrome' (SID) or 'cot death' has received considerable attention. In many infants who die suddenly at home, nothing abnormal is found at post mortem. It is less common in cultures which nurse babies on their backs, so now in the UK mothers are advised not to lie their infants on their fronts. Some consider that SID might be due to a confusion in respiratory control precipitated by a respiratory infection or unexpected regurgitation. Another possiblity is that the infants over-react to a fever, or are unable to lose heat and that hyperpyrexia is an important factor. Some of the infants who die unexpectedly do have evidence of known disease, or non-specific signs of illness at autopsy. A small percentage (under 5 per cent?) have been found to be due to an inherited metabolic disorder. Some studies suggest that as many as 10 per cent are due to 'gentle smothering', that the parents had acted against their infant.

The incidence is higher in families living in poor housing, when the parents are inexperienced or of limited ability, or when there is domestic stress. Early infant death occurs more often in babies born prematurely or experiencing problems in the newborn period. These characteristics can be identified at birth and if the families are given extra advice and support during the early months the number of post-neonatal infant deaths can be reduced.

Deaths over 1 year of age. An unexpected death of a child over the age of one year is rare. Many are due to accidents; others are due to previously diagnosed malignancies. The remainder include children with inherited diseases, for example, cystic fibrosis, muscular dystrophies, and progressive encephalopathies. Acute infections, which used to be a major cause of death, are usually controllable; but occasionally the onset can be so sudden and death follows so quickly that therapeutic measure cannot be introduced in time, for example in meningitis with septicaemia or an intravascular coagulopathy, severe gastroenteritis, acute epiglottitis and fulminating respiratory infections.

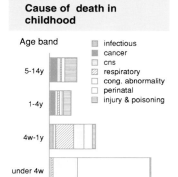

Cause of death in childhood

Age band

- infectious
- cancer
- cns
- respiratory
- cong. abnormality
- perinatal
- injury & poisoning

5-14y

1-4y

4w-1y

under 4w

0   50 100 150 200 250 300

Numbers in Trent Health Region
1983-7

BIBLIOGRAPHY

Committee on Child Health Services 1976 Fit for the future. Report Cmnd 6684,
    Chairman Court S D M. HMSO, London
Forfar B P A (ed) 1988 Child health in society. Oxford University Press, Oxford
Hicks D 1976 Primary health care — a review. HMSO, London
Inequalities in health 1988 (includes the Black Report and the Health Divide). Penguin
    Books, Harmonsworth
MacFaul R 1991 Paediatric outpatient audit study (internal report). British Paediatric
    Association, London
Nottinghamshire County Council 1983. The country deprived area study.
    Nottinghamshire County Council, Nottingham
Polnay L, Hull D (eds) 1993 Community paediatrics, 2nd edn. Churchill Livingstone,
    Edinburgh (in press)
Smith R (ed) 1991 The health of the nation. BMJ, London

Genes

Notation

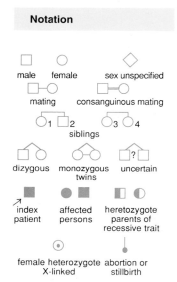

male   female   sex unspecified

mating   consanguinous mating

siblings 1 2 3 4

dizygous   monozygous twins   uncertain

index patient   affected persons   heretozygote parents of recessive trait

female heterozygote X-linked   abortion or stillbirth

Genetic defects may become apparent at any age from conception to senescence, but it is in childhood that inherited disorders make their greatest impact. Approximately 1 in 40 of all babies has a major malformation identifiable at birth and in over half of these infants genetic factors can be implicated. Inherited disorders also account for 50 per cent of all cases of childhood blindness and deafness, and together with congenital malformations are responsible for 25–30 per cent of all hospital admissions and deaths occurring in the paediatric age group.

As a result of continuing progress in obstetrics, community paediatrics and the treatment of both infection and cancer, it is likely that the relative contribution of genetic disease to childhood morbidity and mortality will increase, in parallel with the general public's knowledge of genetics and expectations of good health. Recognition of the importance of genetic disorders in childhood has coincided with a scientific explosion in molecular biology, which has revolutionised understanding of the mechanisms of inheritance and opened up new avenues for the prevention and sometimes the treatment of inherited disease.

CHROMOSOMES AND CHROMOSOME ABNORMALITIES

Genes consist of DNA and are tightly packaged in chromosomes which are present in all nucleated cells. Electron microscopy reveals that the DNA is coiled around histone proteins, the precise function of which is unclear. Normally, each cell contains 46 chromosomes comprising 22 pairs of autosomes and a single pair of sex chromosomes, XY in the male and XX in the female. During meiosis I each pair separates so that each gamete receives a single 'haploid' set consisting of 24 chromosomes. Successful fertilisation results in restitution of the normal 'diploid' complement of 46 chromosomes.

Whereas genes cannot be directly visualised, it is possible to detect alterations in both the number and structure of human chromosomes using a high powered light microscope. Peripheral blood lymphocytes or skin fibroblasts can be cultured in the laboratory. Cell division is arrested during metaphase, the stage of maximum chromosome condensation. The cell nuclei are then swollen by adding a hypotonic solution which separates the individual chromosomes and renders them readily visible by light microscopy. The chromosomes are then stained to facilitate their individual identification and subsequent analysis. The overall chromosome constitution is known as a karyotype and can be illustrated by photographing the metaphase spread down the microscope and then arranging the chromosomes in matching pairs in descending order of size. Normally it takes at least 3 days to obtain a satisfactory chromosome analysis using circulating lymphocytes.

The karyotype of a female infant with Down syndrome resulting from the presence of an additional number 21 chromosome (trisomy 21)

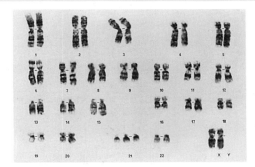

The majority of chromosome abnormalities arise as *de novo* events due to an error in gametogenesis in one of the parents. Many individuals with an autosomal imbalance are unable to reproduce so that the issue of risks to their offspring is largely unimportant. However, autosomal rearrangements may exist in a balanced form such as a translocation or inversion, and carriers of these rearrangements may be at high risk of transmitting the rearrangement in an unbalanced form and therefore of having a handicapped child. This is discussed in the section on Down syndrome.

Any loss or gain (imbalance) of autosomal material is likely to have adverse effects on both mental and physical development. Generally, alterations in the number or structure of the sex chromosomes have a much milder effect than autosomal imbalance, although certain sex chromosome abnormalities such as Turner syndrome and Klinefelter syndrome are associated with a high incidence of infertility.

Spontaneous abortions. At least 15 per cent of all recognised pregnancies end in spontaneous miscarriage. In 40 per cent of these there is a chromosome abnormality consisting most commonly of autosomal trisomy, monosomy X (i.e. 45, X), triploidy or tetraploidy.

Perinatal mortality surveys. In most developed nations, the perinatal mortality rate is around 1 per cent. Approximately 25 per cent of these babies die as a direct consequence of a serious malformation: 5 per cent have a chromosome abnormality such as trisomy 13 or trisomy 18.

Newborn surveys. The pooled results of several surveys show that a chromosome abnormality is present in 0.6 per cent of all newborn infants. In one-third of cases this is present in a balanced form.

Mental retardation. Surveys in the community show that chromosome abnormalities account for at least 30 per cent of all cases of moderate and severe mental retardation. Trisomy 21 and the fragile X syndrome are the most common causes.

COMMON AUTOSOMAL ABNORMALITIES

Down syndrome (T21)

Incidence of Down syndrome

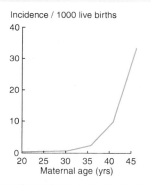

Incidence / 1000 live births

(graph: y-axis 0, 10, 20, 30, 40; x-axis Maternal age (yrs) 20, 25, 30, 35, 40, 45)

Typical facial appearance of an infant with Down syndrome

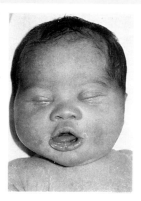

Note the upward sloping palpebral fissures and protruding tongue

Incidence. This condition affects approximately 1 in 700 babies and is found in all ethnic communities. There is a well recognised association with advancing maternal age with the incidence rising to 1 per cent when a mother reaches the age of 40 years. Advanced paternal age has very little effect.

Clinical features. The most striking feature in the neonate is hypotonia, and although the diagnosis is usually evident at this time, it may sometimes be missed if the baby is very premature or his facial features are concealed by ventilatory apparatus. In infants and older children the most characteristic features are upward sloping palpebral fissures and protruding tongue, single palmar creases, mild short stature and mild to moderate developmental delay. IQ scores range from 25 to 70 and social skills often exceed other intellectual parameters. Children with Down syndrome are usually happy and extremely affectionate.

Clinical features in Down syndrome

General	Limbs
Neonatal hypotonia	Fifth finger clinodactyly
Mild–moderate mental retardation	Single palmar crease
Short stature	Wide gap between 1st and 2nd toes
Cranio-facial	**Other**
Brachycephaly	Congenital heart disease (40 per cent)
Epicanthic folds	e.g. common atrio-ventricular canal,
Protruding tongue	ASD, PDA, VSD, Fallot tetralogy
Small ears	Anal atresia
Upward sloping palpebral fissures	Duodenal atresia
Strabismus and/or nystagmus	

Increased incidence of leukaemia (1 per cent)

Life expectancy in Down syndrome has improved dramatically as a result of the widespread availability of antibiotics and advances in cardiac surgery. Approximately 15–20 per cent of Down syndrome children die before the age of 5 years, usually as a result of severe inoperable congenital heart disease. Life expectancy for the remainder is well into adult life. By the age of 40 years almost all individuals with Down syndrome will have developed Alzheimer disease, probably as a direct result of a gene dosage effect, since the gene which codes for the amyloid protein which appears to cause Alzheimer disease is located on chromosome 21.

Cytogenetic aspects. Chromosome abnormalities in Down syndrome are listed below. By far the most common finding is straightforward trisomy 21. Molecular studies have revealed that the additional number 21 chromosome is derived from the mother in 80 per cent of cases. The recurrence risk in these families is approximately 1 per cent. If a female with Down syndrome due to trisomy 21 conceives, then there is a risk of 50 per cent that the baby will also have trisomy 21. Males with Down syndrome have rarely if ever reproduced.

Chromosome findings in Down syndrome

Trisomy 21, e.g. 47,XY,+21	95 per cent
Mosaicism, e.g. 46,XX,/47,XX,+21	2 per cent
Unbalanced Robertsonian translocation, e.g. 46XX,−15,+t(15q21q)*	3 per cent

* This karyotope can be interpreted as showing that the patient is a female (46,XX) with Down syndrome due to the replacement of a normal number 15 chromosome (−15), by a translocation chromosome consisting of the fused long arms of one number 15 chromosome and one number 21 chromosome (+t(15q21q)).

Children with mosaic Down syndrome are usually less severely affected than in the full-blown syndrome, and if only a small proportion of cells are trisomic then these individuals may lead normal lives. In the event of reproduction, there is a relatively high risk that the baby will have full trisomy 21, with the precise risk equalling the proportion of gametes which carry an additional number 21 chromosome.

When a child has Down syndrome as a result of an unbalanced Robertsonian translocation, there is a probability of around 25 per cent that one of the parents will carry this in a balanced form. The remaining 75 per cent of cases arise as *de novo* events and convey a low recurrence risk of approximately 1 per cent. If however, a parent is shown to be a carrier then there will be a significant risk that a future child will be affected, usually of the order of 2–5 per cent for a carrier male and 10–15 per cent for a carrier female. In the very rare event that a parent carries a balanced 21q21q Robertsonian translocation, the risk of Down syndrome in liveborn offspring will be 100 per cent.

Edward syndrome (T18)

Incidence. Trisomy 18 affects approximately 1 in 3000 neonates with a male to female ratio of 1:2. There is a weak association with advanced maternal age: 25 per cent of all cases are conceived by mothers aged 35 years or over.

Lateral view of a baby with trisomy 18 showing prominent occiput and overlapping fingers

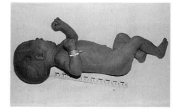

Clinical features. Intrauterine growth retardation is common and the mean birth weight is under 2.0 kg. Characteristic features are listed below; 90 per cent of affected babies have congenital heart disease and 50 per cent die during the first week of life. Almost all cases have died by the age of 1 year. Surviving infants and children show severe retardation of growth and development.

Clinical features in trisomy 18

General	Limbs
Intrauterine growth retardation	Clenched hands with second and fifth fingers
Severe failure to thrive	overlapping third and fourth fingers in survivors
Mental retardation	Small nails especially on fifth finger
	Short dorsiflexed big toes
	Rocker-bottom feet
Cranio-facial	**Other**
Prominent occiput	Cardiac abnormalities
Low set dysplastic ears	Oesophageal atresia
Short narrow palpebral fissures	Tracheo-eosophageal fistula
Small mouth and small jaw	Spina bifida

'Rocker-bottom' foot in a baby with trisomy 18

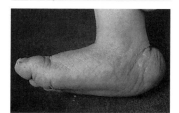

Cytogenetic aspects. Most cases show straightforward trisomy 18. Molecular studies indicate that the additional number 18 chromosome has been inherited from the mother in over 90 per cent of cases. Rarely an unbalanced translocation is found, in which case parental chromosome studies must be initiated. Mosaicism with a normal cell line sometimes occurs and probably accounts for most long-term survivors.

Patau syndrome (T13)

Incidence. This disorder is found in approximately 1 in 5000 newborn babies, and, as with the other autosomal trisomies (18 and 21), there is an association with advanced maternal age.

Clinical features. Almost all babies with trisomy 13 have marked dysmorphic features and major internal abnormalities. Survival beyond a few weeks is very unusual with 50 per cent of affected babies dying within 3 days of birth. Long-term survivors show severe handicap.

Clinical features in trisomy 13

General		Limbs	
Hypertonicity in neonatal period		Polydactyly (post-axial, i.e. on radial side)	
Severe failure to thrive with early death in most cases		Single palmar creases	
		Talipes	
Cranio-facial		**Other**	
Facies type I	Holoprosencephaly, e.g.	Cardiac abnormalities	
	absent nose (premaxillary agenesis)	Exomphalos	
	single nostril (cebocephaly)	Cryptorchidism/hypospadias	
	proboscis (ethmocephaly)	Polycystic kidneys	
	single eye (cyclops)		
Facies type II	Microphthalmia		
	Large bulbous nose		
	Cleft lip/palate		
	Small ears/Scalp defects		

Cytogenetic aspects. In 80 per cent of cases there is regular trisomy 13. Most of the remaining 20 per cent have an unbalanced translocation and occasionally one of the parents is found to carry this in a balanced form. Mosaicism with a normal cell line results in less severe features.

Cri-du-chat syndrome (5p–)

Incidence. This is a very rare condition with an incidence of 1 in 50 000.

Features

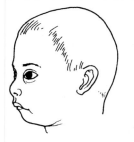

Clinical features. Usually there is a high pitched cat-like cry in the newborn period and early infancy. External anomalies are minimal and may consist of microcephaly only with a round face and abnormal palmar creases. Severe internal abnormalities are very unusual so that most affected children show long term survival. Intellect is severely impaired.

Cytogenetic aspects. Usually there is loss (deletion) of a small portion of material from the end of the short arm (p for 'petit') of one number 5 chromosome. Since this may have resulted from malsegregation of a balanced rearrangement, it is important that parental chromosome studies are undertaken.

COMMON SEX CHROMOSOME ABNORMALITIES

Klinefelter synd. (47,XXY)

Incidence. Chromosome surveys of large numbers of consecutive newborn infants have shown that this condition affects approximately 1 in 1000 males. It is likely that many cases are never diagnosed.

Clinical features. Male infants with Klinefelter syndrome are entirely normal and there is no increase in the incidence of congenital malformations. Intellectual development in childhood may be mildly impaired with average verbal IQ being 10–20 points below that of unaffected siblings and controls. Adults with Klinefelter syndrome tend to be slightly taller than average with long lower limbs. 30 per cent show mild to moderate gynaecomastia, and all are infertile with small soft testes. Otherwise sexual performance in adult life is usually satisfactory. Testosterone replacement therapy should be commenced at adolescence and appears to have a beneficial effect both on psychosexual development and the long-term prevention of osteoporosis.

Cytogenetic aspects. In 80–90 per cent of cases there is a 47,XXY karyotype. Molecular studies have shown that the additional X chromosome is as likely to have come from the father as the mother. The remaining 10–20 per cent of cases show either mosaicism with a normal cell line resulting in only minor problems or the presence of additional X chromosomes (e.g. 48,XXXY or 49,XXXXY) which are usually associated with more marked hypogonadism and mental retardation.

Turner syndrome (45,X)

Incidence. Loss of sex chromosome (i.e. 45,X) is a common finding in abortus material and only around 3–5 per cent of Turner syndrome conceptions survive to the third trimester. The incidence in live-born female infants is 1 in 5000.

Clinical features. During pregnancy Turner syndrome may present with generalised hydrops or localised nuchal swelling which may be mistaken on ultrasonography for an encephalocele. This excess of tissue fluid is due to delayed maturation of the lymphatic drainage system. In surviving babies the vestiges of this intrauterine oedema manifest as residual neck webbing, puffy hands and feet and small hyperconvex nails. Fifteen per cent of cases have coarctation of the aorta.

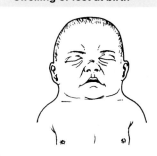

Webbing of neck and swelling of feet at birth

Short stature is the most common presenting feature in childhood when examination may also reveal a low posterior hairline, increased carrying angles, widely spaced nipples (shield chest) and Madelung deformity at the wrists.

Presentation in adult life is with primary amenorrhoea, and infertility. In Turner syndrome the ovaries develop normally during the first half of intrauterine life. Thereafter, they regress ('ovarian dysgenesis') leaving only small strands of ovarian tissue ('streak gonads'). Treatment with genetically engineered growth hormone is beneficial for the short stature seen in Turner syndrome, and oestrogen replacement therapy should be commenced around the time of the onset of puberty. It is important to stress that intellectual development is normal in Turner syndrome.

Cytogenetic aspects. In 50 per cent of cases there is only 1 sex chromosome, ie 45,X. Molecular studies have revealed that this is usually maternal in origin with loss of the X or Y chromosome having occurred in spermatogenesis. In the remaining cases there may be either a deletion of the short arm of one X chromosome, or an isochromosome consisting of 2 long arms with no short arm. Very rarely there may be mosaicism with one cell line showing the presence of a Y chromosome, ie 45,X/46,XY. In these cases there is a small risk of malignant change in the streak gonads which should therefore be removed prophylactically.

Fragile X syndrome

Incidence. Recent studies indicate that this is a relatively common cause of mental retardation affecting 1 in 1000 males. One-third of female carriers show mild mental retardation.

Clinical features. Affected males usually have a long face with large ears and a prominent jaw. Large testes (macro-orchidism) develop after puberty. In childhood autistic behaviour and convulsions may be noted and most affected males are moderately to severely retarded.

Genetic aspects. The diagnosis is made by demonstrating the presence of a gap ('fragile site') at the end of the long arm (q) of an X chromosome. Technically this is difficult and special cultures are needed so that the laboratory must always be informed if this diagnosis is suspected. Although this condition usually shows sex-linked recessive inheritance, the underlying genetic mechanisms are not fully understood. For example, some entirely normal males have been known to transmit the condition to their daughters who have subsequently had sons with the full-blown syndrome. Genomic imprinting — see the next section — is one possible explanation for this curious phenomenon.

Part of a 'metaphase spread' showing the presence of a fragile X chromosome (arrowed)

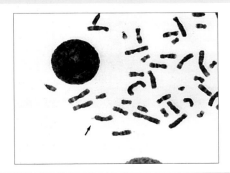

SINGLE GENE (MENDELIAN) INHERITANCE

A condition or trait resulting from a germ-line mutation in DNA is said to show single gene inheritance. Almost 5000 human characteristics or diseases have been attributed to single gene defects. As an alternative, the term Mendelian is sometimes used in recognition of the fact that Gregor Mendel, an Austrian monk, was the first to recognise the underlying principles of single gene inheritance. Ironically the significance of Mendel's work was only recognised long after his death, so that he could have had no idea that his observations would ultimately prove to be of such major importance.

Autosomal dominant

A condition occurring in someone with only a single copy of an abnormal gene located on one of the autosomes is said to show autosomal dominant inheritance. Over 3000 conditions or traits showing this pattern of inheritance have been identified. Some of these disorders, such as polydactyly, may be very mild, whereas others, such as the lethal forms of osteogenesis imperfecta, are very severe.

The fundamental principles of autosomal dominant inheritance are:

1. Each time an individual with an autosomal dominant disorder has a child there is 1 chance in 2 that the child will inherit the disorder. Thus these conditions tend to be transmitted from generation to generation giving rise to the appearance of 'vertical' transmission in a pedigree.
2. Generally males and females are equally affected and each can transmit the disorder to

Dominant inheritance

affected   unaffected

both affected   both unaffected

Example

individuals of either sex. This contrasts with sex-linked inheritance in which male to male transmission cannot occur.

3. When two parents, both with the same autosomal dominant disorder, have a child, risks to the child are:
    1 in 4 for inheriting both copies of the mutant gene.
    1 in 2 for inheriting one copy of the mutant gene.
    1 in 4 for inheriting neither copy of the mutant gene.
    Usually individuals with two copies of the mutant gene (homozygotes) are very severely affected, e.g. early lethality in achondroplasia and ischaemic heart disease by early adult life in familial hypercholesterolaemia.

Genetic counselling is complicated by the fact that many autosomal dominant disorders show quite marked variation in their degree of severity, even amongst affected individuals within a family. For example, some individuals with neurofibromatosis show only cafe-au-lait patches and have no clinical problems: others may be quite severely retarded or have serious illness as a result of tumour formation. This is known as 'variable expressivity'. Occasionally an autosomal dominant disorder may appear to completely skip a generation with the individual who must have transmitted the condition from grandparent to grandchild showing absolutely no clinical abnormality. Such an event represents an example of 'non-penetrance'.

The individual in a family who is the first to be affected is said to represent a 'new mutation'. The recurrence risk to his or her siblings will be very low, whereas the risk to each of his or her offspring will be 1 in 2. For many conditions, such as achondroplasia and Apert syndrome, it has been noted that the mean age of the fathers of children who represent new mutations is greater than average.

As a general rule, autosomal dominant disorders tend to be associated with structural abnormalities, in contrast to autosomal recessive disorders which are often due to defective enzyme activity. There are however, a few notable exceptions, such as several forms of porphyria, which show autosomal dominant inheritance and are caused by a 50 per cent reduction in enzyme activity.

Common examples of autosomal dominant inheritance

Disorder	Chromosomal location
Achondroplasia	NK
Apert syndrome	NK
Familial hypercholesterolaemia	19
Holt-Oram syndrome	?14
Huntington disease	4
Marfan syndrome	15
Myotonic dystrophy	19
Neurofibromatosis	17
Osteogenesis imperfecta	7/17*
Polycystic kidney disease (adult onset form)	16
Polyposis coli	5
Spherocytosis	8
Tuberose sclerosis	9/11*

* These disorders show genetic heterogeneity, i.e. the same phenotype can be produced by mutations at different loci. NK = not known.

Autosomal recessive

An autosomal recessive disorder is one which occurs only in individuals who inherit two copies of an abnormal autosomal gene, one from each parent. Affected individuals are said to be homozygous: carriers are heterozygous. Over 1500 disorders showing autosomal recessive inheritance have been described.

The basic principles of autosomal recessive inheritance are:

Autosomal recessive

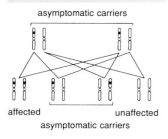

asymptomatic carriers

affected   unaffected

asymptomatic carriers

1. When parents have had one affected child, the risk to each subsequent offspring is 1 in 4. This risk applies equally to males and females.
2. Usually an autosomal recessive disorder affects only members of a single sibship in a family – 'horizontal' transmission. This is because an affected individual can transmit only one of his or her abnormal genes to each child, who in order to be affected would have to inherit another abnormal gene from the other parent.
3. Autosomal recessive disorders, particularly those which are rare, show an increased incidence in the offspring of consanguineous parents. It has been estimated that most humans carry at least one deleterious autosomal recessive gene. Therefore when close relatives marry, there is a risk (usually small) that they may both carry a common ancestor's abnormal gene and transmit it in double dose to a child.

Example

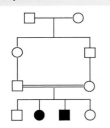

Some autosomal recessive disorders show a particularly high incidence in certain ethnic groups or communities One possible explanation is a 'founder effect' in a population which is restricted in its choice of marital partners by geographical or religious factors. Thus if one of the founding forefathers (or foremothers) of a genetic 'isolate' carried a harmful autosomal recessive gene, it is possible that this could by chance have become widely established in the relevant community. This may be the explanation for the high incidence of Tay-Sachs disease in the Ashkenazi Jewish population in the Eastern United States.

Another is heterozygote advantage. Carriers of some autosomal recessive disorders may be biologically fitter than non-carriers. By far the best known example is sickle-cell disease, carriers of which are relatively immune to infection by malaria. Consequently in areas where malaria is endemic, carriers of the sickle cell gene are at a distinct biological and hence reproductive advantage. This concept may also apply to cystic fibrosis, although no underlying mechanism for carrier advantage has been identified.

Autosomal recessive disorders which have a high incidence in particular ethnic groups

Disorder	Ethinic group
α_1-antitrypsin deficiency	Scandinavians
Congenital adrenal hyperplasia (21-hydroxylase deficiency)	Eskimos
Cystic fibrosis	Western Europeans
Sickle cell disease	Afro-Caribbeans
Tay-Sachs disease	Ashkenazi Jews
α-thalassaemia	Orientals
β-thalassaemia	Mediterranean races and orientals

Sex-linked (X-linked)

Sex-linked disorders are those which are caused by abnormal genes on the X chromosome. If the disease is not manifest in women who have only a single copy of the abnormal gene, then the disorder is said to show X-linked recessive inheritance. Over 300 X-linked recessive disorders have been recognised.

The essential features of X-linked recessive inheritance are:

1. Each time a carrier has a child, there is 1 chance in 2 that she will transmit the abnormal gene, so that for each daughter there is 1 chance in 2 of being a carrier and for each son, 1 chance in 2 of being affected. This is sometimes referred to as a vertical or 'knight's move' pattern of inheritance.
2. When an affected male has children, he will transmit the abnormal gene to all of his daughters who will be carriers and to none of his sons who will therefore not be affected, ie male to male transmission cannot occur.

X-linked recessive

carrier female   male

unaffected   carrier   affected
female   male   female   male

Example

Rarely a woman may be affected with a sex-linked recessive disorder. This may be because she has inherited 2 copies of the abnormal gene, 1 from her carrier mother and 2 from her affected father; or she has Turner syndrome (45,X) or testicular feminization, a very rare condition in which affected 'women' have a 46,XY karyotype with female habitus and external genitalia because of insensitivity to testosterone during embryogenesis; or because Lyonisation (X chromosome inactivation) has not occurred in a random fashion, either by chance or because of an abnormality or rearrangement involving one of her X chromosomes. Most commonly this takes the form of a balanced X-autosome translocation.

One of the greatest problems posed by sex-linked recessive disorders is carrier detection. By definition carriers are usually entirely healthy. Sometimes it is possible to show that a woman is likely to be a carrier using appropriate biochemical tests. For example, serum creatine kinase levels are raised in approximately two-thirds of all carriers of Duchenne muscular dystrophy. Generally however, these indirect measurements of gene activity are not very reliable and this is one of the reasons why the recent isolation of many of the important X-linked genes has proved to be so valuable.

Molecular techniques have also revealed that occasionally a woman may transmit a sex-linked recessive disorder to more than one child, even though tests indicate that the woman does not have the mutation in DNA extracted from her circulating lymphocytes. It is believed

Sex-linked disorders

Sex-linked recessive	Sex-linked dominant
Bruton agammaglobulinaemia	Incontinentia pigmenti
Duchenne muscular dystrophy	Pseudohypoparathyroidism
Factor VIII deficiency (haemophilia A)	Vitamin D resistant rickets
Factor IX deficiency (haemophilia B = Christmas dis.)	
Glucose-6-phosphate dehydrogenase deficiency	
Lesch-Nyhan syndrome	
Red-green colour blindness	

that this is due to the presence of a mutant gene bearing cell line in one of her ovaries (gonadal mosaicism). This phenomenon has also been observed in males, who, though unaffected, may transmit the disorder to more than one daughter.

Sex-linked dominant

A small number of X-linked disorders are manifest in both the heterozygous female and the hemizygous male. An affected female will transmit the disorder on average to half of her daughters and to half of her sons. An affected male will transmit the disorder to all of his daughters and to none of his sons.

Mitochondrial inheritance

Each mitochondrion carries a small amount of DNA which codes for 13 proteins involved in the mitochondrial respiratory chain. Disorders which result from mutations in mitochondrial DNA include very rare forms of encephalopathy and myopathy. Mitochondria are transmitted only by ova and not by sperm, so that mitochondrial inheritance is characterised by transmission exclusively through females.

Genomic imprinting

Studies in mice have shown that apparently identical genes inherited from each parent may sometimes differ in their expression in offspring. This memory or 'imprint' of parental origin is probably due to different patterns of DNA methylation during meiosis and gametogenesis. The effect of this imprint persists throughout life but is altered during gametogenesis in the offspring depending on whether transmission is occurring in the ova or the sperm. It is not yet known how extensively imprinting occurs in humans, nor is it clear how important this mechanism is in causing disease. Observation which may be explained by imprinting are: congenital myotonic dystrophy occurs only in the offspring of affected females and never in the children of affected males, the age of onset of Huntington chorea is often earlier if the transmitting parent is male rather than female, and if a *de novo* deletion occurs on the long arm of the number 15 chromosome inherited from the father, this results in the Prader–Willi syndrome (hypotonia in infancy, mild mental retardation and obesity). If an apparently identical deletion occurs on the maternally inherited number 15 chromosome, Angelman's syndrome (convulsions, ataxia, severe mental retardation and inappropriate laughter) results.

MULTIFACTORIAL (POLYGENIC) INHERITANCE

This is the term used to describe the pattern of inheritance observed for several relatively common conditions which appear to result from the interaction of a genetic predisposition with adverse environmental factors. The genetic susceptibility is determined by the additive effects of many genes and hence is known as polygenic. Conditions believed to show multifactorial inheritance include many of the more common cogenital malformations along with acquired disorders of childhood and adult life.

Various mathematical models have been formulated to explain multifactorial inheritance. The simplest is based on the assumption that there is an underlying 'liability', made up of both genetic and environmental factors, which shows a normal distribution in the general population. Those individuals whose liability falls beyond an arbitrary threshold superimposed on the normal curve develop the disorder.

Hypothetical curves of liability for the general population and for close relatives of affected individuals

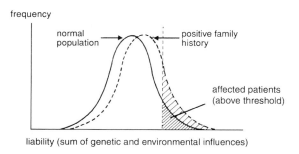

Because of shared genes the liability curve for close relatives of an affected individual will be shifted to the right, so that they will therefore show an increased incidence of the disorder.

The characteristic features of multifactorial inheritance are:

1. Risks to close relatives are generally less than in single gene disorders.
2. Risks to siblings and offspring of an affected individual are roughly comparable.
3. Risks decline sharply as the relationship with the affected individual becomes more distant. For example, the risk to the first degree relatives (siblings and offspring) of someone with a neural tube defect is 4–5 per cent whereas for second degree relatives (nephews, nieces, grandchildren) the risk is 1–2 per cent. For third degree relatives such as first cousins, the risk is close to the general population incidence.
4. Risks to close relatives are greater if more than one family member is affected. For parents who have had two children with a neural tube defect, the risk that a third child will be affected rises to 10–12 per cent.
5. If the index case is very severely affected then the risks to close relatives are greater. This is most noticeable for cleft lip/palate, for which the risk rises from 2 per cent for the sibling of someone with cleft lip to 6 per cent if the index case has bilateral cleft lip and palate.

The concept of multifactorial inheritance is not entirely satisfactory since the underlying mechanisms are not well understood and parameters such as liability cannot be measured. Ultimately it may emerge that at least some of the conditions for which multifactorial inheritance has been proposed are actually caused by mutations at a single locus interacting with a polygenic background and/or environmental factors. Research using molecular techniques suggests that this may be the case for asthma, diabetes mellitus and schizophrenia.

Multifactorial disorders	
Congenital malformations/disorders of infancy	Acquired disorders of childhood and adult life
Cleft lip/palate Congenital dislocation of the hip Congenital heart disease Neural tube defects Pyloric stenosis	Asthma Depression Diabetes mellitus Epilepsy Glaucoma Hypertension Schizophrenia

Neural tube defects

Clinically and embryologically these can be divided into disorders resulting from a defect in neurulation (anencephaly and craniorachischisis) and those resulting from defective canalisation of the neural tube (lumbosacral lesions). There is some evidence that genetically these are distinct and different entities, although both forms have been observed to occur within the same family. Clinical aspects of neural tube defects are described in Chapter 4. Factors known to contribute to the aetiology of neural tube defects include poor socio-economic circumstances, diet, and a Celtic ancestry. Prenatal diagnosis programmes have been established in the United Kingdom and elsewhere based on assay of maternal serum α-fetoprotein at 16 weeks gestation. This is elevated in 60–70 per cent of mothers carrying a fetus with an open lesion. More specific prenatal diagnosis is based on ultrasonography or amniocentesis.

Accumulating evidence suggests that multivitamin therapy taken by the mother around the time of conception prevents the development of a neural tube defect in a genetically susceptible embryo. If substantiated this will provide a universally acceptable means of primary prevention, thereby emphasizing the importance of focusing on the search for potentially treatable or avoidable environmental trigger factors.

RECENT ADVANCES IN MOLECULAR GENETICS

During the last decade new and exciting developments in molecular biology have greatly enhanced understanding of the molecular basis of disease. This has proved particularly valuable for the investigation and diagnosis of inherited disorders both in affected individuals and in their relatives. The following are areas of special relevance for paediatrics.

Gene tracking

This technique can be used to determine whether an individual, who could be an unborn baby, a child or an adult, is likely to have inherited a single-gene disorder known to be running in the family. The underlying principle is relatively complex and relies on study of the cosegregation of the disease with DNA markers known to be linked to the disease locus. These DNA markers are usually identified using the technique known as Southern blotting. This enables detection of randomly occurring polymorphic variation in a portion of DNA close to the disease locus using a combination of a restriction enzyme and a gene probe. The presence or absence of a particular cleavage site results in the generation of different sized fragments, which are known as restriction fragment length polymorphisms (RFLPs). By study of the linkage pattern in the family, it may be possible to determine which DNA marker (ie presence or absence of a cleavage site) is cosegregating with the disease gene.

The principles underlying the use of linked DNA markers in gene tracking

Homologous segments of 2 X chromosomes, each of which contains the locus for the gene (G), at which a disease mutation is present on one chromosome. P represents a radioactively labelled probe which hybridises to the X chromosome very close to the disease locus (G). The vertical arrows represent the cutting sites of a restriction enzyme. Sites a and c are present in both chromosomes: site b is present only in the top chromosome. Presence of this cutting site results in hybridisation of the probe (P) to a 6 kb (kilobase) fragment: absence results in hybridisation to a 9 kb fragment. Presence and absence are denoted as A and B respectively.

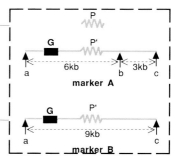

The steps in Southern blotting. In this example, blood from a female who is heterozygous for A and B has been analysed.

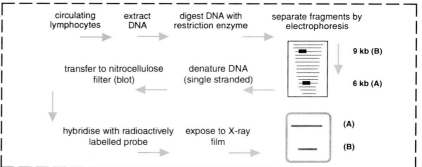

In this pedigree showing segregation of a sex-linked recessive disorder such as Duchenne muscular dystrophy, the disease gene is linked with marker B. Thus if the son in the third generation inherits marker B there is a very high risk that he will be affected. Similarly if his sister inherits marker B there is a very high probability that she will be a carrier.

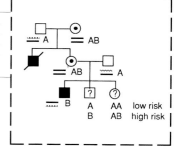

Applications

Prenatal diagnosis. Some parents who are known to be at high risk of having a child with a serious genetic disease may request prenatal diagnosis followed by termination of pregnancy if the baby is found to be affected. Examples of diseases in which gene tracking has been used for this purpose include β-thalassaemia, cystic fibrosis and Duchenne muscular dystrophy.

There are a few situations in which prenatal diagnosis may facilitate early treatment. In congenital adrenal hyperplasia due to 21-hydroxylase deficiency, impaired synthesis of cortisol results in increased secretion of ACTH, which in turn stimulates the fetal adrenal glands to produce excess androgens. This usually leads to virilisation of an affected female fetus. However, if the diagnosis can be made early in pregnancy by analysis of DNA obtained at chorion biopsy, then administration of dexamethasone to the mother may suppress the fetal pituitary–adrenal axis thereby preventing virilisation.

Preclinical diagnosis. Approximately 25–40 per cent of cases of retinoblastoma are hereditary. The risk that a child of someone with hereditary retinoblastoma will develop the condition is close to 50 per cent. It is strongly recommended that regular ophthalmoscopy should be carried out in these children during at least the first 5 years of life. This is not easy in young children and may involve general anaesthesia. If DNA analysis indicates that a child has inherited his or her parent's retinoblastoma gene then obviously very frequent ophthalmoscopy is mandatory. If however, it is shown that a child has almost certainly not inherited the retinoblastoma gene, then it would be reasonable to omit some or all of the ophthalmological assessments.

The same principle applies to diseases of adolescent or adult onset such as polyposis coli and polycystic kidney disease, in both of which it could be argued that early diagnosis might be beneficial to the child's long-term prognosis. However at the present time, the full ethical aspects of this so-called 'predictive testing' in children have not been clarified.

Carrier detection. Women who have close male relatives with a sex-linked recessive disorder may wish to know whether they are carriers and therefore at risk of having affected sons. Until recently for conditions such as Duchenne muscular dystrophy and haemophilia, carrier detection was based upon biochemical assays (creatine kinase and factor VIII levels respectively) which are not always reliable in distinguishing carriers from non-carriers. The availability of DNA markers closely linked to these disease loci has now enabled most female relatives of affected males to be given a very accurate estimate of their carrier status.

Direct mutation analysis

Indirect mutation analysis as outlined in the previous section enables disease status to be predicted based on the study of the cosegregation of DNA markers linked to the disease locus. This method has the disadvantages that DNA has to be obtained from several members of the family, at least one family member has to be heterozygous at the marker locus, there is a small risk that disease status will be predicted incorrectly due to recombination (crossing-over) occurring between the disease locus and the marker locus during prophase of meiosis I.

In contrast, *direct* mutation analysis conveys none of these disadvantages and can be used as a precise diagnostic test for conditions such as cystic fibrosis, which can be difficult to diagnose in neonates using conventional methods. Many techniques for direct mutation analysis have been devised. Some of the simpler approaches are:

Change in a restriction site. A point mutation can be detected easily if it alters a restriction enzyme cleavage site. For example, in the sickle cell gene a thymine to adenine mutation in the sixth codon/residue of the β-globin gene results in loss of an MstII cleavage site, so that the fragments normally produced at Southern blotting are altered in size. This permits very precise diagnosis of heterozygotes (carriers of the trait) and homozygotes (patients with sickle cell disease) by molecular studies.

Use of an oligonucleotide probe. A very short probe will only hybridize to a patient's gene if it is an exact copy. A single base mismatch resulting from a point mutation will prevent hybridization. Oligonucleotide probes of around 20 bases can be used for diagnosing several diseases such as α_1-antitrypsin deficiency and β-thalassaemia.

Ribonuclease A cleavage. In this technique an RNA probe, which is an exact match for the normal gene, is hybridized to the patient's DNA. The resulting hybrid molecule is then exposed to ribonuclease A which will only cleave the RNA probe if there is a mismatch resulting from a point mutation in the patient's gene. Cleavage can be detected by the presence of two bands on a gel instead of one.

Deletion analysis: Southern blotting. It is now known that deletions in the dystrophin gene on the short arm of the X chromosome account for approximately two-thirds of all cases of Duchenne muscular dystrophy. These deletions can be demonstrated in a Southern blot by hybridising the patient's DNA, which has been cleaved into lots of tiny fragments, with a suitable probe. A deletion mutation can be deduced by the absence of several bands on the blot.

Deletion analysis: Polymerase chain reaction (PCR). The PCR technique enables a specific sequence or portion of a gene to be amplified up to 1 million fold. If a deletion is present in the sequence which is amplified, this will result in production of a smaller fragment than that found in unaffected individuals. This approach has proved particularly useful for diagnosing carriers of cystic fibrosis. Approximately 75 per cent of all cystic fibrosis genes in western Europeans show a deletion of codon number 508 (the so-called ΔF508 mutation). Thus if 98 base pairs of the cystic fibrosis gene including codon 508 are amplified, then in an affected patient who is homozygous for the deletion, two fragments, each 95 pairs long, will be generated. Carriers of the deletion will be identified by the presence of one normal 98 base pair band and one truncated 95 base pair band.

Deletion analysis of the Duchenne muscular dystropy gene in 6 affected boys

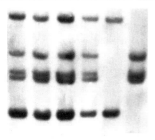

In the 2 right hand lanes, several bands are missing indicating deletion of a portion of their dystrophin gene.

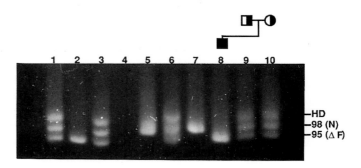

Deletion analysis. Shows separation of the normal (N) and deleted (ΔF) cystic fibrosis genes by polymerase chain reaction followed by electrophoresis. HD represents a heteroduplex band which forms in samples from heterozygotes. The individuals shown in lanes 2 and 8 are homozygous affected, those in lanes 5 and 7 are homozygous normal, and those in lanes 1, 3, 6, 9 and 10 are heterozygous

Oncogenes

These are genes which are normally involved in basic cell functions such as division, proliferation and differentiation, by the production of proteins such as growth factors and growth factor receptors. Overactivity therefore results in uncontrolled cell proliferation with possible induction of maligant transformation.

Mechanisms which may lead to disturbance in the function of an oncogene, a point mutation in a coding exon, a translocation resulting in loss of normal gene suppression or synthesis of an altered gene product, eg Burkitt lymphoma and gene amplification which may be the result of a mutation in a gene controlling DNA synthesis, e.g. neuroblastoma.

Anti-oncogenes are genes which normally control cell turn-over and therefore act as tumour suppressors. Loss of an anti-oncogene in a cell which is already primed by a mutation involving the homologous anti-oncogene results in malignant transformation. The dominantly inherited genes which account for some cases of retinoblastoma and Wilms' tumour are believed to be anti-oncogenes.

Gene therapy

No effective means of gene therapy exists at present, but recent advances in molecular biology have raised hope that direct replacement of an abnormal gene by its normal counterpart may soon be possible. Public unease at the prospect of 'tinkering' with genes has been alleviated by a universal consensus that gene therapy should be used exclusively to cure an illness rather than for eugenic purposes such as increasing intelligence or athletic abilities and that treatment should be directed primarily at altering a body tissue (somatic therapy) rather than altering the heritable underlying genetic constitution (germ-line therapy).

Gene insertion: physical methods. Various strategies have been applied with only limited success. These include microinjection of DNA, exposure of recipient cells to high voltage electric current, and the formation of cell permeable DNA–lipid complexes.

Gene insertion: viral vectors. Retroviruses, which can incorporate up to 7 kb of foreign DNA, can be rendered incapable of replication and then allowed to infect ('transfect') host cells *in vitro*. This may result in the foreign donor DNA being incorporated into the genome of the cells of the recipient tissue, e.g. bone marrow, which can then be returned to the affected individual. This approach is technically feasible, but possible problems include 1) insertional damage in the host such as mutagenesis or oncogenesis, and 2) lack of expression of the donor gene if taken up into an inappropriate region of the host genome.

Gene targeting: homologous recombination. This approach involves the insertion of the donor gene along with flanking sequences into a vector which then aligns with homologous DNA from a host organ *in vitro*. If recombination occurs resulting in equal exchange of DNA between the vector and host, then the donor gene should be correctly sited in the host genome. Technically this method is extremely difficult, but it has the major advantages that insertional damage should not occur and correct gene expression should not be a problem.

Disorders which might be amenable for gene therapy. In order to be a candidate for gene therapy a disorder has to have a well defined genetic or biochemical defect, the relevant gene must have been isolated along with its control sequences, and the target organ has to be easily accessible for manipulation either *in vivo* (e.g. respiratory tract mucosa) or *in vitro* (e.g. bone-marrow, liver, tumour infiltrating lymphocytes). Examples of disorders which might be treatable by gene therapy in the foreseeable future are indicated below. No effective gene therapy exists at yet for any disorder in children and adults.

Disorders which might be suitable for gene therapy	
Haematopoietic	– haemaglobinopathies
	– immunodeficiencies
Hepatic	– α 1 antitrypsin deficiency
Metabolic	– hypercholesterolaemia
	– phenylketonuria
Oncogenic	– solid tumours by insertion of tumour necrosis factor gene into tumour, infiltrating lymphocytes
Endocrine	– diabetes mellitus, growth hormone deficiency
Respiratory	– α 1 antitrypsin deficiency
	– cystic fibrosis

GENETIC COUNSELLING

This can be defined as the process whereby an individual is alerted to the possibility of developing and/or transmitting an inherited illness and how this might be avoided. The key underlying principle is that individuals seeking help should be provided with information rather than advice, thereby enabling them to make their own informed decisions about future child-bearing. It is universally agreed that genetic counselling should be non-coercive with no attempt being made to direct the patient along a particular course of action. If at all possible, the genetic counsellor should also try to adopt a non-judgemental approach.

Much genetic counselling can be and is undertaken by general practitioners and paediatricians. Patients with relatively complex problems can be referred to specialist genetic clinics held at most large hospitals and teaching centres. These are usually located at or close to a regional genetics centre, a large network of which has been established throughout the United Kingdom. These centres are responsible for several tasks including the maintenance of registers of families in which individuals may be at risk of developing or transmitting a genetic disease. The role of these 'genetic' registers is to ensure that a rapid means of two-way communication exists, so that members of these families can seek information at short notice and in turn be alerted to new developments and technical innovations.

BIBLIOGRAPHY

Connor J M, Ferguson–Smith M A 1990 Essential medical genetics, 3rd edn. Blackwell Scientific Publications, Oxford
Emery A E H, Mueller R F 1988 Elements of medical genetics, 7th edn. Churchill Livingstone, Edinburgh
Emery A E H, Rimoin D L 1990 Principles and practice of medical genetics, 2nd edn. Churchill Livingstone, Edinburgh
Harper P S 1988 Practical genetic counselling, 3rd edn. Wright, London
Jones K L 1988 Smith's recognizable patterns of human malformation 4th edn. W B Saunders, Philadelphia
McKusick V A 1990 Mendelian inheritance in man, 9th edn. Johns Hopkins University Press, Baltimore
Weatherall D J 1991 The new genetics and clinical practice, 3rd edn. Oxford University Press, Oxford

3 Fetus

Since the fetus lies hidden, unobserved within the uterus, he can fall ill, lose parts, even die, without the mother being aware of what is happening. In the main, he is protected against diseases which attack the mother, and his favoured status allows him to thrive and grow even though the mother's reserves are under pressure. Paradoxically there are some situations, fortunately rare, when the fetus is seriously harmed by agents which either have little effect on the mother, for example the virus of German measles, or which might even benefit her, for example various drugs. Despite advances in obstetric and perinatal care, fetal life is still a time which carries greater risk of morbidity or mortality than any other period in childhood. Thus in England and Wales each year there are around 700 000 births, of these around 3000 are stillborn and 48 000 are born with a low birth weight due to either growth restraint or premature birth; they are born at a disadvantage.

PERICONCEPTIONAL MEDICINE

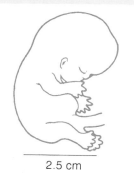

This is the actual size of an 8 week fetus

2.5 cm

Life begins not only before birth but, in a sense, before conception. The health and diet of the parents especially the mother can affect the early development and future well-being of their child. For example folic acid reduces the risk of neural tube defects, large doses of vitamin A may be teratogenic and certain foods are associated with listeriosis; raw eggs, soft or blue-veined cheeses, unpasteurised milk, and pâté. Some of these environmental factors (along with maternal infection and substance abuse discussed later) may contribute to the higher fetal loss rates in areas of social deprivation with high unemployment and sub-standard housing. Risks are also higher if the mother is very young or very old, already has a large family, or if there is a multiple pregnancy. There are also the less common environmental risks to gametes or fetus of radiation or hazardous chemicals, often at the parent's workplace. Microwave cookers and visual display units have not been shown to carry added risks, although lead has been implicated in stillbirths, the commonest source being car exhaust fumes.

Because many of these agents carry the greatest risk around the time of conception, when the mother often does not know she has conceived, appropriate precautions are not taken and this has led to calls for preconceptual clinics to promote healthy diet and behaviour in prospective parents. As a minimum, obesity, smoking, alcohol intake, sexually transmitted diseases, diabetes and hypertension could all be screened for and a history of inherited diseases sought. Ensuring fitness before pregnancy is a cheap and effective way of preventing ill health in the next generation of children.

THE PLACENTA

The tissues of the mature human placenta, unlike many other mammalian species, are derived entirely from the fetus. The placenta starts to develop shortly after the blastocyst implants in the uterine wall. Despite being antigenically different from the maternal tissues, the placenta is immunologically privileged and is not rejected. It is situated outside the body of the fetus, and is connected to it by a cord of blood vessels.

The placenta in a single structure combines many functions which are performed by separate organs after birth. It acts as a fetal lung and a fetal kidney; it transfers nutrients and substrates essential for growth and metabolism, a role the gut later fulfils, and allows heat loss, a function of the skin post-natally. It is a barrier to the transfer of cells from mother to fetus, and vice versa, which would be damaging and allow the cell mediated immunity of the maternal 'host' to reject the fetal 'graft'; it prevents uptake of large molecules, such as hormones which would interfere with fetal homeostasis, and yet selectively transfers IgG; it is an important site of hormone production. It grows rapidly early in gestation, the placental to fetal weight ratio changing from 4:1 at 10 weeks to 1:5 at term. Finally it is a disposable organ with a finite lifespan which naturally separates from the fetus at birth and is safely expelled despite its very vascular structure. The loss of this low-resistance bed triggers the circulatory changes which occur after birth.

Towards the end of pregnancy fetal demands for oxygen and nutrients reach a point where they may challenge the capacity of the uteroplacental unit to supply them. At this stage, any disturbance of that supply line might interfere with fetal growth or damage, sometimes permanently, the delicate rapidly growing tissues, particularly in the brain.

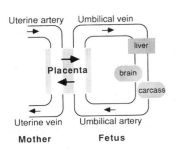

The blood supply to the placenta

Uterine artery Umbilical vein

liver

Placenta brain

carcass

Uterine vein Umbilical artery

Mother **Fetus**

EXAMINATION OF THE FETUS

In the past, the assessment of fetal growth depended on a knowledge of the date of the last menstrual period and an estimation of fetal size by

Measurement of fetal head growth by antenatal ultrasound scan

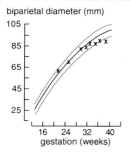

biparietal diameter (mm)

gestation (weeks)

palpation; now ultrasound techniques provide a more accurate means of measuring growth.

Most women in the UK have a dating scan at 16–18 weeks to measure fetal head size and determine gestation. Serial measurement of biparietal diameter, abdominal circumference and crown–rump length allow detection of microcephaly or hydrocephaly, ascites and intrauterine growth retardation. Symmetrical growth retardation from early pregnancy suggests an intrauterine infection or dysmorphic syndrome whereas asymmetrical growth retardation, with relative preservation of head growth, in the final trimester is usually the product of fetal 'starvation' due to utero-placental dysfunction. Evaluation of fetal health is more difficult. Maternal serum concentrations of human chorionic gonadotrophin, a protein derived from the placenta, reach a maximum at 12 weeks and seem to relate to fetal well-being in early pregnancy. In late pregnancy, hormone tests for fetal well-being, such as oestriol concentration in the mother's urine or human placental lactogen in maternal blood, have fallen from favour because of the wide normal range and considerable variability within an individual. Biophysical tests have largely superceded these biochemical profiles.

Although the placenta functions as the fetal kidney in terms of excretion of waste products, the fetal kidney itself produces urine from early in gestation which contributes in amniotic fluid volume and is swallowed and reabsorbed from the gut of the fetus. Hence, fetal renal disease (absence of the kidneys, obstructive uropathy) is associated with oligohydramnios, as is premature rupture of the fetal membranes, whereas atresia of the gastrointestinal tract and large diaphragmatic hernias are associated with polyhydramnios. Amniotic fluid volume can be estimated from ultrasound scans.

In fetal life, the respiratory tract is also filled with amniotic fluid and it appears that fetal 'breathing' activity, an important determinant of fetal lung development, is affected by the absence of amniotic fluid. As a result, pulmonary hypoplasia is a serious complication of oligohydramnios. Limb and facial deformities occur, and so can the fetal inertia syndrome, since the fetus is squashed rather than floating within a fluid filled container. Amniotic fluid volume, fetal 'breathing' activity and lung volume can be assessed by ultrasound scan and used to estimate the likelihood of lung hypoplasia.

Fetal diagnosis

A detailed ultrasound scan is done if there is a previous history of congenital abnormality or fetal loss and can reliably detect structural abnormalities such as spina bifida, exomphalos and renal abnormalities and the presence of abnormal collections of fluid. Early dysmorphic features can sometimes be seen, for example in Down or Turner syndrome, and a four chamber view of the fetal heart can detect half of the 8/1000 incidence of congenital heart disease. Fetal arrhythmias can also be diagnosed.

Ultrasound guidance is also used to direct amniocentesis, cordocentesis and chorionic villus biopsy. Amniocentesis carries approximately 1 per cent risk of abortion and chorionic villus sampling slightly

Amniocentesis

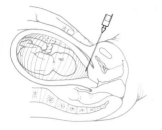

Some abnormalities which may cause a raised alpha-fetoprotein in maternal blood

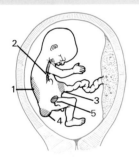

1 open neural tube defect
2 oesophageal atresia
3 exomphalos
4 sacrococcygeal teratoma
5 bladder neck obstruction
6 fetal–maternal haemorrhage

Fetal therapy

higher. Cell-free amniotic fluid can be used for biochemical measurements (eg alpha-fetoprotein in neural tube defects and metabolic markers of a number of organic acid and mucopolysaccharide disorders) whilst the fetal cells within amniotic fluid obtained at 16 weeks can be cultured for subsequent karyotyping, molecular biological techniques or assay of enzyme activity in suspected inborn errors of metabolism.

As the human placenta is derived entirely from fetal tissue chorionic villus biopsy, either by the transabdominal or transcervical route, provides a source of fetal cells as early as 10 weeks which can be subjected to the same enquiry as amniotic cells but with more rapid results. Early sexing of the fetus enables the parents to choose selective termination of male fetuses if there is a history of sex-linked disorders. Cordocentesis is used to obtain fetal red cells to diagnose haematological disease, such as thalassaemia, to monitor severity of rhesus haemolytic disease, or to obtain fetal white cells for rapid karyotype or enzyme assay. Some inborn errors of metabolism can only be diagnosed antenatally from fetal tissue and fetal liver biopsy may then be necessary.

Early detection of fetal abnormalities may allow the parents to opt for termination or enable the paediatric staff to anticipate problems at delivery and ensure correct follow-up. Occasionally, fetal therapy is recommended. The velocity of blood in the umbilical artery can also be measured non-invasively using an ultrasound scan and the Doppler principle. It appears that absent or reversed diastolic flow indicates a worse prognosis for the fetus and may therefore help in the timing of active delivery of a fetus.

Once labour starts, some indication of the likelihood of fetal hypoxia can be gained by analysis of the fetal heart rate, measured either non-invasively by transabdominal ultrasound or, once the presenting part can be reached, from a fetal ECG electrode. Normally, the fetal heart rate shows variability due to sympathetic and parasympathetic innervation, chemoreceptor activity, sleep patterns and circulating catecholamines. Loss of variability, prolonged decelerations or sustained bradycardia are all sinister changes but a normal trace does not exclude serious fetal compromise. A more direct estimate of fetal hypoxia and acidosis is measurement of fetal pH, or lactate, from capillary blood samples obtained from the presenting part.

Medicine. Fetal medicine is based on the premise that certain drugs may, if given to the mother, cross the placenta and exert desirably pharmacological effects in the fetus. Digoxin has been given to treat fetal supraventricular tachycardia which, if untreated, results in fetal heart failure, hydrops (oedema, ascites, pericardial and pleural effusions and hepatomegaly) and intrauterine death. In families with a child previously affected by congenital adrenal hyperplasia, maternal administration of dexamethasone in a subsequent affected pregnancy will suppress ACTH release, by negative feedback, and hence limit the accumulation of adrenogenic steroids. Glucocorticoids given to the mother in the latter half of pregnancy mature the fetal lungs and induce surfactant production and should be used whenever premature labour threatens with

Ultrasound: normal head

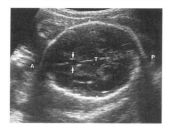

Ultrasound: normal spine

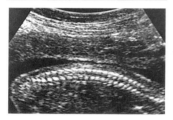

Ultrasound: heart arrow points to a ventricular septal defect

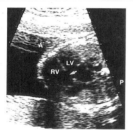

the risk of respiratory distress syndrome. Maternal parenteral nutrition has been shown to improve feto-placental biochemical function in fetuses who were growth retarded and maternal gamma globulin infusion may ameliorate fetal alloimmune thrombocytopenia. Maternal intrapartum ampicillin reduces the risk of neonatal Group B streptococcal infection.

In theory, intra-amniotic administration of drugs is feasible and absorption could occur across fetal skin, lung or gut. Amnio-infusion of saline has been tried in an effort to combat the pulmonary hypoplasia resulting from oligohydramnios.

Surgery. Non-pharmacological fetal interventions have also been attempted, the intrauterine treatment of severe rhesus haemolytic disease being the most successful. The fetus can be given rhesus negative red cell transfusions either intraperitoneally or by cordocentesis. Such therapy allows the pregnancy to continue to a safe gestation without the development of hydrops although the fetal bone marrow is suppressed for some months and postnatal anaemia may require further transfusions. Platelet transfusions can be given to correct fetal thrombocytopenia in iso- or alloimmune thrombocytopenia but obviously the risks of an invasive procedure are greater.

Needle aspiration of cysts, bladder, hydrothorax or ascites may be performed for diagnostic or therapeutic purposes, and vesico-amniotic or pleuro-amniotic shunts can be inserted to prevent reaccumulation of fluid. Fetal renal function can be assessed by quantification of urine flow and urine biochemistry and these complement estimation of liquor volume and the appearances of the kidneys on ultrasound scan. However, the long-term benefits of these intervention strategies remain controversial. Fetal surgery for diaphragmatic hernia has been undertaken following formal hysterotomy and the fetus then returned to the uterine cavity to continue the pregnancy. Theoretically, fetal bone marrow transplantation may one day be feasible to cure severe thalassaemia and storage disorders *in utero*. The last decade has seen great advances in the technology available to undertake fetal diagnosis and therapy. Hopefully, the next decade will shed more light on when these techniques should be used and whether they confer real, long-term benefits on the infant to be.

DRUGS WHICH CROSS THE PLACENTA

There is no doubt that some drugs cause embryopathy. There is some suspicion that many others may under some circumstances have harmful effects, but it is very difficult to establish beyond doubt that they made a contribution to the production of an abnormality in one particular child. Difficulty in establishing the association is due in part to the fact that the drug may only occasionally have this harmful effect, and in part to the fact that the end pathology may not be specific.

Drugs affecting the embryo

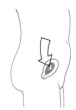

thalidomide
antimitotic
alcohol
anticonvulsants
ethisterone
warfarin

Maternal smoking in pregnancy increases the risk of miscarriage, stillbirth, premature birth, cot death, and possibly cleft palate and neural tube defects. As little as 10 cigarettes a day will lower birth-weight.

Cytotoxic agents can kill the fetus, but if the pregnancy continues the fetus may survive with many deformities. Progesterone preparations will masculinise the female fetus. Alcohol can cause facial abnormalities, growth retardation and mental handicap and the risk starts to increase once more than 7 units of alcohol per week are consumed, ie one drink per day. A single 'binge' in the first 8 weeks may also be significant. Anti-convulsant drugs, for example phenytoin and primidone and the anticoagulant warfarin, have been associated with dysmorphic features and a variety of abnormalities. Certainly there is sufficient evidence to recommend that they are not given during pregnancy unless there are sound clinical indications.

Drugs administered to the mother during the time prior to delivery may affect the baby's behaviour immediately after birth. Obviously sedatives and anaesthetics which cross the placenta will make the baby sleepy and inactive. This is the reason why many babies after Caesarean section used to require resuscitation. Mothers who are on long-term anticonvulsant therapy may have babies with withdrawal symptoms. The babies on the second and third day become hyperactive and difficult to feed and some have 'jittery' episodes. It is important to reassure mother of the nature of these episodes as she may fear that her baby is going to have fits like herself. Mothers who are heroin addicts have babies who are undersized but their maturation may be advanced so that they have a lower incidence of respiratory distress syndrome. However, the babies may show severe withdrawal symptoms and require careful management over the first few weeks of life. Maternal addiction to codeine and cocaine can also lead to neonatal withdrawal problems.

Drugs which cross the placenta and affect the newborn infant

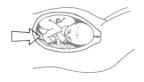

anaesthetics
sedatives
opioid analgesics
narcotics
anticonvulsants
antihypertensives
prostaglandin-synthetase
inhibitors

Any drugs that the obstetrician uses to accelerate labour may interfere with the baby after birth. For example, prostaglandin and anti-prostaglandin agents may interfere with the balance between patency and closure of the ductus arteriosus. Oxytocin administered to control labour causes a small increase in bilirubin levels in the infants after birth and if administered in large volumes of intravenous dextrose can cause dangerous neonatal hyponatraemia.

FETAL TRANSPLACENTAL INFECTIONS

The list of organisms that have been proven to cross the placenta and affect the fetus is relatively short. It is possible that a much larger number might on rare occasions cause fetal disease or death, but gathering evidence for this relationship is difficult.

Rubella

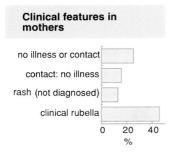

Clinical features in mothers

no illness or contact

contact: no illness

rash (not diagnosed)

clinical rubella

0   20   40
%

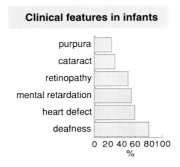

Clinical features in infants

purpura

cataract

retinopathy

mental retardation

heart defect

deafness

0 20 40 60 80100
%

A small percentage of women have their first attack of german measles during early pregnancy, and they may or may not have a suggestive rash. The risks to the fetus are considerable, particularly if a viraemia occurs in the first trimester; a large percentage of pregnancies abort or the surviving fetus is seriously damaged. The viraemia may persist throughout pregnancy and the infant may continue to excrete virus for many years afterwards. During this time the disease process continues. It is because of these terrible consequences of this otherwise trivial infection, that rubella immunisation was offered to all teenage girls. Nevertheless, fetal damage due to rubella continued to occur because some girls were missed or declined immunisation and therefore, in an effort to eradicate all rubella from the community, rubella immunisation is now recommended for all children, boys and girls, at 15 months and the incidence of congenital rubella has fallen dramatically.

Clinical features. A surviving fetus may be left with congenital heart defects, defects of the ears with deafness, and eye disorders, particularly cataracts. A small percentage present at birth with purpura, thrombocytopenia, hepatosplenomegaly and have X-ray evidence of bony lesions. Many have an associated encephalopathy and are subsequently mentally retarded. 85 per cent of infants infected during the first 8 weeks of pregnancy will have detectable defects, usually multiple, in contrast to only 15 per cent of infants infected at 16–20 weeks (usually sensorineural deafness only). There appears to be no risk of exposure after 22 weeks.

If a pregnant woman has contact with suspected rubella it is essential to determine whether she is vulnerable to primary infection or whether she has protection from previous exposure. If the diagnosis is suspected, blood is taken and tested for serum haemagglutinin inhibition antibodies (HI) for rubella. If antibodies are high within the incubation period, the patient can be considered to be protected by a previous infection. If they are low, a further sample should be taken 7 to 10 days and if possible 17 to 21 days after first exposure. A rise in titre confirms primary infection and the risk of fetal damage and many consider this grounds for a therapeutic abortion. Diagnosis in the newborn is confirmed by the presence of a specific rubella IgM antibody.

Cytomegalovirus disease

CMV is the commonest congenital infection in the UK and occurs in 3 per 1000 live births. In common with rubella virus, CMV produces a mild disease in adults. It is also widespread in the community; 50 per cent of pregnant English women have antibodies to CMV. It has been estimated that between 1 and 5 per cent of pregnant women contract CMV infections and that the fetus is affected in around 50 per cent. Infection in early pregnancy may cause abortion or a spectrum of malformations including growth failure, microcephaly, mental retardation and deafness. CMV may be a significant cause of mental handicap, epilepsy and nerve deafness, which manifest in later life when the relationship with intrauterine infection is less likely to be appreciated. CMV infection in late pregnancy may produce a systemic illness comprising purpura, hepatosplenomegaly, pneumonia and encephalitis.

Overall, about 5 per cent of infected infants will have clinical signs at birth, and this group invariably has long term sequelae. Another 5 per cent develop severe handicaps later (particularly sensorineural deafness) despite an asymptomatic neonatal period.

Due to the absence of clinical illness in the adult, the infection in the mother often passes undetected. Even routine screening of the newborn for raised CMV specific IgM levels can be misleading. However, the presence of virus in the urine of the newborn with raised cytomegalovirus specific IgM antibody confirms the diagnosis. At present there is no reliable vaccine available for the protection against CMV infections.

Unlike rubella, routine serological screening for CMV in pregnancy and the option of termination cannot be justified because fetal infection can occur following primary or recurrent CMV infection in pregnancy, damage can occur following infection at any time in pregnancy, and 90 per cent of infants will be unaffected.

Human immunodeficiency virus

HIV may be transmitted from mother to child before, during or after birth but because transplacental maternal antibodies persist until up to 18 months of age, neonatal diagnosis is difficult in asymptomatic infants. Tests to detect viral antigen are not yet widely available. Postnatal infection via breast milk may occur.

Approximately one-third of infants born to HIV-positive mothers will ultimately be shown to be infected. The prognosis for this group is variable from rapid progression to full-blown AIDS with serious opportunistic infections in the first year of life to mild or non-specific features such as lymphadenopathy, hepatosplenomegaly, chronic diarrhoea, failure to thrive, fever or parotitis presenting up to school age.

Parvovirus B19 infection

70 per cent of adults are seropositive for this virus which causes slapped cheek syndrome and erythema infectiosum (5th disease) in children. Infection is often subclinical. In pregnancy, the risk of transplacental transmission is estimated at 33 per cent with an increased incidence of abortion and hydrops fetalis. However, there is no evidence of damage in the 85 per cent of infants who survive maternal infection and therefore termination of pregnancy is not indicated.

Herpes varicella zoster infection

85 per cent of women have antibodies to HZV and therefore, whilst they may develop shingles in pregnancy, the fetus will not be at risk from maternal chickenpox. Although chickenpox early in pregnancy rarely affects the fetus, the complications are severe (the 'varicella syndrome' — scarring skin lesions, chorioretinitis, cataracts and CNS damage). The greatest risk to the infant is if the mother develops the rash between four days before delivery and four days after delivery, in which case there is no time for protective transplacental antibodies to be acquired and neonatal mortality is high. The transplacental transmission rate to the fetus of this late-onset maternal HZV is 25 per cent and these infants should be given passive immunisation with zoster immune globulin as soon after birth as possible. Acyclovir is usually reserved for those infants who show clinical features of neonatal HZV but these may take up

to two weeks to appear. In view of the high mortality rate, a mother developing the rash perinatally should be isolated and should barrier nurse her infant and not breast-fed until all the skin lesions have crusted over.

Listeria monocytogenes

Maternal infection with these Gram positive bacteria may result in abortion, premature labour or fetal infection, which is acquired predominantly transplacentally although other rare routes are by inhalation of infected liquor or by ascending infection from the genital tract. The organism has been isolated from under-cooked chickens or 'cook-chill' meals, unpasteurised milk and soft cheeses and gives rise to a mild 'flu-like' systemic illness in the mother.

Infants infected prenatally present soon after birth with a generalised septicaemic illness which may include pneumonia, meningitis and a rash. The liquor is usually foul smelling and there may be placental abscesses. There is a 30 per cent mortality. Those infected during vaginal delivery present after 1–8 weeks, usually with meningitis, and have a better prognosis. Ampicillin and gentamicin are synergistic and maternal treatment may improve prognosis for the fetus.

Toxoplasmosis

Toxoplasma gondii, a protozoon parasite, is found around the world and affects animals as well as man. In the UK, only 20 per cent of women are protected by antibodies. Again, the maternal infection may not produce any clinical symptoms. Only a small percentage of women contract the infection in the first part of pregnancy but when they do so the organism may invade the placenta and spread to the fetus. Infection occurs from ingestion of undercooked meat or of oocysts excreted in cat faeces. Pregnant women should not empty cat litters and should wear gloves for gardening and wash hands after touching soil.

The risk of transplacental transmission is about 40 per cent but only 10 per cent of these show clinical features at birth. Toxoplasmosis has widespread effects on the developing brain, causing hydrocephalus or microcephaly with cerebral calcification and a chorioretinitis. There is usually resultant mental handicap with other neurological abnormalities. The major risk to the other 90 per cent appears to be chorioretinitis which may only appear in adulthood.

A diagnosis is made on the basis of rising antibody titres. In the newborn, the toxoplasma specific IgM fluorescent antibody test will be positive in those infants who have been infected, but the absence of antibodies does not rule out the possibility of a congenital infection. Infants thought to have the disease should be followed up both clinically and serologically.

If infection is confirmed in the first trimester, when the risk to the fetus is greatest, termination may be considered or the mother treated with spiramycin which reduces the risk of fetal infection.

Fetal infections

Treponema pallidum (syphillis)

rubella virus

herpes varicella & zoster

cytomegalovirus

plasmodia (malaria)

Toxoplasma gondii

human immuno-deficiency virus

parvovirus

Others

Syphilis used to be the most commonly recognised organism that attacked the fetus but happily it is now very rare in the UK. The same is true for congenital tuberculosis. Malaria commonly affects the placenta and may interfere with the fetal growth. Mothers with malaria have babies of relatively low birth weight. Occasionally the parasites cause fetal disease.

INFECTIONS ACQUIRED DURING PASSAGE THROUGH THE BIRTH CANAL

A sterile infant passing through the birth canal is at risk of contracting a wide range of infections, particularly from pathogenic organisms in the maternal bowel. If the membranes have ruptured prematurely, the infant may be infected 2 or 3 days prior to birth by organisms entering the uterus via the birth canal. There has been some concern that, even without rupture of the membranes, infection can pass up the birth canal to produce an infection of the placenta and the fetus.

Gonococcal ophthalmia

Infection due to *Neisseria gonorrhoea* acquired during the birth can lead to a purulent conjunctivitis, which if not treated promptly, results in corneal ulceration and perforation. Frequent irrigation with antibiotic eye drops is recommended together with a course of systemic penicillin or, if the organism is insensitive to penicillin, a broad spectrum antibiotic.

Chlamydia

The endocervix is the site most frequently infected by *Chlamydia trachomatis* in women, and chlamydia is a common cause of conjunctivitis in the newborn in the first month of life. Chlamydial pneumonia is rarer and difficult to diagnose as symptoms appear 4–6 weeks after birth and the infant may be apyrexial. Chest X-ray shows widespread pneumonitis.

Pneumonia and meningitis

So-called congenital pneumonia is in most instances not due to a bacterial infection. However, occasionally listeria or group B streptococcal organisms in the birth canal can be drawn into the respiratory tract and produce a bacterial pneumonia in the first few days of life. The possibility needs to be recognised and vigorous antibiotic therapy given for septicemia and meningitis may quickly follow. All infants with respiratory distress are given penicillin because of the very high mortality from group B streptococcal infection.

Herpes simplex infections

Herpes virus Type 2 infection (HSV) is a sexually transmitted disease. The cervicitis is frequently asymptomatic but it creates a major risk for the fetus. Ascending infection may result in abortion or, in later pregnancy, premature birth. There is a high (40 per cent) risk of direct infection during the infant's passage through the birth canal. Neonatal herpes infection is frequently fatal and obstetricians regard active herpetic cervicitis as an indication for elective Caesarean section. The risk to the fetus is less if the lesions represent reactivation rather than primary infection. The risk of post-natal spread to a baby from a parent with a 'cold sore' is very low but topical treatment should be given.

Neonatal disease usually presents at a week with localised, vesicular skin lesions or with a generalised viraemia with hepatosplenomegaly, jaundice, petechiae, encephalopathy and seizures. There may be chorioretinitis or cataract and increased white cells in CSF. Rapid diagnosis is by electron microscopy or antigen detection of fluid from blisters and all neonatal HSV should be treated with intravenous acyclovir.

Heptatitis B virus

Hepatitis B is a major health problem in developing countries. It contributes to a high mortality from cirrhosis and hepatocellular carcinoma. The pool of chronic carriers is perpetuated by maternal-child transfer at birth. Screening for HBs, a surface antigen, is carried out in all non-Caucasian women and Caucasian women with previous hepatitis, drug abuse or with a sexual or occupational lifestyle suggestive of increased exposure to HBV. If the mother is also positive for the E antigen of HBV, her blood is highly infective whereas if the anti-HBe antibody is present, the infectivity is much lower. Although HBV can be transferred to the fetus at any time during pregnancy or delivery, or to the baby post-natally, the combination of active immunisation (with HBV vaccine) and passive immunisation (with anti-HBs immunoglobulin) shortly after birth and active immunisation again at 1 and 6 months appears to reduce the risk of subsequent HBV carriage, cirrhosis and hepatoma.

MATERNAL IMMUNOGLOBULINS

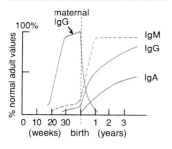

Immunoglobulin levels before and after birth

The immune defence mechanisms develop early in fetal life, but in the absence of stimulation, specific antibodies are not produced. The human fetus gains some specific protection by the transfer of maternal IgG across the placenta. In general the maternal immunoglobulins confer benefit but they can produce disease. The commonest example is the transfer of maternal antibodies against the fetal blood cells as in rhesus and ABO incompatibility.

Less commonly, mothers suffering from the so-called autoimmune diseases may transfer damaging antibodies to the fetus. Thus, mothers with platelet antibodies, who may or may not themselves have clinical features of idiopathic thrombocytopenia, may have babies who develop purpura in the first two to three days of life due to the transfer of platelet antibodies across the placenta. Similarly, mothers with systemic lupus erythematosis may have infants who have either systemic disease, which is usually lethal, or transient lupus rashes on the face. Likewise, babies of mothers with myasthenia gravis may have transient but severe hypotonia, and infants of mothers with ulcerative colitis may have transient melaena. Finally, mothers with circulating thyroid antibodies, irrespective of whether they are thyrotoxic or even in a hypothyroid state during pregnancy, may have infants who develop all the signs of thyrotoxicosis after birth including exophthalmos. There may be little indication that the baby is affected until they develop

Transient disorders in the newborn caused by maternal immuno-globulins

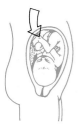

rhesus incompatibility

thrombocytopenia

lupus erythematosis

myasthenia gravis

thyrotoxicosis

heart failure in the second week or so of life. It is as well to keep an eye on all infants at risk.

Fetal determinants of adult disease. The state of pregnancy can be associated with illness in the mother as well as the fetus and some of this morbidity appears to be generated by the feto-placental unit. It has long been known that pre-eclampsia is cured by delivery of the fetus and placenta but it now appears that the propensity of a woman to develop pre-eclampsia may be determined by a gene on a fetal chromosome. Multiple sclerosis, congenital heart disease and insulin dependent diabetes are examples of pre-conceptual maternal diseases which may become worse during pregnancy.

Some of the risks of disease in adult life appear to be manifest in fetal life. Systolic blood pressure in men at retirement is inversely related to birth weight and the risk of ischaemic heart disease is greater the lower the fetal/placental weight ratio.

Birth: a reminder

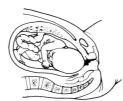

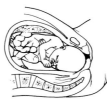

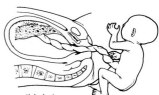

first stage:
contractions begin
and cervix opens

second stage:
cervix opened and
baby descends

third stage:
baby born and
placenta seperates

BIBLIOGRAPHY

Allan L D 1989 Diagnosis of fetal cardiac abnormalities Archives of Diseases in Childhood 64: 964–968

Barker D J P, Bull A R, Osmond C, Simmonds S J 1990 Fetal and placental size and risk of hypertension in adult life. British Medical Journal 301: 259–262

Battaglia F C, Meschia G 1986 An introduction to fetal physiology. Academic Press, London

Beard R W, Nathanielsz P W (eds) 1984 Fetal physiology and medicine, 2nd edn. Butterworths, London

Best J M 1987 Congenital cytomegalovirus infection. British Medical Journal 294: 1440–1441

Cleary M A, Wraith J E 1991 Antenatal diagnosis of inborn errors of metabolism. Archives of Diseases in Childhood 66: 816–822

Logan G S, Pekham C 1991 Congenital infections. Hospital Update 17 (7): 586–591

Pattison J R 1988 Diseases caused by the human parvovirus B19. Archives of Diseases in Childhood 63: 1426–1427

Polin R A, Fox W W 1992 Fetal and neonatal physiology. WB Saunders, Philadelphia

Rosevear S K 1989 Placental biopsy. British Journal of Hospital Medicine 41: 334–348

4 Newborn

In our concern to provide every mother and her child with a safe birth we may overlook the importance of their first meeting face to face. They have a deep basic need to 'recognise' and respond to each other. Fascinating research has demonstrated how very aware and responsive the human newborn is to his new environment. If the mother is ill or the delivery is difficult or the newborn infant is sick or weak it is even more important for the caring staff to encourage the establishment and the strengthening of the bond between mother and child. Failure to do so may lead subsequently to poor feeding patterns, failure to thrive, and the longer term consequences of maternal neglect. When mother and infant have failed to establish a mutually satisfying relationship there is an increased risk of child abuse and post-neonatal infant death.

ROUTINE EXAMINATION OF THE NEWBORN

'Is my baby all right?' is often the first question that mothers ask after delivery and it is so difficult to answer if he is not! As soon as the baby is born a quick but careful scrutiny of the face, eyes, mouth, chest, abdomen, spine and limbs should exclude major abnormalities; a lusty cry and the development of a suffuse pink blush over the face and body denote satisfactory immediate adjustment to independent existence. Together they are sufficient to answer the mother's pressing question. If you are not sure of the sex of the infant do not make a guess. Explain to the parents that occasionally it can be difficult to tell immediately and that tests may be necessary. If there is difficulty establishing adequate breathing, then the appropriate steps in resuscitation should be taken. If the baby is small, immature or injured, he must be given extra support and protection. If the mother has had hydramnios then a firm tube must be passed into the stomach to exclude oesophageal atresia, a congenital abnormality which is usually associated with a trachea-oesophageal fistula.

Over the next 48 hours all infants should be examined thoroughly and at leisure, preferably in the mother's presence, ideally with both parents, and only after the details of the medical history of the family,

The average newborn!

body weight	3.5 kg
body length	50 cm
head circumference	35 cm
Hb	18 g/dl
blood volume	300 ml

Incidence of the commoner malformations in Great Britain (these figures are approximate)

Malformation	per 1000 livebirths
Anencephaly	1.0
Spina bifida	1.5
Cleft lip/cleft palate	1.4
Club foot	1.2
Congenital hip dislocation	1.5
Congenital heart mal.	6.0
Down syndrome	1.6
Pyloric stenosis	3.0

the pregnancy and labour are known. This first medical examination is a screening procedure, and its aim is to discover disorders which are open to early management. The baby should be naked in a warm room, and the mother should be able to see clearly what you are doing. The examination should be thorough and in a logical sequence; first assess overall size, proportions and maturity, then look for structural abnormalities, starting with the head and eyes and then the ears, mouth, chest, abdomen and limbs, hands and feet. Note any accessory tags, digits and dimples. Many abnormalities follow failure of complete union in the midline, and so a quick check along the midline is worthwhile, and this should include a close look at the palate and anus. Respiratory disorders are more easily seen than heard. Palpating the peripheral pulses may suggest, if full, a ductus arteriosus, or, if weak, a major defect causing poor systemic cardiac output. The presence or absence of femoral pulsations must always be noted. Abnormal heart sounds and murmurs are more difficult to interpret; if there is doubt, it is better to find an opportunity to re-examine the baby later. If the murmur persists but the baby is otherwise well, then the parents are told of the finding and a follow-up examination is arranged. Two other conditions are specifically sought; congenital dislocation of the hips, and in boys, the presence of testes in the scrotum.

The third stage of this examination is to assess the baby's behaviour and responsiveness. The mother and the midwife will usually be quick to tell you about the baby's feeding, behaviour, crying and sleeping patterns. An unduly floppy or sleepy baby, an irritable or restless baby, or a poor 'suckler' all call for more careful evaluation, particularly in relation to the establishment or otherwise of satisfactory breast feeding. Parents should be reassured about minor anomalies. Finally give the parents an opportunity to ask any other questions.

Minor anomalies

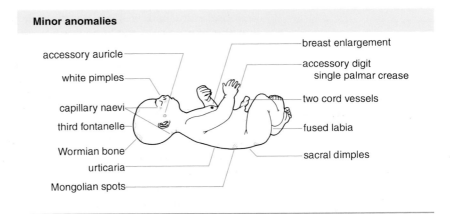

- accessory auricle
- white pimples
- capillary naevi
- third fontanelle
- Wormian bone
- urticaria
- Mongolian spots
- breast enlargement
- accessory digit
- single palmar crease
- two cord vessels
- fused labia
- sacral dimples

Capillary or macular haemangioma (stork bites, salmon patch) around the eyes and at the nape of the neck are seen in 30 to 50 per cent of babies. Those around the eyes usually disappear in the first year. Those at the nape may persist.

Blue–black pigmented areas (Mongolian blue spots) at the base of the back and on the buttocks are unimportant and are common in infants of dark skinned parents but can also occur in Caucasian infants. They usually fade over the first year or so.

Urticaria of the newborn is a fluctuating, widespread, erythematous rash with a raised white dot at the centre of the red flare. It is usually most marked on the trunk and is most evident on the second day. It disappears spontaneously, requiring no treatment.

Heat rash (miliaria) is seen in mature infants nursed in warm humid atmospheres. Both red, macular patches and superficial, clear vesicles may be seen, most evident on the forehead and around the neck. The lesions clear in a cool environment.

Breast enlargement. Both girl and boy infants may develop breast enlargement and even secrete small amounts of milk (witch's milk). Girls may discharge a mucous plug from the vagina and there may be a little vaginal bleeding on about the fourth day.

White pimples (milia) on the nose and cheeks are very common and are found in about 40 per cent of infants. They are blocked sebaceous glands and clear spontaneously.

Cysts in the mouth occur on the palate near the midline (Epstein's pearls) and larger ones on the gums (epulis) and on the floor of the mouth. Epstein's pearls and most of the others resolve spontaneously. Teeth may be present at birth: some are loose and have to be removed.

Accessory skin tags on the face, anterior to the ears (accessory auricles) or loosely attached, vestigial, extra digits can usually be dealt with easily but this should preferably be done by the surgical team.

Sacral dimples should be explored gently to exclude underlying sinuses.

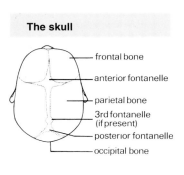

The skull

frontal bone
anterior fontanelle
parietal bone
3rd fontanelle (if present)
posterior fontanelle
occipital bone

Some anomalies, although relatively unimportant in themselves, may be associated with more important abnormalities. The fontanelles (head 'soft spots') are occasionally wide and extra bones may float in the space, Wormian bones. If skin defects overlie the posterior fontanelle chromosomal abnormalities should be considered. A third fontanelle is occasionally found between the anterior and posterior fontanelles and is common in trisomy 21.

Oddly shaped ears and two cord vessels may be associated with renal abnormalities. A single palmar crease, instead of the usual two, may sometimes be associated with other abnormalities, including Down syndrome. Abnormalities of the face, jaws and ears, including accessory auricles, may be associated with varying degrees of deafness, and a newborn hearing screening test should be arranged.

Congenital postural deformities

The posture of the infant after birth often reflects his position *in utero*. However, with more freedom, the infant soon chooses to curl into a compact shape with arms and legs flexed. If there is less than an average amount of amniotic fluid to cushion the fetus, then towards the end of gestation the infant may be so tightly packed within the uterus that deformations of the musculo-skeletal system develop. These congenital postural deformities may mould the head into odd shapes (dolichocephaly, plagiocephaly), suppress or distort the chin, resulting in its being unduly small (micrognathia), or cause mandibular symmetry or neck muscle contractures and torticollis. The shoulders may be dislocated, the chest wall compressed, the hands and feet distorted (club hand, club foot). These effects are usually multiple and are seen in their extreme form when the kidneys are absent in renal agenesis, and very little amniotic fluid is present (oligohydramnios). The presenting part is often the most deformed. One special example of postural deformity associated with intrauterine position is dislocation of the hip, which is more common in breech presentation.

Intrauterine postures

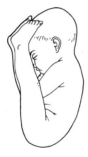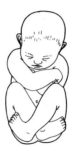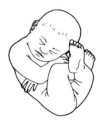

Biochemical screening

The number of inherited biochemical disorders or variations which can be recognised by relatively simple and cheap biochemical tests increases yearly. It is the simplicity and cheapness of the test which makes it feasible to test the blood of every newborn infant. The tests are primarily intended to screen for phenylketonuria (the Guthrie test), hypothyroidism and cystic fibrosis, but other conditions including galactosaemia, maple syrup urine disease and homocystinuria may be identified. The blood test is performed when milk feeding has been established, between the sixth and eighth day of life.

BIRTH INJURIES

The short journey down the birth canal is not without hazards for the infant but fortunately the risks are becoming less as the techniques for

Caput succedaneum (common)

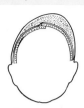

Cephalhaematoma (occasional)

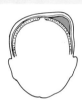

Subaponeurotic haemorrhage (rare)

recognising fetal distress improve. Infants who are judged to be too big for the birth canal or who fail to advance during labour and become distressed are delivered by Caesarean section, making heroic obstetric manipulations to achieve vaginal birth rarely necessary. The risk of birth trauma is greater in breech deliveries, in premature births, in precipitate deliveries and when the baby is unexpectedly large.

Some of the damage caused by the birth is unsightly but quickly resolves. Inevitably, the presenting part becomes oedematous and bruised. This caput succedaneum is commonly found on the back of the head and happily it clears spontaneously in a few days. However, the swelling looks uncomfortable when it involves the breech and scrotum and very unpleasant in a face presentation. The face also looks bloated, blue and bruised when the cord is pulled tightly around the neck (an appearance called 'traumatic cyanosis'), and there may also be retinal and conjunctival haemorrhages. As the fetal head is pushed down the birth canal it rotates and the apex of the parietal bones may catch the ischial spines and be dented like a ping pong ball or the outer shelf may be cracked and crepitus may be felt, or the periosteum may separate and a cephalhaematoma form beneath the periosteum producing a lump the size of a small hen's egg. Again, these injuries are of little import although the cephalhaematoma may take many months before it finally disappears. Rarely a bleed may occur under the aponeurosis (sub-aponeurotic haemorrhage) when the bleeding is not confined to a single cranial bone like a cephalhaematoma but spreads rapidly over the head and down towards the eyes. A significant fraction of the blood volume may be lost into this haematoma.

Birth injuries

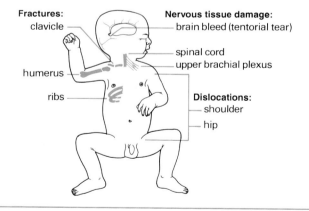

Fractures: clavicle, humerus, ribs. Nervous tissue damage: brain bleed (tentorial tear), spinal cord, upper brachial plexus. Dislocations: shoulder, hip

Severe compression with extreme moulding of the skull can tear the tentorium cerebelli and its accompanying vein. The resulting haemorrhage is likely to cause permanent damage or death. The baby may be born in a state of shock and may not respond to resuscitative procedures.

Manipulation of the spine and arms, which is most likely to be required for breech deliveries, may damage the cervical spinal cord with residual palsies in arms and legs, or lead to stretching and damage of the upper part of the brachial plexus causing weakness or paralysis of abduction at the shoulder, flexion at the elbow and extension and supination of the wrist (Erb's palsy). The arm is dropped into the position a waiter adopts in the expectation of a tip. The weakness usually resolves spontaneously in a few weeks.

Rough handling may lead not only to fracture of the skull but also of the clavicle, humerus or ribs. These injuries may pass undetected immediately after birth, but can be recognised when a lump appears due to callus formation around the fracture.

Forceps blades may compress the facial nerve as it leaves the parotid gland. Usually the resultant facial palsy is transient, but occasionally the pressure causes overlying fat necrosis with permanent scarring and a residual palsy.

BIRTH ASPHYXIA

The fetus, floating in the amniotic fluid, 'breathes', 'feeds' and 'excretes' through the placenta. The fetal lungs are filled with fluid secreted by the alveolar cells to a volume close to the functional residual capacity found after birth. Following delivery, the placenta is discarded and 'dies' whilst the independent infant activates his own system for obtaining oxygen and nutrients and discarding waste.

The most urgent requirement is to breathe. To do this the lung liquid must be displaced by air. During a vaginal birth the thorax is squeezed in the birth canal and the lung liquid can sometimes be seen pouring out of the baby's nose when his head is just emerging from the birth canal. Once the infant gasps, air is drawn into the lung and lung liquid disappears to the periphery of the respiratory tree. From there it is cleared by the pulmonary circulation and lymphatics. Failure to complete this process satisfactorily is one factor leading to transient tachypnoea.

As the infant passes down the birth canal his head is squeezed and then released and exposed to the cooling air. His limbs are pushed, pulled and finally allowed to drop into positions they have never occupied before. His umbilical cord is intermittently obstructed, stretched and finally clamped. His arterial concentration of oxygen falls and that of carbon dioxide rises. Many of these stimuli provoke a gasp.

On average, newborn infants gasp after 6 seconds and the majority have done so by 20 seconds. With these efforts the lungs rapidly fill with air and a residual lung volume is formed. Once this is achieved, tidal breathing begins. It occurs on average after 30 seconds and the majority of infants are breathing regularly by 90 seconds.

As the lungs expand and fill with gas, the pulmonary vascular resistance falls, the pulmonary blood flow increases and the pressure in the

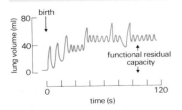

Onset of breathing

left atrium rises closing the foramen ovale. As a consequence of these changes, oxygenated blood passes through the ductus arteriosus; oxygen has a direct effect on the muscle of the ductus causing contraction and physiological closure, anatomical closure proceeds more slowly over the following weeks.

Circulatory adjustments after birth

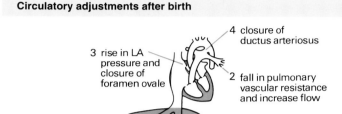

3 rise in LA pressure and closure of foramen ovale

4 closure of ductus arteriosus

2 fall in pulmonary vascular resistance and increase flow

1 interruption of placental flow and closure of ductus venosus

Occasionally, in cyanosed infants, the ductus may remain open or the physiologically closed ductus may reopen, and so add to the infant's problems sometimes to the point of precipitating heart failure.

Infants may be asphyxiated *in utero* for a variety of reasons. If the disorder is not reversed they will be asphyxiated at birth and they must be resuscitated immediately. Many of the babies who appear all but dead at birth but who respond promptly to active resuscitation may make a full recovery. More commonly, infants are reasonably oxygenated at birth but due to previous asphyxia or sedative drugs given to the mother they fail to begin adequate ventilation, and then become asphyxiated and require resuscitation. Many factors are associated with birth asphyxia including the general well being of the mother and the maturity and nutrition of the infant.

Causes of intrauterine asphyxia

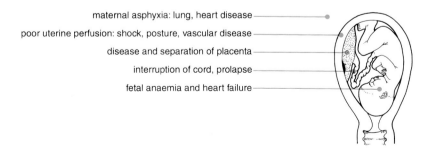

maternal asphyxia: lung, heart disease

poor uterine perfusion: shock, posture, vascular disease

disease and separation of placenta

interruption of cord, prolapse

fetal anaemia and heart failure

With increasing asphyxia the infant becomes blue and then white, hypotonic, unresponding, and the heart rate begins to fall. These features: colour, tone, response to stimulation, respiration and heart rate were arranged into a scoring system by an American anaesthetist, Dr Virginia Apgar. The main features to watch are the infant's attempts to breathe and the rate and strength of the pulse. Those who fail to breathe and become asphyxiated should be actively resuscitated when the heart rate begins to fall.

Assessment of neonatal asphyxia

	Apgar score		
	0	1	2
Response to stimulation	None	Facial grimace	Cry
Respiration	Absent	Gasping	Regular
Heart rate	0	< 100	> 100
Colour of trunk	White	Blue	Pink
Muscle tone	Flaccid	Some flexion	Normal with movement

Resuscitation

The newly born baby is gently dried and wrapped in a warm towel. The time of birth is noted. The upper airway is cleared by gentle suction of excess fluid and any inhaled vernix, blood or meconium. If during this procedure the infant fails to make any respiratory effort then a gasp may be provoked by blowing cold oxygen on the nose. If this is not effective then the other bizarre methods used in the past, for example pinching, slapping, injecting respiratory stimulants, or putting champagne or pepper on the nasal mucosa, are not likely to work.

The next step is to expand and ventilate the lungs. Often inflation of the lungs itself will initiate a gasp with spontaneous breathing. If it does not, the lung should be ventilated at a rate between 20 and 30 inflations per minute with pressures limited to 30 cm H_2O. The majority of infants will quickly become pink and begin breathing within 2 or 5 minutes.

Steps in resuscitation: watch the clock

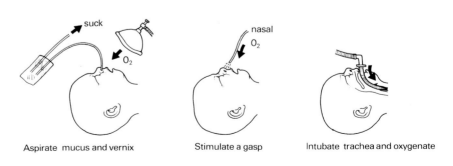

Aspirate mucus and vernix   Stimulate a gasp   Intubate trachea and oxygenate

The most effective method of inflating the lungs is via an endo-tracheal tube. To insert the tube, the infant's head must be carefully positioned in slight extension, the small finger of the hand holding the endoscope pushes the larynx into view. If either the skill or the equipment is not available for intubation then the infant can be resuscitated nearly as well with a face mask, which fits snugly over his mouth and nose, and a bag which delivers small volumes of gas. It is essential to hold the lower jaw forward to ensure a clear airway. Over-inflation of the stomach can be avoided by passing a nasogastric tube and putting gentle hand pressure on the upper abdomen.

If the infant fails to become pink with good expansion of the lung then he is probably in a state of shock. If the apex rate is less than 60 and falling, start cardiac massage using two finger pressure on the lower half of the sternum at 100–120 beats per minute. Metabolic acidosis can be corrected by giving 4.2 per cent sodium bicarbonate 4 ml/kg into the umbilical vein. It is important to flush it through.

If the lungs do not expand then either there is a rare abnormality of the airways or lungs, or the endotracheal tube is not in the trachea. Clumsy insertion of the tube can damage the upper airways; energetic and faulty inflation may damage the lungs. Occasionally, the difficult decision of whether to resuscitate or not has to be made. If the baby is physically normal and can be resuscitated then recent reports suggest that he will probably survive intact, although he may have a stormy few days rather like an older child after a head injury. If the baby is physically abnormal then one must ask oneself firstly, could this child survive even if resuscitation is successful, and secondly, has the infant's brain developed adequately? If the answer to either is no, then resuscitation is not justifiable. If there is uncertainty, call a colleague, remembering that in general parents would wish us to respond to their offspring as we would wish others to respond to our own.

Reasons for failure to resuscitate

Brain damage:
   haemorrhage: ischaemia
Upper airway obstruction:
   laryngeal spasm
   laryngeal stenosis
Lung pathology:
   pneumothorax
   hypoplasia
   effusion
   diaphragmatic hernia
Small chest cage
Shock due to ruptured viscera

Effects of asphyxia

Birth asphyxia may have both immediate and long term effects. Acute total asphyxia seen, for example, with cord prolapse, may by haemorrhage and oedema, damage and interfere with brain function, causing profound hypotonia followed by irritability and fitting; there may be an abnormal cry and poor sucking patterns. The breathing pattern may be so disturbed as to suggest a primary respiratory problem. Loss of homeostatic control may lead to hypoglycaemia, hypocalcaemia and hypothermia. But asphyxia may damage many other organs as well: in the lungs it causes oedema; in the myocardium changes resembling an infarct; in the bowel it causes an ileus or ischaemic perforations; in the kidneys it may result in renal vein thrombosis or tubular necrosis; and in the liver disorders of metabolism and haemostasis may result. In premature infants, birth asphyxia increases the risk of idiopathic respiratory distress syndrome and of two types of intracranial damage: intraventricular haemorrhages and periventricular leucomalacia (softening of the white matter around the ventricles).

The immediate postnatal effects of chronic intermittent prenatal asphyxia are more difficult to assess for invariably asphyxia is not the only

Immediate effects of severe birth asphyxia

Brain:
   fits, irritability
   abnormal tone
   hypo and hyperventilation
   hypoglycaemia
Lungs:
   aspiration, RDS
   haemorrhage
Kidneys:
   vein thrombosis
   tubular necrosis
Bowels:
   ileus, perforation

noxious factor affecting the infant.

Cerebral oedema, haemorrhage or ischaemia may lead to permanent brain damage and resultant cerebral palsy and mental handicap. That less severe degrees of asphyxia can lead to less severe evidence of brain damage, for example, fits, hyperactivity and learning problems, is generally accepted but the extent to which it is responsible for these disorders in the community is difficult to assess.

We are still left with the problem of trying to determine which infants asphyxiated before or during the birth are likely to be permanently affected. Some infants make remarkable recoveries so parents should be encouraged to be reasonably optimistic. It has been estimated that only 1 in 10 infants showing evidence of brain asphyxia in the week or so after birth are subsequently found to have evidence of brain damage.

SIZE AT BIRTH

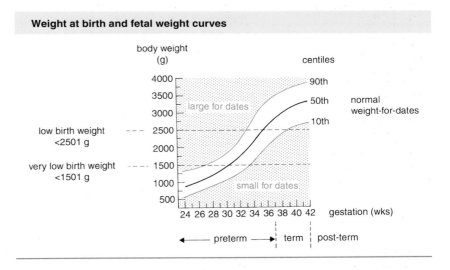

Weight at birth and fetal weight curves

The birth weight plotted on growth charts of body weight against gestational age help us to define groups of babies. Those whose birth weights are between the 10th and 90th centile lines are 'normal weight for dates'. Those babies with birth weights over the 90th centile are called 'large for dates', and those with weights under the 10th centile are 'small for dates'. Small-for-dates babies also described as 'small for gestational age', 'light for dates', and dysmature. It is important to determine whether a baby is 'large for dates' or 'small for dates' or premature or postmature, for each has special problems which can be anticipated and treated.

Large-for-dates infants

The infant of a diabetic mother is large and obese. Not many years ago many of them were stillborn. Now with improved antenatal care the majority survive but they are still at a slightly greater risk of having a congenital abnormality; their broad shoulders may give problems during the birth (shoulder dystocia) and after birth they are more likely to develop hypoglycaemia, respiratory distress and to become jaundiced. Their hyperexcitability, jitteriness and immaturity may initially cause feeding difficulties. With meticulous control of the diabetic state during the whole of pregnancy, many if not all these problems can be avoided. The exciting question is whether or not good control in early pregnancy will reduce the incidence of congenital abnormalities.

Low birth weight

About 7 per cent of UK births are low birth weight, defined as all those weighing 2500 g or less, at birth. The incidence is lower in Scandinavian countries and higher in Third World countries. The low birth weight group includes a disproportionate number of the babies with problems. In the UK about 60 per cent of stillbirths and 70 per cent of first week deaths are of low birth weight. Low birth weight is associated amongst other things with poor socioeconomic conditions, congenital abnormalities, intrauterine infections, multiple pregnancies, poor placental function, and maternal starvation, illness, smoking, drug and alcohol abuse. Low birth weight may be due to premature birth, before 37 weeks (preterm infant), or poor fetal growth ('small-for-dates' infant). Although they may be of the same weight, preterm and 'small-for-dates' infants look different and have different problems. Some babies are both preterm and small for dates and are at risk of the problems of both groups.

Small-for-dates infants. It is important to recognise these infants preferably before birth for they are more likely to be in trouble during delivery and be in need of prompt and skilful resuscitation. They are particularly susceptible to damaging hypoglycaemia in the first days of life. Four hourly estimations of blood glucose concentration should be made and early generous feeding commenced. Should the blood glucose concentration fall below 1.5 mmol/l, intravenous glucose therapy is necessary.

Small-for-dates babies have a lower perinatal mortality rate than babies of similar birth weight born preterm, but their eventual outlook may not be so good. Those who are small but perfectly proportioned, suggesting intrauterine growth retardation early in the pregnancy, may remain small, and their abilities are more likely to fall below the average. The situation is complex because of the association with poor socioeconomic status.

Preterm infants. The survival rates of preterm babies have improved over the years. Much of this progress is due to the better management. Neonatal care is provided at two levels. Special care is for well preterm infants who need to be carefully watched and monitored in a relatively stable environment and where special expertise is available to help them establish and maintain adequate nutrition. Intensive care is for sick and very immature infants who require a strictly controlled environment, respiratory support and parenteral nutrition.

Structurally normal babies of 32 weeks or more with good birth weights (over 1.5 kg) and without major birth damage now survive and

Characteristics of term small-for-dates infants

Wasted
White or pale pink
Length > 50 cm
Head circumference > c.35 cm
Thick, dark hair
Skin: dry, loose, thick
Ears, breast tissue, genitalia — all mature
Good muscle tone

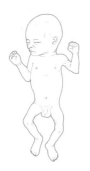

Problems of small-for-dates infants

Respiratory:
  birth asphyxia
  meconium aspiration
  pulmonary haemorrhage
Hypothermia:
  large surface area
Infections *in utero*:
  toxoplasma, rubella, CMV, herpes virus
Metabolic:
  symptomatic hypoglycaemia
Congenital anomalies

Characteristics of preterm infants

Small but plump
Red or very pink
Length < 50 cm
Head circumference < c.35 cm
Lanugo hair
Skin: shiny transparent, thin, oedematous
Ears, breast tissue, genitalia—all immature
Hypotonic (floppy)

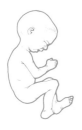

Problems of preterm infants

Respiratory:
respiratory distress syndrome
apnoeic attacks
Hypothermia:
immature control system
Infections after birth:
reduced maternal antibodies
Metabolic:
jaundice of prematurity
Feeding problems:
poor suck and swallow
functional ileus
Necrotising enterocolitis
Intraventricular haemorrhage
Late anaemia

survive intact. The same is true of the majority of babies between 28 and 32 weeks (1.0–1.5 kg). Below 28 weeks (under 1.0 kg) an increasing number of babies are surviving but 15–25 per cent are left with a serious handicap. Premature birth brings with it a number of immediate problems.

Nutrition. As the ability of the weak preterm infant to suckle is limited they often require to be fed for some weeks after birth using a nasogastric tube. Breast milk and various artificial milks have been given with success but recent work suggests that milks formulated specially for low birth weight infants result in better growth and development. The immature bowel adjusts surprisingly well, although there may be a functional ileus for the first few days of life.

Thermal stability. Premature babies have high surface area to body weight ratio and little subcutaneous fat, and over the first few days they lose water rapidly through their skin (transepidermal water loss). These physical characteristics make it difficult for them to maintain thermal stability. As cold exposure jeopardises their survival, great attention must be paid to keeping them warm. To provide a controlled ambient temperature it is current practice to nurse premature infants in incubators or under radiant warmers but it is also important to reduce heat losses by insulating the infant with clothing and a thermal blanket.

Respiratory difficulties. Because of their immaturity many preterm babies have difficulty expanding their lungs and the work of breathing is greatly increased due to the idiopathic respiratory distress syndrome. Also their respiratory drive varies, and this is apparent in their periodic breathing pattern which becomes troublesome when it leads to long apnoeic spells.

Liver immaturity. Physiological jaundice is often more marked and more prolonged in immature infants but with careful nursing and early establishment of feeding and the use of phototherapy, exchange transfusions should rarely be necessary. It is thought that the preterm brain is more at risk from damage due to high bilirubin levels.

Infections. Because of their delicate surfaces and limited immunological competence, premature babies are more susceptible to infections. Because of their weak defence systems, they do not show the symptoms and signs that are seen in older infants. Their clinical state changes rapidly from bacteraemia, to septicaemia, to death. Associated meningitis can easily pass undetected. Therefore in any infant suspected of having an infection, it is necessary to perform a 'septic screen' including culture of urine, blood and cerebrospinal fluid and to commence therapy with broad spectrum antibiotics before the results come back.

Intraventricular haemorrhage (IVH). Small haemorrhages into the germinal layer lining the lateral ventricles in the brain are commonly seen on ultrasound scanning of preterm babies, especially those who have experienced asphyxia or severe respiratory problems. These may extend into the ventricular system and a few infants subsequently develop hydrocephalus. However, the majority have small haemorrhages and seem to recover without serious long-term effects.

Periventricular leucomalacia (PVL). Ischaemia of the brain parenchyma may lead to changes recognised initially as 'flare' on cranial ultrasound examination. Sometimes this resolves, but in other babies these damaged areas of brain break down to form cysts. Cystic periventricular leucomalacia has a much poorer outlook than haemorrhage confined to the ventricles, with about 9 out of 10 of the children developing spastic cerebral palsy.

X-ray of NEC

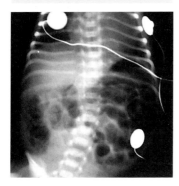

Necrotizing enterocolitis (NEC). This is a serious condition affecting the bowel during the first 3 weeks. It is much commoner in the smallest preterm infants. The cause is not known but hypoxic damage to the bowel wall possibly associated with umbilical catheterisation, apnoeic spells, and septicaemia, and the colonization of the bowel with certain organisms are probably precipitating events. Isolated cases occur but so do worrying outbreaks within neonatal units. The baby vomits bile-stained fluid, the abdomen distends and blood and mucus appear in the stools. The diagnosis is confirmed by abdominal X-ray which shows thickened bowel wall containing intramural gas. Perforation may occur. Oral feeds are stopped for at least a week, and intravenous feeding is used. Broad spectrum antibiotics and metronidazole are given intravenously. Surgical resection of perforated and necrotic bowel may be needed.

Retinopathy of prematurity

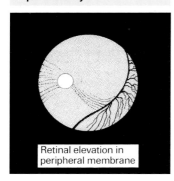

Retinal elevation in peripheral membrane

Retinopathy of prematurity (ROP). In the 1960s it was found that preterm infants who inhaled gas mixtures with high oxygen concentrations were at risk of developing abnormal vascularisation at the back of the eye (retrolental fibroplasia or retinopathy of prematurity). Some of these babies became blind. Whilst it was clear, even from these early studies that oxygen excess was not the only cause of ROP, nevertheless it seems wise not to give extra oxygen to preterm infants when they do not need it. However many do, and then it is important to measure the percentage of oxygen in the inspired gas (FiO_2) and the partial pressure of oxygen in arterial blood (PaO_2), if it is at all possible, so that oxygen is not given in excess. However even with strictly controlled oxygen levels some very immature infants develop retinopathy of prematurity and a few go on to partial or complete blindness. Associated disorders include intraventricular haemorrhage, apnoeic attacks, patent ductus arteriosus, septicaemia and metabolic acidosis and any or all may play a part in its causation. Oxygen, it seems, is neither the only nor a necessary aetiological factor.

Nutritional deficiencies. Once they have adjusted to extra-uterine life and feeding has been established, preterm babies can grow at a rate similar to that which they would have achieved *in utero*. This high growth rate can lead to vitamin deficiency, so vitamin supplements are given. Significant iron transfer takes place across the placenta during the third trimester of pregnancy. Preterm infants are commonly given iron supplements from the fourth week. Calcium, phosphorus and vitamin D supplementation all appear to be necessary to avoid oesteopathy of prematurity, a condition that develops in some preterm infants in the first months and is characterised by pathological fractures and rickets.

Other hazards. Premature babies are often born unexpectedly and are therefore more likely to experience asphyxia during birth and their delicate tissues are more likely to be damaged. They are susceptible to hypoglycaemia, metabolic acidosis, peripheral oedema, and irritability and fits due to birth injury and asphyxia. The delicate preterm infant is also more easily damaged by nursing and medical procedures. For example, if hypertonic solutions like 10 per cent glucose, calcium or amino acid preparations leak out of a peripheral vein they quickly cause necrosis which can result in a permanent scar.

A chemical burn

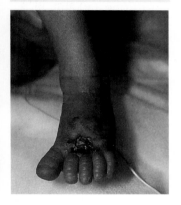

Prognosis. The outlook of prematurely born infants, particularly those with only moderate problems adjusting to extrauterine life, is good. The majority reach their expected size and ability level. Until recently infants born before 26 weeks were thought not to be viable. It was exceedingly rare for infants weighing less than 750 g to survive. Now, with intensive care, including if necessary artificial ventilation and intravenous nutrition, more and more are surviving. It is important to follow them all. Five to 10 per cent of babies with birth weights below 1500 g are found to have a major handicap such as cerebral palsy, developmental delay, blindness or deafness. Within this group those weighing less than 1000 g at birth have a major handicap rate of about 20 per cent.

Survival rates in preterm infants (Nottingham 1990)

gestation (wks)							
12	16	20	24	28	32	36	term / 40

approximate survival rates (%) 1991					
100 / 0		67	90	96	99.8

Inevitably intensive neonatal care interferes with the normal establishment of the parent–child relationship and this, with adverse social factors, is probably responsible for the fact the immature babies are at increased risk of cot death and child abuse.

RESPIRATORY PROBLEMS IN THE NEWBORN

Respiratory distress in newborn babies is recognized by tachypnoea (a respiratory rate of more than 60 per minute); recession of the intercostal spaces, sternum and subcostal areas; expiratory grunting, and cyanosis or the need for oxygen to remain pink. Respiratory failure may be due to a wide variety of both pulmonary and extrapulmonary causes.

Lung disorders due to aspiration

An infant may aspirate foreign material before, during and after birth.

Intrauterine pneumonia. Occasionally babies are born with lung consolidation due to material aspirated from the amniotic fluid. This 'congenital pneumonia' is associated with prolonged rupture of the fetal membranes, amnionitis and fetal asphyxia. If organisms are present they are usually *E. coli*, *Staph. aureus* and *epidermidis*, and the beta-haemolytic streptococcus group B. The latter can produce a particularly vicious infection leading to septicaemia and meningitis. The babies develop respiratory distress in the first few hours after birth. A chest X-ray shows patchy shadowing. Broad spectrum antibiotics should be given on suspicion. Group B streptococcus can also cause a fulminating septicaemia and meningitis in the 2–6 week postnatal period. Less common but important lung infections are caused by *Listeria monocytogenes* and by chlamydia.

Lung disorders

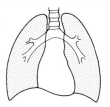
ground-glass appearance
+ air bronchogram:
idiopathic respiratory
distress syndrome

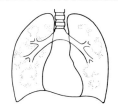
patchy collapse with overinflation.
meconium aspiration

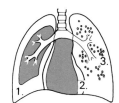
1. pneumothorax
2. pneumomediastinum
3. interstitial emphysema

Meconium aspiration. Asphyxia during birth will provoke mature infants to make vigorous efforts to breathe in. If there is meconium in the amniotic fluid, or if the baby's head is in the birth canal surrounded by vernix, meconium and blood, these tenacious materials may be drawn into the upper airway and then into the respiratory tree. They may result in patches of lung collapse, and other areas of over-inflation, due to a ball valve effect of the meconium plug allowing air in but not out. The infants may have severe respiratory difficulties for some days, and complications like pneumothorax and pneumomediastinum are common and may be fatal. Oxygen will be needed, and any tension pneumothorax must be drained. Supportive ventilation is difficult. A new technique which can help the most severely affected babies is extra-corporeal membrane oxygenation (ECMO). An oxygenator takes over the function of the baby's lungs until spontaneous recovery of the aspiration occurs. But it is better to try to prevent the meconium reaching the lungs by clearing the airways promptly at birth. If meconium is seen around the larynx, the baby is intubated and suction applied directly to the endotracheal tube as it is withdrawn. In skilled hands this can be repeated.

Milk aspiration. It is quite a challenge to the newborn infant to separate in the pharynx the air breathed in through the nose and milk sucked in through the mouth. They often get it wrong and swallow air; and they occasionally get it wrong and inhale milk. Obviously the latter is the more dangerous and every effort must be made to anticipate and avoid it. Aspiration of feeds is quite a common occurrence in preterm babies and in full term babies with a neurological or cardiorespiratory problem. Those with structural anomalies of the nose, mouth and oesophagus are particularly at risk, for example cleft palate, choanal atresia and oesophageal atresia. Management of these babies requires considerable nursing skill and judgement. A nasogastric or nasojejunal feeding tube may be needed, or even total parenteral nutrition for a while.

Transient tachypnoea of the newborn. This is not so much an aspiration as a delay in the clearance of lung fluid which is naturally present *in utero*. The rapid breathing usually settles within a few hours of birth, and chest X-ray shows the fluid as streaky shadows spreading out from the mediastinum and in the greater fissure on the right.

Disorders due to lung immaturity

Idiopathic respiratory distress syndrome. The more immature the infant the greater is the risk of respiratory distress and the lower the survival rate. In the adult, alveolar spaces are clustered around the terminal bronchioles; in the infant at term a single, simple sac is found at the end of each bronchiole. The alveolar epithelium has two types of cells. The Type II pneumocytes secrete a complex of lipoproteins, surfactant, which has the property of lowering surface tension. In some preterm infants these cells seem unable to release or produce enough surfactant, with the result that the air sacs collapse each time the infant breathes out, and the work of breathing is greatly increased. The pulmonary capillaries ooze liquid and red cells into the interstitial space causing oedema and haemorrhage. The protein leaked into the alveolar sacs form 'hyaline' membranes which can be clearly seen on light microscopy. This finding led to the disorder being called hyaline membrane disease, but in early severe forms membranes may not have had sufficient time to form.

The ability of the Type II cells to release surfactant can be assessed before birth by measuring the ratio in the amniotic fluid of two of the lipoproteins which make up surfactant, lecithin and sphingomyelin. Certain stimuli, including maternal ill health, uterine contractions and drugs may induce the cells to begin secreting earlier in gestation. Steroids given to the mother at least 48 hours before a preterm delivery have been shown to reduce the incidence and severity of the respiratory distress syndrome. Perinatal asphyxia, acidosis and hypothermia have the opposite effect and inhibit surfactant synthesis. Within a few days of birth, whatever the gestation, the cells begin to function and produce adequate surfactant.

As the affected infants have difficulty forming and maintaining a functional residual capacity, they are recognised clinically by their struggle to draw in air and to hold it. Each diaphragmatic tug pulls in the lower rib cage and soft tissues of the neck. An expiratory grunt accompanies each effort. The signs appear at birth or soon after, with apparent increasing severity. If the infant survives then improvement is usually seen after the second or third day and the lungs appear to recover fully. It might be deduced from the pathogenesis that the disorder will vary in severity and this is true; at one extreme it produces an unimportant transient disturbance in the respiratory pattern, at the other it leads to increasing cyanosis, acidosis and death in the first hours of life.

The diagnosis is confirmed by the chest X-ray which shows a diffuse ground glass appearance with an air bronchogram. The management requires considerable medical and nursing skill and involves continuous monitoring of many features of the baby (HR, RR, PaO_2) and of his environment (T, FiO_2) as guides for respiratory support, nutrition programmes, and intravenous therapy. Initially oxygen can be given in a headbox, and then as additional support is needed, by a nasal tube delivering a continuous positive airways pressure (CPAP) and finally by intermittent positive pressure ventilation (IPPV) via an endotracheal tube.

X-ray in IRDS

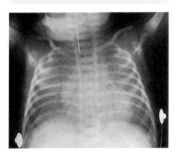

Bronchopulmonary dysplasia (BPD). Forcing the lungs open when they are not ready by using high inflation pressures from a mechanical ventilator together with raised inspired oxygen concentrations can result in the development of chronic lung disease in some preterm infants with respiratory distress. The X-ray reveals areas of patchy collapse and fibrosis interspersed with areas of cystic change and overdistension. The infants may remain dependant on IPPV for many days, but it has now been shown that giving dexamethasone can significantly reduce the duration of assisted ventilation. The babies can be weaned down onto CPAP and then onto added oxygen alone over a period of weeks. Many recover well but others continue to need respiratory support and die of chronic respiratory failure, cor pulmonale or added infections.

X-ray in BPD

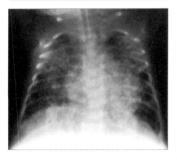

Pulmonary haemorrhage may complicate asphyxia and atelectasis, or occasionally appear to be a primary problem. It also occurs during recovery from hypothermia.

Apnoeic attacks are a common problem in sick and preterm newborn infants. The respiration of infants at risk must be continually monitored. Physical stimuli are sufficient to provoke a gasp and the recommencement of breathing. Occasionally CPAP or intubation and supportive ventilation may be required. Respiratory stimulants like theophylline may help.

Pneumothorax may occur spontaneously but is also a common complication of respiratory distress syndrome and of meconium aspiration, especially when CPAP or IPPV are being used. The air leak can be confirmed by transilluminating the affected side with a powerful fibreoptic light or by X-ray. The air can be aspirated with a syringe and needle, but it will usually require placement of a chest drain.

Extra-pulmonary causes of respiratory distress. Three non-lung diseases may present with respiratory symptoms. Cerebral anoxia can produce bizarre respiratory patterns mimicking dyspnoea though more commonly cerebral asphyxia leads to hypoventilation. If lung expansion matches respiratory effort this possibility should be considered. Metabolic acidosis, frequently an outcome of disorders of amino acid metabolism, presents with hyperventilation, deep and effective breaths. Congenital heart disease is perhaps the most difficult to exclude. Auscultation may not help or be positively misleading; assessment of peripheral perfusion, an electrocardiograph and chest X-ray are often more helpful. Babies with cyanotic heart disease will not improve on breathing 100 per cent oxygen, whereas babies with a respiratory cause for cyanosis will respond with a clear rise in PaO_2 ('the nitrogen washout test'). Sometimes there is no structural heart defect but the baby's circulation continues in the fetal pattern by-passing the lungs and causing cyanosis. This 'persistent fetal circulation' can be treated with the drug tolazoline which improves oxygenation. Babies who fail to respond can be treated with extra-corporial membrane oxygenation(ECMO).

JAUNDICE IN THE NEWBORN

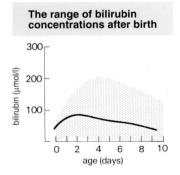

The range of bilirubin concentrations after birth

bilirubin (µmol/l)

300

200

100

0 2 4 6 8 10
age (days)

Many healthy normal newborn infants develop jaundice after birth. *In utero,* bilirubin crosses the placenta and is excreted by the mother. After birth, the infant must activate his own excretory systems but there is usually some delay and blood bilirubin concentrations rise. This 'physiological' jaundice appears at 2–3 days of age and begins disappearing towards the end of the first week; the bilirubin is largely unconjugated and the baby remains generally well. There is considerable variation from one infant to another. The condition is more severe and prolonged in preterm infants; if hypoxia and hypoglycaemia further limit bilirubin conjugation; and if the infant has an ileus or bowel obstruction then there may be increased enteric reabsorption of bilirubin. The diagnosis of physiological jaundice is made by the typical presentation, and by excluding other more serious causes.

Kernicterus

Unconjugated bilirubin is lipid soluble and travels in the circulation largely bound to albumin. It is the small fraction of free bilirubin which escapes from the vascular compartment and enters the cellular lipid fractions of the brain cells, which may cause transient or permanent damage, kernicterus. When this happens the infant behaves abnormally, feeds badly and may fit and develop opisthotonus when the back is arched and the head thrown back. If the infant recovers there is usually residual brain damage, often with severe choreoathetosis and mental handicap. High-tone deafness is common after hyperbilirubinaemia, and hearing should be tested carefully in early life.

In healthy full term infants unconjugated bilirubin concentrations above 380 μmol/l are considered dangerous, but much lower thresholds apply to preterm babies and those who are sick. The risks are greater when albumin levels are low or when there is competition for albumin binding by, for example, free fatty acids and drugs like sulphonamides. Various diseases can cause unconjugated bilirubin to rise to dangerous levels, and these are best considered chronologically.

Causes of neonatal jaundice, by time of appearance

First 24 hours of life	2nd–5th day	End of 2nd week onwards
Haemolytic diseases	Physiological	Breast milk jaundice
Rhesus incompatibility	Infection	Hypothyroidism
ABO incompatibility	Bruising	Hepatitis
G6PD deficiency	Galactosaemia and other	Biliary atresia and other
Spherocytosis	metabolic diseases	biliary tract problems
Congenital infections	Familial non-haemolytic jaundices	Pyloric stenosis
	Infants of diabetic mothers	

Jaundice: first 24 hours

A few babies who are jaundiced at birth are suffering from one of the congenital infections which can cross the placenta and may severely damage the fetus: toxoplasmosis, rubella, cytomegalovirus, herpes virus and syphilis. The jaundice is usually mixed conjugated and unconjugated, and the babies have other abnormal signs of the infection. Most jaundice appearing in the first 24 hours is however due to excess haemolysis.

Haemolytic diseases of the newborn. Haemolysis of the newborn red cells may be caused by antibody from the mother. This will only happen if the maternal and fetal blood are incompatible. The haemolytic jaundice which causes some of the most severe problems is due to rhesus incompatibility. The problems occur after the mother has been sensitised by either a mismatched blood transfusion, or from fetal blood entering her circulation during a miscarriage or, more commonly, at the end of a previous pregnancy during labour and delivery. She reacts to the fetal blood by producing antibodies. The concentration of the antibodies are measured serially during pregnancy in affected mothers. It is these globulin antibodies which cross the placenta in increasing concentrations during the pregnancy, and which attack and haemolyse the red cells in the fetal circulation.

Exchange transfusions

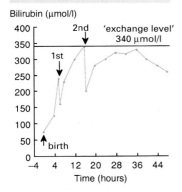

Bilirubin (µmol/l)

When the condition is mild, the fetus and newborn tolerate the small increase in haemolysis rate, although after birth the baby may become moderately jaundiced and have mild anaemia. With higher rates of haemolysis, the bilirubin levels in the fetus may still stay low because the unconjugated bilirubin passes back across the placenta and the fetus can tolerate moderate anaemia, but after birth the bilirubin concentrations rise rapidly and dangerous bilirubin levels may be reached within 24 hours. In the severe forms with high rates of haemolysis the fetus is unable to maintain his haemoglobin and becomes severely anaemic, and this with an associated general disturbance in fetal metabolism leads to severe oedema (hydrops fetalis), a condition which is usually fatal.

The aim of obstetric management is to deliver the baby before the anaemia becomes critical. A measure of the state of the fetus can be gained by serial analysis of amniotic fluid, taken by amniocentesis, for bilirubin products. If the fetus is very severely affected and too immature to be delivered, fetal blood transfusions can be given *in utero* to correct the anaemia. Rhesus incompatibility is now far less common, following the discovery that administration of anti-D antibodies to the mother immediately after birth destroys any red cells which might have leaked into the maternal circulation and so reduces the risks of the mother producing antibodies.

Incompatibility of the ABO system is more common, and produces a similar but usually milder clinical picture. The mother is usually group O and the baby A or B. There is a marked rise in the titres of the naturally occurring anti-A or anti-B haemolysins, but these drop back to normal levels after the pregnancy, and the next pregnancy is not at greater risk, unlike rhesus disease.

Haemolysis due to a deficiency of one of the red cell enzymes. Many Asian and Negro babies have relative lack of glucose-6-phosphate dehydrogenase. This can be found with a screening test. Those affected have to avoid a number of drugs which precipitate haemolysis. Finally abnormalities of the red cell shape, such as spherocytosis, can result in increased osmotic fragility and haemolysis.

Jaundice: 2 to 5 days

Before jaundice at this age is labelled 'physiological', the baby has to be examined carefully to exclude any infection. Bruising, especially in forceps or breech deliveries, may be exacerbating the jaundice. The urine is checked for reducing sugars to exclude galactosaemia, and sent for a metabolic screen if the baby is acidotic and ill.

Jaundice: 2 weeks on

Many babies who are being breast fed have a prolongation of their jaundice. This does not rise to harmful levels, and the mother is encouraged to continue breast feeding, but the diagnosis can only be made by exclusion. Thyroid function tests are needed to exclude cretinism. Distinguishing between neonatal hepatitis and binary atresia is both difficult and important, because early surgery is essential in the atresia but would exacerbate hepatitis.

Management.   Having established the cause of the jaundice, bilirubin levels can be measured serially. This is especially important in the haemolytic diseases since the bilirubin level may rise rapidly. Good hydration and an adequate calorie intake help the liver to conjugate the bilirubin efficiently. The hyperbilirubinaemia can be treated by using phototherapy. Light of wavelength 450 nm from the blue-band of the visible spectrum (*not* ultraviolet) converts unconjugated bilirubin by photodegradation to a biliverdin-like pigment which is water soluble and harmless. Light of the correct wavelength is produced by fluorescent tubes or more specialised blue lamps. Care is needed with temperature control and fluid balance. If there is a risk of the bilirubin rising to dangerous levels in spite of phototherapy and the measures above, then an exchange transfusion is performed. During this procedure blood is alternately withdrawn and transfused in 10 to 20 ml aliquots via a catheter in the umbilical vein, until 60 to 70 per cent of the infant's red blood cells have been replaced. In rhesus incompatibility an exchange transfusion is often needed shortly after birth, even before bilirubin levels have had time to rise, in order to remove from the baby's circulation the antibodies which are causing the haemolysis.

Haemorrhagic disease of the newborn

This coagulation disturbance arises from vitamin K deficiency and the resulting impairment of hepatic production of factors II, VII, IX and X. Early onset disease develops between the 2nd and 4th days of life and presents with gastrointestinal bleeding. Late onset, 4 to 8 weeks, is rarer but often presents with intracranial bleeds. Breast fed, premature and infants experiencing asphyxia are most at risk. The occasional tragedy due to this readily preventable condition merits the prophylactic administration of vitamin K to all newborn infants shortly after birth.

GASTROINTESTINAL PROBLEMS

Oesophageal atresia

Tracheo-oesophageal fistula

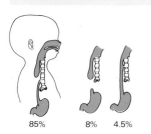

85%   8%   4.5%

Oesophageal atresia (incidence 1:2500) is usually associated with a tracheoesophageal fistula. In every infant born to a mother with hydramnios, it should be excluded by passing a firm, large-bore (12 G) tube through the mouth into the stomach. After birth, the affected infant is unable to swallow his own saliva and bubbles fluid from the mouth, another sign requiring investigation. It is always a sad event when the diagnosis is made only after the child has choked over his first feed. It is the condition of the lungs as well as the extent of the abnormality which dictates the success of surgical correction.

The diagnosis is confirmed radiologically by passing a firm, radioopaque tube into the upper pouch and taking a lateral film of the chest, and an antero-posterior film of the chest and abdomen. Air in the stomach confirms the presence of a fistula. Associated anomalies may include ano-rectal agenesis and cardiac defects, particularly Fallot tetralogy.

Congenital diaphragmatic hernia

Diaphragmatic hernia

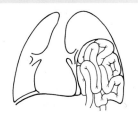

Often associated with bilateral lung hypoplasia

Duodenal atresia

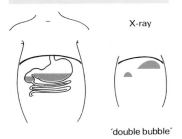

X-ray

'double bubble'

Ileal atresia

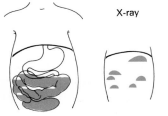

X-ray

fluid levels

Congenital diaphragmatic hernia (incidence 1:2200) is due to a defect of the hemidiaphragm, usually the left. Fetal ultrasound can make the diagnosis before birth, and allows for delivery and management in a unit experienced in neonatal surgery.

Where the diaphragmatic defect is the only anomaly, the baby may appear well at birth, but observation will show a deep chest and a scaphoid abdomen. Respiratory distress develops as the child swallows air, which passes into the small bowel within the chest cavity. The resulting mediastinal shift leads to compression of the previously unaffected lung. The diagnosis is confirmed by X-rays of chest and abdomen. A nasogastric tube should be passed to empty the stomach and small bowel. Endotracheal intubation and ventilation may be necessary preoperatively.

Babies with diaphragmatic hernias may have severe pulmonary hypoplasia which either prevents initial resuscitation and preparation for surgery, or leads to profound hypoxia postoperatively. Extra-corporeal membrane oxygenation (ECMO) may save some of these infants. Other associations include heart defects and gut malrotation.

Small bowel obstruction. The most common form of organic obstruction of the small bowel is meconium ileus. Other causes of small bowel obstruction in the neonatal period include atresia, stenosis and diaphragms of the duodenum, jejunum or ileum, midgut volvulus 'volvulus neonatorum', Ladd's band associated with failure of caecal descent, enterogenous cyst and milk curd obstruction. Meconium ileus and atretic lesions will present very early with distension and vomiting within hours of birth. The other lesions may not produce symptoms for some days or even a week or two after birth.

Vomiting of green rather than yellow bile-stained material suggests organic obstruction. Meconium may or may not have been passed in the early hours of life. The area of distension will depend on the level of the obstruction; in duodenal obstruction it is confined to the upper abdomen, in ileal obstruction it is generalised. Erect X-rays of the abdomen should be taken, and may be diagnostic, for example, the double-bubble of duodenal atresia, the ground-glass appearance of some cases of meconium ileus, and the calcification of an ileal atresia with prenatal perforation. In other cases fluid levels may be present but do not necessarily indicate mechanical obstruction. They will be present in functional ileus, and in a baby with ileus secondary to septicaemia.

Large bowel obstruction. In the neonate there are two main causes of large bowel obstruction, Hirschsprung's disease and ano-rectal agenesis. The former is the more common, and it is suggested by delay in the passage of meconium beyond 24 hours. The baby may appear otherwise well for a few days but is liable to become suddenly and acutely distended, with peripheral circulatory collapse, a feature of a 'Hirschsprung's enterocolitis'. Ano-rectal agenesis is an all embracing name for a very large number of anatomical anomalies. Basically there are two types of ano-rectal agenesis, high and low, depending on whether the bowel ends above or below the pelvic floor. All low anomalies are easily treated at birth by a perineal procedure. High anomalies require a temporary colostomy; in boys there is always a fistula to bladder or urethra; in girls there may be a fistula to the vagina. Most babies with ano-rectal agenesis have no visible anus at birth: it is extremely rare for the anal canal to be present but not communicating with the upper bowel.

Rectal agenesis

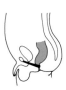 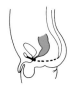 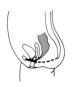 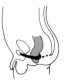 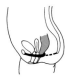

normal   'high' agenesis with or without fistula into urogenital tract   ' low' agenesis—covered or anterior ectopic anus, both usually with stenosis

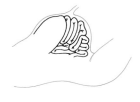

Exomphalos major

Exomphalos is a persistence of the herniation of the gut into the extra-embryonic part of the umbilical cord which is normally present between the sixth and fourteenth weeks of intrauterine life. Occasionally complete return of the gut into the abdominal cavity does not occur, the bowel which remains outside will be obvious at birth. In its mild form one or two loops of bowel are seen in the base of the cord, exomphalos minor; at its most severe a huge swelling occurs in the centre of the abdomen containing most of the abdominal contents (exomphalos major). The gut is covered by membrane.

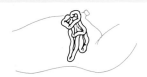

Gastroschisis

In **gastroschisis** there is a protrusion of gut through a defect in the abdominal wall which is usually to the right of an otherwise normal umbilical cord. Gastroschisis also differs from exomphalos in that there is a much lower likelihood of associated chromosomal and other major malformations. The gut is however uncovered and is therefore exposed and vulnerable to damage which can complicate early management.

It is now relatively common for exomphalos and gastroschisis to be diagnosed by fetal ultrasound. It is important to differentiate the two conditions because the former merits fetal chromosomal analysis and further detailed scans to determine whether other major problems should influence the continuation of the pregnancy and postnatal management.

NEURAL TUBE ANOMALIES

The neural tube should be completely formed and closed throughout its entire length by the end of the third week of intrauterine life. The process starts at the 14th day with thickening of the dorsal ectoderm to form the neural plate. The neural plate starts folding into a groove and by about 22 to 23 days complete fusion of the groove has occurred to form the neural tube. Fusion commences in the mid dorsal region and extends towards the head and tail of the embryo.

In the early 1970s neural tube defects occurred in 2–3/1000 live births and formed a large percentage of the admissions to paediatric surgical wards. The incidence has now fallen to below 1/1000, in part due to antenatal screeening with termination of fetuses with severe defects and in part to a natural decline possibly due to better maternal nutrition.

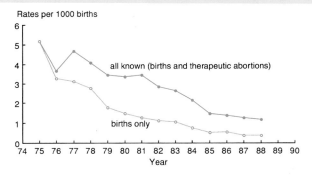

The fall in incidence of neural tube defects in Scotland (Davis & Young 1991)

Rates per 1000 births

all known (births and therapeutic abortions)

births only

Year

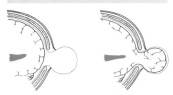

Cranial meningocele and encephalocele

Anencephaly is a tragic deformity in which most of the infants are still-born, but if liveborn survive only a few hours.

Cranium bifidum defects are relatively uncommon. The minor lesions are eminently treatable; all that is required is a good skin cover, and the prognosis is excellent, for there is no associated spinal neurological lesion, and the incidence of hydrocephalus is low. An occipital meningocele, even when very large, is also treatable, although hydro-cephalus is more likely. The overall prognosis is still good. On the other hand, a large encephalocele is not open to treatment, for surgery usually means either excision of a mass of brain tissue or a closure which results in raised intracranial pressure.

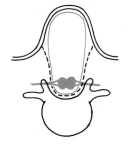

Meningocele with skin cover

Spina bifida cystica defects vary from a meningeal sac full of cerebro-spinal fluid with a normal placement of the spinal cord (a meningocele), to the exposure and complete unfolding of the spinal cord on the surface of the child's back (a myelomeningocele).

Meningoceles are less common and have a good prognosis. Neurologi-cal problems with the lower limbs and hydrocephalus are rare, but par-tial neurological deficit affecting the bladder is not uncommon. Virtually all babies with a meningocele will be treated surgically in the first days of life. During infancy they may develop minor foot problems and bladder dysfunction but they usually can cope well. Children with meningoceles should be followed up throughout the whole of their growing period since neurological problems may develop with growth of the spine.

Myelomeningocele

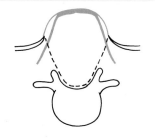

Myelomeningoceles are both more common and more serious. They are usually located in the lumbo-sacral region. The range of severity varies considerably. A child with a small lumbo-sacral myelomeningocele, which is closed on the first day of life, may with careful attention have good mobility, normal bladder function and intellect. On the other hand, a baby with an extensive thoraco-lumbar myelomeningocele is likely to have no functioning motor or sensory nerves distal to his nipple line. His skin will be completely anaesthetic and therefore at risk of trauma; his trunk and limbs will be paralysed and either completely flaccid or deformed as a result of reflex activity. Involuntary movements may be seen. The bladder and bowel will be paralysed and insensitive. Hydrocephalus is present in 80 per cent of infants with myelomeningocele.

Early management

Every baby with spina bifida cystica should have full and expert assessment as soon as possible after birth to determine the extent of neurological deficit; the presence or otherwise of hydrocephalus, the extent of bony deformity of the spine; and the coexistence of any other congenital abnormality. This permits an estimate to be made of his potential. The decision to operate can only be taken after a full and open discussion between surgeon and parents. Many babies with extensive defects will die within a short time whether their lesions are covered with skin or not. Early surgery is not justified. On the other hand, a baby with a lesser lesion is still at risk of infection and the complications of hydrocephalus even after surgery. It is a mistake to think that all babies will survive if operated upon and that those with uncorrected lesions will always die. One can only say that the majority of babies with minor lesions and a good prognosis will survive with treatment to adult life, and that most babies with very major lesions will die without treatment.

Long term management

Once active treatment is commenced the child's management should be directed by a team consisting of an orthopaedic surgeon, a paediatric surgeon, and a physiotherapist. The facilities of an assessment unit are useful, and close contact with local schools for the physically handicapped is essential. Orthopaedic problems are particularly common in those children with unbalanced lower limb function. Bladder stasis may lead to problems of infection and reflux. Intermittent bladder catheterisation is a relatively simple and effective and has largely replaced surgical procedures. A ventriculoperitoneal or atrial shunt is usually required to control hydrocephalus. The complications of these shunts are blockage and infection, and they may be very troublesome. The anaesthetic skin is also a problem especially in the more mobile child; pressure sores and accidental burns are likely to occur. Learning and psychological problems may add to the child's troubles in the school

Spina bifida occulta

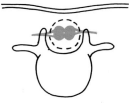

years but their unhappiness may be most profound when they begin to realise the full meaning of their handicap, with regard to job prospects, sex and marriage.

The quality of life in children over 5 after surgery for myelomeningocele (after Lorber)

18% mild/moderate physical handicap and normal IQ
49% severe physical handicap and normal IQ
33% severe physical handicap and borderline or subnormal IQ

Split notochord syndrome (diastematomyelia) with meningocele

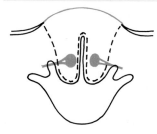

Spina bifida occulta is a common anomaly, said to occur in up to 20 per cent of normal individuals. Most people with an occult deficit are asymptomatic. Occasionally the bony defect is associated with a hairy patch or a birth mark on the back. A few children with spina bifida occulta develop a mild spastic gait, or bladder problems with spinal growth due to tethering of the cord, a split notochord syndrome, or an associated intraspinal dermoid or lipoma.

Hydrocephalus without spina bifida. This may result from a congenital abnormality of the brain, for example aqueduct stenosis, or acquired as the result of intracranial haemorrhage or infection. Premature infants with severe intracranial haemorrhage are at risk. Early child abuse with shaking injury is another cause and it appears to be increasing. The prognosis of a child with hydrocephalus is dependant on the underlying cause and the residual integrity of the brain tissue. It is important to recognise hydrocephalus early either by careful measurement of the head circumference or by serial cranial ultrasound in infants at risk. Detailed ultrasound studies can demonstrate not only the size of the ventricles but also the flow of CSF. Ultrasound and other imaging techniques guide the neurosurgeon to the correct placement of the shunt.

The treatment of hydrocephalus (ventriculo-peritoneal (A) and ventriculo-atrial (B) CSF shunts)

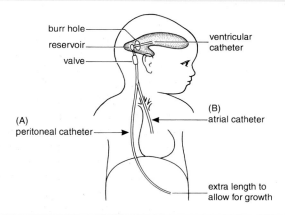

CLEFT LIP AND PALATE

The middle third of the face develops as the result of migration and fusion of mesodermal folds covered by ectoderm. The earlier or primary palate creates the olfactory pits, and failure of fusion results in unilateral, bilateral or, rarely, median cleft lip. The secondary palate originates from folds on either side of the tongue. These rise above the tongue and fuse in the mid-line to form the true palate. Cleft palates occur when tissue migration is disorganised or obstructed by the tongue. It is sometimes the result of a small mandible.

Malformations of soft and hard palate

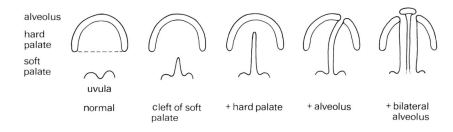

alveolus
hard palate
soft palate
uvula

normal | cleft of soft palate | + hard palate | + alveolus | + bilateral alveolus

Cleft lip and palate are common, 1 in 700 births. The majority are isolated abnormalities but they may be part of a chromosomal or other malformation syndrome. The family history is often positive, and most clefts are determined by polygenic inheritance which influences the threshold to ill-defined environmental factors. Occasional cases have been linked to maternal corticosteroid or anticonvulsant therapy. One-third of clefts are limited to the lip, one-quarter to the palate and the remainder involve both.

Management. The alarming facial appearance calls for prompt counselling of the parents, preferably with 'before and after' photographs to emphasise the successful outcome of corrective surgery. Feeding problems can usually be overcome by using a soft teat with an enlarged hole and by nursing the baby erect. Those with a cleft lip may cope with breast feeding. The baby should have a newborn hearing screening test. The aims of surgery are to provide a good cosmetic result and an adequate speech mechanism. The usual practice is to repair the cleft lip at 3 months of age and the palate at 6 months or later. Too early a repair may interfere with mid-facial growth. In the later years additional specialist help is required to overcome Eustachian tube obstruction, speech delay and dental problems.

Pierre-Robin syndrome refers to severe micrognathia with a secondary

Feeding of infants with micrognathia

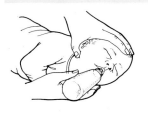

Feeding position—thumb holding mandible forward

cleft palate. The affected infants are susceptible to feeding and respiratory problems, and require expert nursing until the mandible grows.

Treacher-Collins syndrome encompasses a spectrum of ear and facial malformations caused by first and second pharyngeal arch developmental failure.

Abnormal development of the face

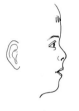 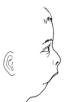 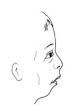 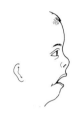 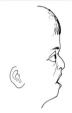

normal

Pierre-Robin
hypoplasia of
mandible
cleft palate

Treacher-Collin's
hypoplasia of
mandible
deformed ears (80%)
deafness (40%)

facio-auriculo–
vertebral anomalies
unilateral (70%)
hypoplasia of
maxilla and mandible
deformed ears
deafness

Crouzon's syndrome
ocular ptosis
hypoplasia of maxilla
craniosynostosis

CLUB FOOT p. 252   DISLOCATED HIP p. 248

NEONATAL INFECTIONS

Newborn babies can die from infections before anyone is aware that they are ill. The signs of a systemic infection are generalised and often not specific to a particular system. Apparently trivial infections can rapidly lead to systemic sepsis, especially in the preterm baby.

Systemic infections

If an infant goes 'off his feed', handles badly, has an unexpected body temperature up or down, or develops unusual respiratory patterns, fits or apnoeic spells, he should be thoroughly examined at all sites for signs of possible infection. A 'septic screen' is performed in which samples of blood, urine, and cerebrospinal fluid are taken for examination and culture, together with swabs from eyes, ears, throat, umbilicus and rectum. While awaiting the results of the investigations the ill baby should be started immediately on an antibiotic combination parenterally to cover the common pathogens of the newborn period such as Group B streptococcus, *Staphylococcus aureus*, *Escherichia coli*, and the Gram negative organisms pseudomonas, klebsiella, proteus. Widely used combinations are gentamicin and penicillin G in the first week of life, and gentamicin and flucloxacillin thereafter; others prefer third generation cephalosporins. When the results of the septic screen are known, the length of treatment can be decided, and the antibiotics altered to cover a particular organism more thoroughly or in accordance with the antibiotic sensitivities of the organisms grown. Serious infections include septicaemia, meningitis, pneumonia, urinary tract infections, gastro-enteritis, and osteomyelitis. Further investigations and follow-up will be needed depending on which of these is present.

Neonatal meningitis

Neonatal meningitis has high mortality and morbidity rates. Penicillin is used to cover the possibility of Group B streptococcal meningitis, and a third generation cephalosporin such as cefotaxime or ceftazidime can be combined with gentamicin to cover the other organisms. Fits or irritability are controlled with phenobarbitone. Treatment of meningitis must continue for 3 weeks. Ultrasound scanning is used to identify any developing hydrocephalus.

Superficial infections

Conjunctivitis. Sticky eye is a common problem. Usually there is no underlying infection and, after taking swabs for culture, saline washes are all that is required. Sometimes, conjunctivitis is due to a staphylococcal infection, less commonly streptococcal or pseudomonal organisms. It may also be caused by organisms acquired from the mother's birth canal, in particular *Neisseria gonorrhoeae* and *Chlamydia trachomatis*. Both are sexually transmitted diseases. The latter is also responsible for the eye disease, trachoma. If conjunctival inflammation and pus is present, then swabs should be taken into standard and into chlamydial transport medium for Gram and Giemsa staining and appropriate cultures. Scrapings should also be taken from the inside of the lower eyelid with a swab on a stick, smeared on to glass slides, allowed to dry and examined in the laboratory for chlamydial inclusion bodies. Gonococcal eye infections can involve the cornea and damage the whole eye very rapidly, and, to prevent this, significant eye infections on the first day or two, should be presumed to be gonococcal until proven otherwise and treated vigorously with penicillin given parenterally, as well as very frequent cleaning and eye drops. Chlamydial infections are now common and must be treated with both 1 per cent tetracycline eye drops and oral erythromycin. Ordinary bacterial infections such as caused by staphylococci are treated with chloramphenicol eye drops or ointment.

Septic spots. Small septic spots and blisters are not unusual, especially in the skin creases, and are commonly due to staphylococcal infections. The baby can be washed with a soap containing an antibacterial agent such as chlorhexidine. If there are only a few lesions, they can be cultured and cleaned with a spirit swab. More extensive lesions should be treated with systemic flucloxacillin.

Umbilical infections. The umbilical cord dries and usually drops off after a few days. The residual sticky stump can be treated with local antiseptic powder but if the surrounding area becomes inflamed with an offensive discharge, swabs and a systemic antibiotic are needed.

Thrush. This is a fungal infection. Inside the mouth it is recognized by adherent white plaques on the buccal membranes and the tongue. Treatment is with nystatin oral suspension or miconazole oral gel. On the perineum the candida produces a rash with red areas around the anus and in the groins. Nystatin cream is used. The mouth should be checked for involvement.

NEONATAL CONVULSIONS AND JITTERS

Causes of convulsions in childhood

Asphyxia
Birth injury with haemorrhage
CNS infections
CNS malformations
Hypoglycaemia
Hypocalcaemia
Hyponatraemia
Inherited metabolic disorders

Timing of two common causes

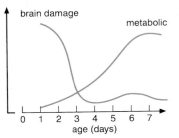

Many normal newborn babies react to minor physical stimuli or loud noises with startle responses. It can be difficult to distinguish these normal 'jitters' from intermittent focal fits (twitching) and generalised tonic spasms. If the jitteriness seems excessive a blood sample is taken to exclude hypoglycaemia, and low levels of calcium, magnesium, or sodium. If the baby also seems unwell an infection screen including a lumbar puncture must be carried out. If the cause is still not determined a search is made for less common inherited metabolic disorders, congenital infections and CNS malformations.

Treatment. Treatment is directed at the cause. If the blood glucose is reduced below 2.0 mmol/l (1.5 mmol/l in preterms), the hypoglycaemia is corrected urgently with 25 per cent glucose (2 ml/kg) followed by a 10 per cent dextrose infusion. Hypocalcaemic fits are uncommon since the introduction of low phosphate milks, and normal levels vary considerably making interpretation difficult, but if fits are thought to be related to low plasma levels, 0.5 ml/kg of 10 per cent calcium gluconate can be given intravenously, slowly and under ECG monitoring, followed up by oral supplements added to the feeds. If an infant's hypocalcaemia seems resistant to correction he may well have hypomagnesaemia as well, and this can be treated with 0.1 ml/kg of 50 per cent magnesium sulphate intramuscularly or very slowly intravenously. Hyponatraemia responds to fluid restriction if it is dilutional, or to sodium supplements if there is a true deficiency.

If life-threatening convulsions are continuing in spite of these metabolic corrections they should be stopped with diazepam infusion 0.4 mg/kg given intravenously slowly, followed by a high loading dose of phenobarbitone 20 mg/kg and maintenance at 2 mg/kg 12-hourly. Rectal paraldehyde in arachis oil can be helpful if breakthrough fits still occur. Meanwhile meningitis must be excluded and investigations set in train to find any other underlying cause. The management is particularly difficult where the fits are due to severe birth trauma or asphyxia. The large doses of anticonvulsants required severely depress the baby's respiration. Surprisingly the prognosis in neonatal convulsions is favourable in the absence of meningitis and obvious cerebral damage, with 70 per cent having normal development at long-term follow-up.

BIBLIOGRAPHY

Curnock D A 1986 Neonatal resuscitation. Hospital Update 12:679–692
Davis J A, Richards M P M, Roberton N R C 1983 Parent–baby attachments in premature infants. Croom Helm, London
Fleming P J, Speidel B D, Marlow N, Dunn P M 1991 A neonatal vade-mecum, 2nd edn. Edward Arnold, London
Levene M I, Bennett M J, Punt J 1988 Fetal and neonatal neurology and neurosurgery. Churchill Livingstone, Edinburgh
Levene M I, William J L, Fawer C 1985 Ultrasound of the infant brain. Clinics in Developmental Medicine No. 92. MacKeith Press, London
Lister J, Irvine I M 1990 Neonatal surgery, 3rd edn. Butterworths, London
Macfarlane A 1977 The psychology of childbirth. Fontana, London
Remington J S, Klein J O 1990 Infectious diseases of the fetus and newborn infant, 3rd edn. W B Saunders, Philadelphia
Roberton N R C 1986 A manual of neonatal intensive care, 2nd edn. Edward Arnold, London
Roberton N R C 1992 Textbook of neonatology 92, 2nd edn. Churchill Livingstone, Edinburgh
Taeusch H W, Ballard R A, Avery M E 1991 Schaffer and Avery's diseases of the newborn, 6th edn. W B Saunders, Philadelphia

5 Nutrition

The nutrients supplied to the young in early development are uniquely and sensitively adjusted to their requirements. During intrauterine life a mixture of water, salts, proteins, carbohydrates and fats, which are drawn from the maternal blood stream and processed by the placenta, enters the fetal circulation and determines the substrates that are available for growth and energy metabolism. After birth, the breast produces a specialised total food in an acceptable and digestible form. Breast milk production is a characteristic of mammals. The mixture of nutrients in their milk varies widely from one species to another and this is to be expected for the rates of growth of the young at birth and their motor activities are very different.

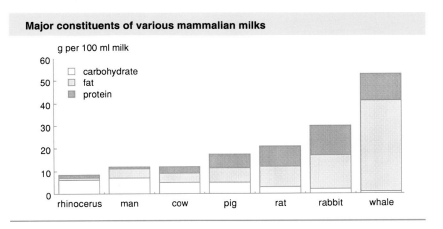

Major constituents of various mammalian milks

g per 100 ml milk

□ carbohydrate
□ fat
■ protein

rhinocerus man cow pig rat rabbit whale

In view of this it is perhaps surprising that the young of one species can be reared effectively on the milk of another. But this is so, for some decades now it has been a common practice to rear human infants on cow's milk. So successful has it been in western societies that the advantages of human breast milk are being questioned! Breast feeding benefits both mother and child in many ways and therefore mothers should be given every encouragement to breast feed their infants; however for those who are unable to do so it is important to reassure them that there are other ways of rearing their infant successfully.

BREAST FEEDING

During pregnancy many endocrine agents prepare the breast for lactation. These include lactogen (human chorionic somatomammotropin), which is secreted by the placenta, and prolactin which is released by the pituitary gland and is important not only in initiating milk secretion but also in maintaining milk production after birth. Suckling is a powerful stimulus both to prolactin release from the anterior pituitary gland and to the secretion of oxytocin from the posterior pituitary gland. Oxytocin stimulates the ejection or 'let down' of milk by acting on the myoepithelial cells which surround the alveoli and ductules.

Hormonal involvement in lactation

Preparation

oestrogens
progesterone
placental lactogen

Milk production

suckling releases
ant. pituitary
hormones
especially prolactin

suckling releases
post. pituitary
hormone oxytocin

Milk ejection

Technical problems

Even from this brief outline, it is obvious that breast feeding is a complex process which might break down at a number of stages. For example, the breast and nipple may be ill-formed, although appropriate care during pregnancy can do much to encourage adequate development. Milk production may not be initiated and maintained at a rate fast enough to suit a hungry baby or may flow too quickly for an ill or sleepy infant. If the full breast is not emptied then it may become engorged and inflamed, and the resulting pressure and pain will inhibit further milk production. Gentle manual expression of milk will avoid this complication. Finally, the unhappy, nervous, drowsy or sick mother may not be able to 'let down' her milk as she would wish or a lethargic, sick, newborn baby may not stimulate her to do so.

Breast feeding does not seem to be a basic instinct; many mothers who have not seen others breast feeding need considerable guidance initially. A simple explanation of how the breast works is often very helpful and avoids unnecessary anxiety. Should it be desirable to discontinue breast feeding, this can be achieved most simply by firm breast support and analgesia.

Constituents of breast milk

As a food, milk has some remarkable characteristics. Most of the carbohydrate is in the form of a disaccharide, lactose, which requires a specific disaccharidase for its digestion. The fats are present mainly as triglyceride in globules surrounded by lipoproteins which are probably

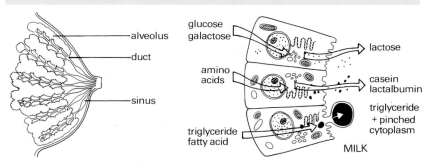

Breast anatomy and milk production

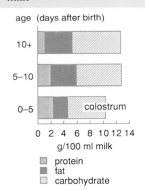

Constituents of breast milk

age (days after birth)

protein
fat
carbohydrate

remnants of the walls of the alveolar cells. The individual fatty acids reflect the mother's diet and her fat stores. If mothers are on low fat diets then the alveolar cells themselves make saturated fatty acid with chain lengths of 12 to 16 carbons. The protein content of human milk is surprisingly low but a large percentage is in the form of the more easily digestible whey, rather than indigestible curds. Whey contains in addition to lactalbumin, proteins which influence the infant's bowel bacterial flora, namely lactoferrin, lysozyme and IgA. Breast milk also contains vitamins, minerals, enzymes, especially lipase, and cells. The latter are predominantly macrophages and act either to keep the lacteals free from infection or to assist in the defence of the intestinal tract.

The relative amounts of the constituents vary. The first milk produced after birth, colostrum, is rich in protein and cells but the volume is small. When feeding is established, the mature milk constituents vary diurnally and from day to day. The milk at the end of a feed, hind milk, has a higher fat content than fore milk. The content of milk is also modified by the maternal diet and wellbeing, and by the mother's general level of nutrition.

Advantages of breast feeding

If a mother wishes and is able to breast feed, then she should be supported in this and given every encouragement to do so. Human milk is an excellent nutrient mixture which also gives the baby some protection against infection. Its protein content is less likely to induce allergic reactions and the infant may be less at risk from unexplained sudden death. The process of breast feeding usually gives satisfaction and pleasure to mother and child and this in itself will be of lasting benefit to both. Technically, breast feeding is easier than bottle feeding in as much as the mother is not required to make up the mixture according to instruction, and sterilising bottles is not a problem. In western societies breast feeding may be economic, but elsewhere it certainly is.

Some mothers are anxious that breast feeding or, alternatively, not breast feeding may alter the contour of the breast but there is little evidence one way or the other. Under non-lactating conditions the shape of the breast is largely determined by fat cells rather than the mammary gland. However, pregnancies and age are certainly two major factors leading to change. Approximately 9 out of 10 women who are feeding their babies do not ovulate; but nevertheless breast feeding should not be regarded as a method of contraception. Cancer of the breast is less common in women who have borne children and breast fed them.

Why mothers do not breast feed?

Mothers give a variety of reasons when asked why they have chosen not to breast feed. Some women just do not like the thought of breast feeding and, given an alternative, they take it. Others are embarrassed or uncertain and fear that they will fail or develop sore nipples and swollen, painful breasts. Some mothers obviously believe that bottle feeding is an easier and more certain way of ensuring their baby grows well and sleeps regularly. Others feel that bottle feeding offers greater freedom by, for instance, making it possible for them to return to work and to take the contraceptive pill. They might, perhaps, feel differently if they were better informed and more carefully prepared during the antenatal period; for example, once lactation is established, the contraceptive pill can be taken without it influencing breast feeding.

Contraindications

Maternal: technical. For some mothers, breast feeding is just not possible or may be contraindicated. For example, successful breast feeding is difficult with twins and virtually impossible with triplets; and in a premature birth, neither breasts nor baby, are prepared for feeding. It is possible with manual techniques to establish breast feeding for these infants who initially are unable to suckle satisfactorily, but it requires a great deal of resolve on the mother's part.

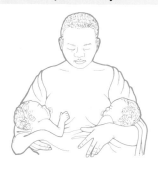

Twins: double productivity?

Maternal: health. If the mother has been chronically ill, severely undernourished, subject to severe asthmatic episodes or has limited renal function, breast feeding may be an unacceptable drain on her reserves. Similarly, mothers with diabetes may find that the metabolic challenge of producing milk upsets their diabetic state. Active tuberculosis in the mother is a contraindication to breast feeding until the infant has been immunised. HIV infection can be transmitted by breast feeding.

Drugs. Most drugs taken by the mother enter the milk. For practical purposes it can be estimated that one-tenth of the dose given to the mother enters the milk so that the possibility that a drug given to a breast-feeding mother may affect her baby must always be kept in mind.

Infant: technical. Some babies with abnormalities of the mouth, particularly cleft palate, are unable to suckle satisfactorily and breast feeding is virtually impossible. Tongue tie, unless it is in a very extreme form with forking of the tongue, should not interfere with the baby's ability to suckle.

Infant: health. Babies with inherited disorders of digestion or metabolism may not be able to tolerate the nutrients in human or other milks and special formulae are required. The inherited mono- and disaccharide intolerances, galactosaemia and phenylketonuria fall into this group.

ARTIFICIAL FEEDING

Artificial feeding in babies who suck well is usually by the bottle, but a spoon, cup, or plastic feeding tube may be used. The currently fashionable bottle sits on its base and has a wide neck surmounted by a rubber teat or nipple. Between feeds it must be washed with cold and then warm water and sterilised. The hole in the teat must be large enough to allow the baby to take his feeds in under 15 minutes but not so large that the feed flows so quickly as to cause the baby to splutter and choke. If a baby is unable to suck or swallow, or too weak or breathless to complete the feed, then he can be fed via a fine plastic nasogastric tube. This procedure properly performed is simple, safe and well tolerated by the infants. It has probably saved more lives than any other innovation in neonatal care. In certain situations the end of the tube may be advanced into the duodenum or jejunum.

Disadvantages of cow's milk

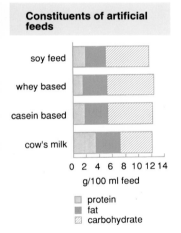

Constituents of artificial feeds

soy feed
whey based
casein based
cow's milk

0 2 4 6 8 10 12 14
g/100 ml feed

☐ protein
■ fat
▨ carbohydrate

The feed is usually cow's milk modified in some way. Many babies have been reared successfully on ordinary pasteurised or sterilised cow's milk, reconstituted evaporated liquid, or dried powdered cow's milk, but there have been problems. Some have been due to the way cow's milk differs from human milk. Cow's milk contains more protein, in particular more curd protein or casein, and these thick curds being less easy to digest have caused bowel obstruction. Cow's milk contains more fat and phosphorus. In the early weeks of life, particularly from 5 to 15 days of age, this may lead to hypocalcaemia with subsequent fitting. Cow's milk has a relatively high sodium content and this, with the tendency of mothers to make strong or concentrated feeds from powdered or condensed milks leads to hypernatraemia, which may cause fits and brain damage, complications which are more likely during superimposed episodes of infection, particularly gastroenteritis. Some infants are allergic to cow's milk protein; they may react to feeding with perioral rashes and oedema or by vomiting or passing frequent loose stools which usually contain blood.

Makers of infant feeds now prepare a variety of modified cow's milk formulae, which have been 'humanised' in that the mixture more closely resembles that found in average mature human milk. This has posed considerable problems for manufacturers, for milk is a complex colloid mixture and, as such, it is very sensitive to any attempts to change it. In addition, manufacturers can only modify and supplement cow's milk to resemble human milk as far as their knowledge of the constituents of human milk permits. Pyridoxine was added to formulae only after its deficiency had led to fits in artificially fed babies. They cannot of course add the 'living elements', cells and enzymes, and at the moment we do not know how important these are.

Each manufacturer markets four standard products, a whey based formula with a whey:casein ratio of 60:40 like human milk, a casein based formula with a whey: casein ration of 20:80 like cow's milk, a soy protein based formula with no milk constituents at all, and a 'follow-on' milk for weaning infants with a higher protein content.

Nutritional requirements

If a breast-fed child is content and growing, one need not trouble to consider the volume and nutrient value of each feed. There are, however, many reasons why an adequately breast-fed child may not be content or may not be growing satisfactorily. The nutrient intake of artificially fed infants is as much determined by the giver as the receiver and is more easily assessed. It is this facility which tempts some mothers whose infants are not thriving on the breast to change to bottle feeding, for then she and her health advisers can at least see the feed going in! Thus, it is essential in both breast and artificially fed infants to be able to assess their nutrient intake and their nutritional status.

Daily milk intake of healthy, thriving, free-feeding babies

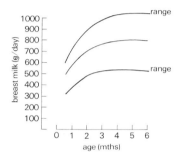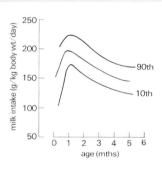

Just for interest, breast milk consumption is expressed per baby, artificial feeding is given per kg body weight.

Nutrient intake in breast-fed babies may be assessed by weighing the baby before and after feeds, that is by carrying out a test feed. In artificially-fed babies it is advisable to watch the mother make up and give at least one feed before calculating a daily intake from the history of feed volume and frequency. Nutritional status is usually assessed from the infant's weight, a visual evaluation of the quality of the skin and by the amount and distribution of subcutaneous fat. More information can be gained by measuring length or height and skin fold thicknesses. Appetite and metabolic efficiency vary from infant to infant, much as they do in adults. The average intake of healthy infants can be used as a guide, but it must be remembered that the range is wide and each infant's needs must be assessed individually.

FEEDING PROBLEMS

New mothers often wish to be reassured that their babies are feeding normally. If there are problems, they may seek advice from more experienced members of the family or from shop keepers who sell milk foods, or midwives, community nurses and health visitors and it is to be expected that they will be given differing opinions. Occasionally, the problem is of such magnitude that medical advice is sought. The doctor must be aware of, or take advice about, the general abilities, approach and attitudes of the parents, the mother's feeding technique and the infant's nutrient intake, before considering the possibility of more serious underlying conditions.

Vomiting

Most babies swallow air with their milk. Gentle patting or massage of their backs helps them bring back the 'wind'. Most babies bring up a little milk as well; this is called poseting and is unimportant.

Occasionally, infants regurgitate large amounts of milk, either immediately after a feed or between feeds. It is rare for this to be sufficiently severe to affect the infant's nutrition but it does distress his mother and, apart from other considerations, it makes all her clothes and furnishings smell and it fills her washing basket. Various strategies may be tried. By not allowing the baby to cry or become too upset before a feed and using good feeding technique, excess air swallowing can be avoided. Using agents which thicken the feed like cornflour or carob seed flour also reduces the baby's ability to bring them back. Propping the baby up after a feed may also help.

Some babies enjoy bringing their feeds back, 'ruminating' like a cow. This habit may be difficult to break but it will become less of a problem as the infant's diet, abilities and interests change.

There is no clear distinction between regurgitation and vomiting. An underlying cause *must* be sought if a baby suddenly starts to be sick, if the vomit contains blood or bile, if the vomiting persists to the point of dehydration or malnutrition, or is associated with other signs and symptoms. Vomiting may be the first indication of a general infection; it may be the only clue to an infected throat; it is common in pyelonephritis and is usual in meningitis and gastroenteritis. Certain disorders of the oesophagus and stomach must also be considered.

Gastro-oesophageal reflux

Gastro-oesophageal reflux is very common in infancy. The lower oesophageal valvular mechanism is made up of two main components: the intra-abdominal segment of the oesophagus, and the length of the muscular component of the sphincter. Both may be relatively deficient in early life allowing for free reflux. This is regarded as innocent or physiological when it does not interfere with weight gain or health. It becomes pathological when secondary oesophagitis causes symptoms such as irritability or feeding difficulty, or results in blood loss and iron deficiency anaemia. The reflux may also lead to episodes of aspiration pneumonia, or may produce apnoea or vagus nerve mediated bradycardia. The latter can lead to apparent life-threatening events or 'near miss cot-death'. Diagnosis of significant reflux is provided by a careful history supported by barium swallow or oesophageal pH studies. Endoscopy and biopsy establish the severity of the oesophagitis.

The majority of mild to moderate cases are managed conservatively in expectation that time and the development of a more competent lower oesophageal sphincter will resolve the problem. Appropriate management includes increased time spent in a baby chair, thickening the milk feeds, addition of an alginate preparation (Gaviscon) and, if indicated by pH studies, the use of H_2-receptor antagonists. A small number of refractory cases and those threatening to produce an oesophageal stricture need surgical repair of the hiatus and a fundoplication. Children with severe developmental delay and mobility problems are especially liable to have reflux. Unfortunately their handicaps often delay the recognition of their reflux symptoms.

There is now less emphasis on the diagnosis of hiatus hernia of infancy. This is regarded as part of the spectrum of gastro-oesophageal reflux. Occasionally delayed gastric emptying due to mild pyloric stenosis manifests as severe reflux; the appropriate management may therefore be pyloromyotomy or pyloroplasty.

Oesophageal reflux

oesophagael incoordination

oesophageal reflux

hiatus hernia

Oesophageal incoordination

Oesophageal incoordination leads to dribbling, choking and aspiration of milk as well as regurgitation and vomiting. It may be due to a wide variety of conditions all of which are rare, or sometimes it may be an isolated problem. It can be recognised by cine radiography.

Oesophageal incoordination can be a major problem in infants with cerebral palsy, and should be considered and excluded in all of them. Until recently this problem has not been addressed as thoroughly as it should have been and as a consequence such children have suffered unnecessarily and their growth and development has been compromised.

Pyloric stenosis

Pyloric stenosis is due to hypertrophy and hyperplasia of the pyloric muscle, mainly the circular fibres. It usually develops in the first 4 to 6 weeks of life. The condition is inherited by the multifactorial mode and is commonest in first-born, male children. Characteristically, the vomiting is projectile and may be so persistent that the baby becomes undernourished or even dehydrated. Being hungry, the baby is eager to feed again soon after he has vomited.

On examination, stomach wall peristalsis may be visible and a rubbery tumour is felt by gentle deep finger palpation in the area half way between the mid-point of anterior margin of the right rib cage and the umbilicus. The diagnosis is primarily clinical but useful confirmation is provided by ultrasound imaging of the pylorus. Contrast X-ray studies are seldom necessary. The plasma biochemistry is also characteristic with hyponatraemia, hypokalaemia, hypochloraemia and a metabolic alkalosis. It is essential that the dehydration and biochemical disturbance are corrected before general anaesthesia and surgery. Intravenous administration of half-normal saline solution with added potassium and dextrose provides for initial correction. Surgery aims to divide the pyloric muscles without penetrating the mucosa, pyloromyotomy (Ramstedt procedure).

Palpation

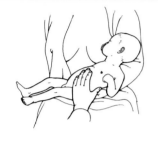

Pyloric stenosis: signs and surgery

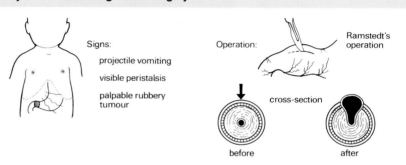

Failure to thrive

Mothers are naturally anxious if their infants do not appear to be growing fast enough. In most western societies now, babies are measured at regular intervals and if they fail to grow satisfactorily compared with the average for that community, further enquiry is made.

Failure to thrive can be the first indication of a serious underlying problem, such as chronic renal failure and congenital heart disease, but this is rare. More often than not, it reflects difficulties in the home, limitations in the parents, unhappiness in the relationship between mother and child or uncertain feeding methods. Many women feel 'down' after pregnancy and their unhappiness and nervousness may be communicated to their babies who in turn become irritable and restless

Failure to thrive

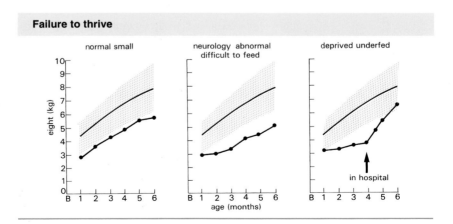

so that a vicious spiral is begun which ultimately leaves both mother and child exhausted. Bringing one or both of them into hospital to permit both to have a good night's sleep may go a long way to easing the problem. This condition is perhaps more appropriately described as 'failure to rear'.

If a baby is undersized, and it has been established that he was of normal birth weight, that he is receiving an adequate diet in a settled home and that he has no obvious serious underlying disorder, then investigation should be made for the various causes of malabsorption. These will include food intolerence, low grade infections, cystic fibrosis (lest it has been missed by the sceening procedures), and gluten enteropathy.

A crying baby and 3 month colic

Babies cry when they are hungry. They also cry for other reasons, such as cold or discomfort and as they get older they cry when they are cross or frustrated. With experience their mothers are usually able to distinguish a cry for food and a cry in pain, but it can be difficult. Not many parents can stand a baby crying intermittently throughout the night and the temptation is to feed him, not so much for his nutrition as to keep him quiet. He may react to this by vomiting.

Some babies, particularly at feeding time, but at other times as well, may have inconsolable outbursts of crying, sometimes to the point of screaming, for no obvious reason. During the attacks they may draw their knees up and go red in the face. It is difficult to believe that they are not having colic. It is possible that some infants have inflamed Peyer's patches and resulting painful bowel contractions. Drug therapy is seldom justified for they do not appear to come to any harm. This so-called '3 month colic' may last well beyond 3 months of age.

Diarrhoea, constipation and nappy rashes

There is no doubt that what an infant eats influences the frequency and nature of his stool and the effect the stool has on the skin of the buttocks. It is normal for a baby to have a loose yellow bowel motion with every feed, and it is equally acceptable that he has a bowel action every other day passing a firm large brown stool. But it is not acceptable that he passes frequent stools which are green and watery, or large stools which are pale and oily, or very occasional stools which are hard enough to tear the anal mucosa causing pain and bleeding.

All require investigation. They may respond to simple dietary adjustments. Stool gazing is a dying art, for the information it yields is disappointingly small, but occasionally it can be instructive.

NUTRITIONAL DEFICIENCIES

When unexpected symptoms or signs appear in infants and children on odd diets or with major feeding problems, the possibility of a vitamin or mineral deficiency should be considered. Clinical syndromes due to deficiency of most vitamin and many trace elements have been reported.

Vitamin A

Xerophthalma due to vitamin A deficiency is a common serious nutritional disorder in the third world and leads to blindness. Dark green leafy vegetables are the main source of vitamin A in the developing world.

Scurvy

Scurvy is due to vitamin C deficiency. Cow's milk contains little vitamin C and most of this may disappear if the milk is stored or heated. Before artificial milks were fortified with extra vitamin C to a level similar to that in human milk, artificially-fed babies were at risk of developing scurvy. In this disorder connective tissues and structural membranes break down, small vessels bleed and wounds are slow to heal. The infants present with bruises, painful periosteal bleeds or persistent superficial haemorrhages.

Rickets

Rickets is due to vitamin D deficiency. The body obtains the vitamin by the action of ultraviolet light on the ergosterols in the deeper layers of the skin or from certain foods, including fish, eggs, butter and margarine. Lack of sunshine, a pigmented skin or a poor diet leaves a child at risk. It is important that lactating mothers have adequate vitamin D so that her milk will contain sufficient for her rapidly growing infant.

Vitamin D aids the absorption of calcium from the bowel and the formation and calcification of bone. Deficiency leads to softening and deformity, particularly of the long bones. In early life rickets may be suspected if the skull bones are soft, craniotabes; in the 3 to 6 month old child the enlargement of the ends of ribs produces a rachitic 'rosary'. In a child 12 to 18 months of age just beginning to walk, the ends of the long bones may be bowed either in or out by the strain. This is a tragedy if it occurs because the deformity is easily and cheaply avoided by vitamin D supplementation of the diet.

Clinical picture

Craniotabies

Rickety rosary

Swelling of ends of long bones

Delay in walking

Curvature of ends of long bones

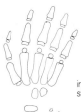

X-ray appearances in rickets

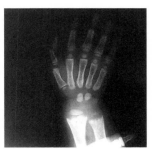

irregular metaphysis causing swelling of wrist

Secondary rickets

Vitamin D deficiency may be secondary to other disorders. It occurs in the very immature when they begin to grow and can be reversed by extra vitamin D, calcium and phosphate supplements. Rarely it develops during recovery from malabsorption (rickets occurs only in the growing child) and in children with chronic liver disease when the first hydroxylation step, vitamin D to 25 (OH) D, fails. It is not uncommon in chronic renal failure when the second hydroxylation step, 25 (OH) D to 1,25 (OH) D, fails. This step is also limited in vitamin D dependent rickets, a rare recessively inherited disorder. In vitamin D resistant rickets (familial hypophosphataemic rickets, a sex-linked dominant condition) there is thought to be a defect in renal tubular transport of phosphate. Rickets also complicates more general disorders of tubular function, like Fanconi syndrome, renal tubular acidosis and cystinosis.

Classification of rickets and vitamin D metabolite levels

	Vitamin D	25 (OH)D	1,25(OH)D
Deficient synthesis and supply – no sunlight – poor diet – immaturity	↓	↓	↓
Malabsorption	n	↓	↓
Liver disease	n	↓	↓
Chronic renal failure	n	n	↓
Vitamin D dependent rickets (recessively inherited)	n	n	↓
Vitamin D resistant ricket (sex-linked dominant)	n	n	n
Renal tubular disorders (defect of phosphate reabsorption)	n	n	n

Dental caries

Dental caries is due to progressive decay of teeth by organic acids produced locally by bacteria that ferment dietary carbohydrate, particularly sucrose. Fluoride reduces the incidence and severity of caries, by converting the enamel mineral, hydroxyapatite, to fluorapatite which is more acid resistant, by promoting remineralisation, and by antibacterial effects which reduce acid production. Thus, tooth decay can be considered to be a nutritional disorder, in part due to a deficiency of fluoride and in part due to excess of simple sugars. The risks of dental

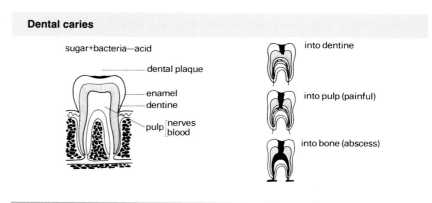

Dental caries

sugar+bacteria—acid

dental plaque

enamel

dentine

pulp [nerves / blood]

into dentine

into pulp (painful)

into bone (abscess)

caries may be reduced by avoiding food between meals, particularly sticky sweets or sweet drinks in nursing bottles or pacifiers; by regularly cleaning the teeth; and by an adequate intake of fluoride either in the water, toothpaste or if necessary by tablet.

MALNUTRITION

Many children in some parts of the world simply do not get enough to eat. Following a political or natural disaster, the news media have been quick to make us more aware of the severe forms of childhood malnutrition which are prevalent during famine.

A WHO Expert Committee divided the protein-energy deficiency syndromes into marasmus, where failure to grow is associated with emaciation and a fair appetite; kwashiorkor, where malnutrition is associated with oedema and loss of appetite; and 'unspecified' where growth retardation and undernutrition are evident without frank emaciation or oedema. These terms describe the various ways by which starvation can affect the growing child. With starvation of whatever degree comes misery and an increased risk of infections. Both add to domestic problems and increase the risk of death or permanent damage.

Marasmus

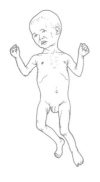

Marasmus in western societies may be seen in infants born severely undernourished, or after severe chronic illnesses, particularly affecting the bowel. In poorer communities, nutritional marasmus commonly occurs due to failure of lactation in people who just cannot afford artificial milks. Thus it is more common in low-birth-weight infants, twins and in infants after infection, particularly gastroenteritis.

The infant's survival depends on the mother's ability to maintain lactation, even if the infant is unable to suckle for a few days. If food can be found, the prognosis of these infants is good. During a famine children of all ages may become marasmic and the recovery of older children may take longer. The risk of death due to superadded infection during the recovery phase is also higher.

Kwashiorkor

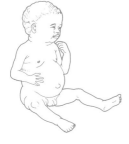

Kwashiorkor is a colourful word that gives the impression of a specific disease entity but it is but one end of a spectrum. Most commonly, it occurs in children 18 to 24 months old at the time of weaning. The marasmic child receives a little of a balanced diet; in the child with kwashiorkor the energy intake may be just about adequate but the protein content is insufficient for growth. As a consequence there is muscle wasting but preservation of some subcutaneous fat.

The infant is oedematous, listless and irritable. There may be a 'flaky paint' dermatitis of a depigmented skin and the hair is sparse and friable. The liver may be large due to fatty infiltration and the serum albumin concentration may be reduced.

The complications include hypothermia, hypoglycaemia, drowsiness, severe diarrhoea, cardiac failure and all these are compounded by superimposed infections.

An inadequate supply of food is not primarily a medical problem. However the health service can help in the following ways:

1. By encouraging and supporting the lactating mother; there is no reason why breast feeding should not be continued for 18 or 24 months.
2. By advising parents about weaning.
3. By recommending those local foods which will meet the protein needs of the growing child.
4. By the early recognition of children in difficulties so that limited food resources can be optimally deployed.
5. By the treatment of associated infections and vitamin deficiency states.

OBESITY

Obesity is a common health problem when food is in abundance. Fat parents tend to have fat children for there is a genetic component in the aetiology. Fat children tend to but do not invariably become fat adults. Fat people die on average at a younger age than thin people. In particular, fat adults are more likely to develop diabetes and hypertension; they weather chronic chest disease, heart failure and abdominal operations badly; and they have more problems with varicose veins, piles and skin crease ailments.

Obesity can be assessed reasonably well just by looking at the child and by plotting body weight on a centile chart. The height:weight ratio and skin fold thicknesses can be measured if more accurate analysis is required.

Prevention. As obesity is so difficult to treat it is best to avoid it. There is some evidence that bottle-fed babies are more likely to become overweight than breast-fed infants. This may be because the baby is less

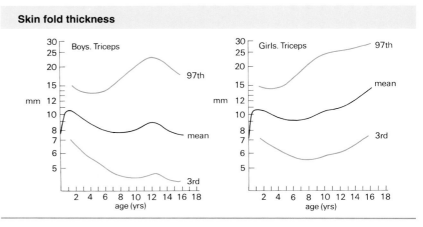

Skin fold thickness

able to resist pressures to finish the bottle. Obesity may develop in the months after weaning when clearing the plate or emptying the cup becomes a virtue. Early weaning encourages this development. There is little virtue in commencing weaning before 4 or 5 months of age. One big meal a day appears to be more fattening than many small ones amounting to similar caloric value. Thus, the best prophylaxis for infants at risk of obesity because of fat parents is for them to be breast fed and weaned late; overfeeding should be avoided, particularly during the weaning period and the habit of taking regular exercise and eating small frequent meals should be established.

Treatment. Obese children may be referred for medical advice for a variety of reasons. The child may be concerned because of his appearance or the clothes he is required to wear or because he is teased. His parents may be concerned for the same reasons but also because they fear it may affect his health in other ways. His teachers may be concerned because of his lack of physical fitness. If the child really wants to be thinner and his parents are prepared to put themselves out to help him then there is some hope that a diet and exercise regimen will work. However, occasionally over-eating is an outward sign of inner confusion and unhappiness. This needs to be recognised and discussed. But in the majority of cases a detailed enquiry brings little to light except bad parental dietary attitudes and practices. One mother still gave her child aged 7 years a breast feed at night; another considered that a bumper gorge was a high treat; a third used food to settle a particularly active and demanding baby.

Who is for dieting?

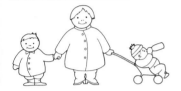

BIBLIOGRAPHY

Francis D 1987 Diets for sick children. Blackwell Scientific Publications, Oxford
McLaren D S, Burman D, Belton N R, Williams A F (eds) 1991. Textbook of paediatric nutrition, 3rd edn. Churchill Livingstone, Edinburgh
Taitz L S, Wardley B 1989 Handbook of child nutrition. Oxford University Press, Oxford

6 Infection

Infections can spread readily among children. Acute respiratory infections, gastroenteritis and the main subject of this Chapter, the infectious 'fevers' account for a large part of childhood illness, although scourges of the past, such as diphtheria and poliomyelitis, have now virtually disappeared from many countries. Infections are most likely to occur when the child first mixes with others, at a nursery, a playgroup or at primary school, and he may bring them home to his younger siblings. Usually the infectious fever is diagnosed by the mother, and the child is not very ill and can be looked after at home. If hospital admission is required it is often for social rather than medical reasons, though occasionally complications arise which are potentially damaging or life threatening.

Child infectious disease morbidity 1987 for England and Wales (selected data from OPCS and General Registrar Office)

	0–4 years	5–14 years	Adults
Measles	41 379	39 478	5143
Food poisoning	6176	3756	29 772
Whooping cough	3164	1710	243
Scarlet fever	2905	3013	31
Acute meningitis	1457	419	1111
Dysentery	827	663	2202
Infective jaundice	295	1672	3095
Tuberculosis (all) *	124	253	4784
Malaria	45	142	1080
* Excluding chemoprophylaxis			

Deaths (infants under 29 days age excluded) due to infectious diseases in UK 1988 (data selected from OPCS and General Registrar Offices)

	0–1 years	1–4 years	5–9 years	Total
Pneumonia	134	36	11	181
Other bacterial disease	86	50	16	152
Acute bronchitis/bronchiolotis	76	15	3	94
Meningococcal infection	53	40	9	102
Meningitis	40	33	4	77
Septicaemia	25	5	6	36
Viral disease	23	17	11	51
Intestinal infectious disease	14	3	1	18
Viral disease of the nervous system	9	6	1	16

MEASLES

Measles is a common and very infectious viral disease. The incubation period is followed by a prodromal illness with fever, coryza, conjunctivitis and cough. Generalized lymphadenopathy may be found, and tiny white spots on a bright red background, Koplik's spots, are present on the buccal mucosa of the cheeks. After 3 or 4 days a florid rash appears, and spreads downwards from the head and neck to cover the whole body. The earlier lesions are more numerous and become confluent and blotchy. The rash begins to fade by the third day and the child's general condition improves steadily.

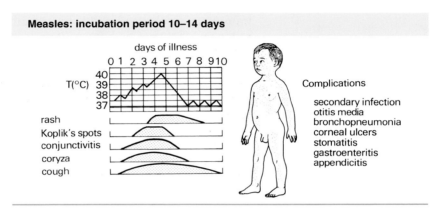

Measles: incubation period 10–14 days

Respiratory complications, particularly bronchopneumonia and otitis media are common. Encephalitis occurs in about 1 in 5000 affected children and is manifested by headache, drowsiness and vomiting. Convulsions and coma begin 7 to 10 days after the onset of the illness. The course of encephalitis is unpredictable but about 15 per cent of cases die, and 25 per cent suffer brain damage resulting in mental retardation, fits, deafness, or behaviour disorders. Measles may be associated with a disturbance of immune mechanisms, especially lymphopaenia. Defective immune response may also be the basis of the rare late complication, subacute sclerosing panencephalitis (SSPE) which occurs 4 to 10 years after an attack of measles and is characterised by slow progressive deterioration. There are very high levels of measles antibody in the blood and cerebrospinal fluid, and measles virus antigen has been demonstrated in brain tissue.

In developing countries, measles carries a high morbidity and mortality. It tends to occur in younger children than in the UK (median age 17 months in Nigeria, 52 months in England and Wales). Reported mortality rates range from 5.5 per cent in East Africa to between 20 and 40 per cent in a selected hospital series in West Africa. In the malnourished child, a severe form of measles may occur with a confluent rash that darkens to deep red or purple, and then desquamates. This is followed by depigmentation of the skin which lasts for several weeks and may be associated with pyodermia. A sore mouth is common during the acute illness and may lead to cancrum oris; invariably breast feeding is disturbed. Diarrhoea is common and may persist for a long time, further aggravating any underlying malnutrition. Measles mortality rate is directly related to socio-economic conditions, and there is a strong correlation with the distribution of kwashiorkor. In young susceptable children measles itself causes loss of weight. In a village in Nigeria almost 1 in 4 children lost more than 10 per cent of their weight following an attack of measles, and the average time to regain the previous weight was 7 weeks. It is therefore important to maintain the child's hydration and nutrition during the illness and afterwards. In the weeks and months following measles there is an increase in mortality from other illnesses. Another group particularly vulnerable to severe measles is the immunocompromised child. Encephalitis and viral pneumonia can occur and there is a high mortality rate.

There is a live attenuated vaccine which is used in many countries. It was introduced in the UK in 1968. If sufficient children are immunised (perhaps 95 per cent) epidemics of measles should cease, but for many years only about half the children in the UK were immunised. In recent years this has risen to about 88 per cent but the distribution across the country is uneven. In the USA where measles immunisation has been widely accepted for some time, measles was virtually eliminated, but there is concern that measles continues to be seen in young children before they are immunised and in young adults.

RUBELLA

Rubella, or German measles, is usually a mild illness, and may pass unrecognised. The incubation period is 14 to 21 days and there may be little or no fever or malaise before the appearance of the pink macular rash which lasts for about 3 days. Generalised lymphadenopathy, especially involving the suboccipital nodes, may be present. A rising haemagglutinin inhibition titre confirms the diagnosis. This test is seldom necessary in children but is essential when the possibilty arises of

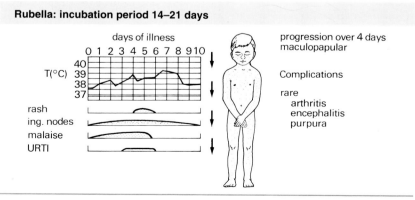

Rubella: incubation period 14–21 days

days of illness
0 1 2 3 4 5 6 7 8 9 10

T(°C) 40 39 38 37

rash
ing. nodes
malaise
URTI

progression over 4 days
maculopapular

Complications

rare
  arthritis
  encephalitis
  purpura

rubella in early pregnancy. Complications of rubella, such as thrombocytopaenia and encephalitis, do occur but they are rare. Arthritis may occur in adolescents.

The importance of this disease lies in its devastating effect on the developing fetus if the mother contracts the infection during the first 3 months of pregnancy. A generalised viraemia may lead to fetal death and spontaneous abortion, or may affect the growth and development of the fetus resulting in a severely handicapped child with multiple congenital defects, classically including cataracts, deafness and congenital heart disease. All women should be tested for rubella immunity preferably before or in early pregnancy.

There is a live attenuated vaccine against rubella and its value is in preventing rubella during pregnancy. In the UK between 1970 and 1988 the vaccine programme was aimed at girls in early adolescence. However a significant number of girls did not get the immunisation and still caught rubella in pregnancy, because there were still regular epidemics of rubella. Since 1988, the vaccine has been given at the age of 12 to 18 months to girls and boys to stop epidemics occuring and protect even those who have not or cannot be immunised. The vaccine is combined with measles and mumps vaccines.

MUMPS

Mumps is caused by a paramyxovirus. Subclinical infection is common. A long incubation period of 16 to 21 days is followed by fever, malaise and enlargement of one or both parotid glands, which develop over a period of 1 to 3 days. The child may complain of earache and difficulty in swallowing, and the glands may be painful and tender. The submandibular glands may also be affected. The swellings settle in 7 to 10 days and there is no specific traetment. Other causes of parotitis are rare in children and the distinction from cervical lymphadenopathy should not be difficult after careful examination.

Differential diagnosis of mumps and cervical adenitis

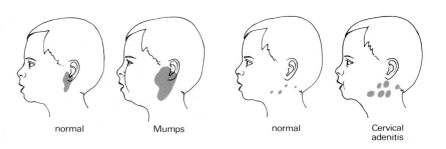

normal   Mumps   normal   Cervical adenitis

Meningitis is a common complication, but is usually mild and characterised by headache, photophobia and neck stifness. The cerebrospinal fluid contains an increased number of lymphocytes and a raised concentration of protein. Recovery is almost always complete. Sensorineural deafness, usually unilateral, can occur; mumps is thought to be the commonest cause of unilateral severe deafness in children Pancreatitis and epididymo-orchitis also occur, but epididymo-orchitis is much more common after puberty.

A live attenuated vaccine has been available for some years and was introduced in the UK in 1988 combined with measles and rubella vaccines, given at 12 to 18 months. There has been a noticeable fall in mumps illness since then.

CHICKEN POX (VARICELLA)

Chicken pox is a common and highly infectious disease but is usually mild in children. The same virus produces herpes zoster. The incubation period is 14 to 16 days. There may be no symptoms apart from the rash and a low grade fever. Chicken pox spots appear in crops, progressing rapidly from macule to papule to vesicle. The vesicle soon dries and crusts and the scabs separate without scarring. Lesions may also occur on mucous membranes, especially in the mouth where they quickly produce shallow ulcers. Now that smallpox has been erradicated from the world, problems of differential diagnosis are rare.

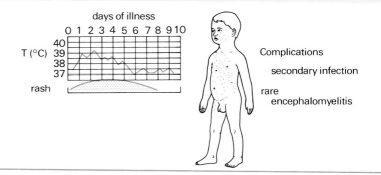

Chicken pox: incubation period 14–16 days

Complications of chicken pox are uncommon in healthy children. Encephalitis is rare but when it does occur there is often cerebellar involvment. The child presents with ataxia 3 to 8 days after the onset of the rash. At least 80 per cent of affected children make a complete recovery. Pneumonia is a rare complication in children, but it may be part of the very severe form of the illness when the rash is haemorrhagic. This is more likely to occur in children with immune deficiency, in particular children treated for leukaemia. Between 1967 and 1985 there was an average of 19 deaths a year from chicken pox in the UK, often in adults and immunocompromised people.

A vaccine is available, but is not licensed for use in the UK and at present is not routinely used.

HERPES SIMPLEX INFECTIONS

Infection with this virus is extremely common and usually asymptomatic, less than 10 per cent of children with primary infections becoming clinically ill. Herpes virus Type 1 is spread by infected saliva and transmission therefore requires close personal contact. Primary infection may affect the mouth, skin or eyes. Herpes virus Type 2 is a genital infection usually spread by sexual contact.

Newborn infants may be infected during delivery by maternal genital herpes infection (Type 2) or, less commonly, by the usual Type 1 virus in the postnatal period. Infection may result in a severe, disseminated disease characterised by lethargy, vesicular rash, hepatosplenomegaly, bleeding and neurological symptoms. Mortality is about 70 per cent and there is a high morbidity rate among the survivors. The risk of this severe illness is about 40 per cent if the mother has active genital herpes at the time of delivery, and an elective Caesarean section should be considered.

Acute gingivostomatitis is common, particularly in preschool children from poor socioeconomic circumstances. It is characterised by high fever, swelling and bleeding of gums and extensive ulceration of buccal mucosa, tongue and palate. The cervical glands are enlarged. Eating and drinking are painful, and the child may become dehydrated. The illness lasts about 10 to 14 days. A vulvovaginitis may result from transfer of the infection from the mouth by the child's finger.

Keratoconjunctivitis is associated with severe oedema of the eyelids and dendritic ulcers of the cornea which may lead to scarring and loss of vision. Primary infection of the skin with vesicular lesions tends to develop in older children, often at the site of trauma. In children with eczema, an extensive vesicular rash which later scabs may occur on the eczematous skin. The child may be febrile and sometimes there is generalised infection due to blood stream spread, which is potentially fatal. Secondary infection of skin lesions is a complication. The diagnosis of local infection is not difficult, as the vesicular lesions are characteristic. Rapid confirmation can be obtained by culture of the vesicular fluid or microscopic examination of scrapings for inclusion bodies. Topical treatment with idoxyuridine is partially effective.

Cold sores. Recurrent herpes simplex infection is common and usually occurs as 'cold sores' round the mouth. The recurrence rate is very variable and though the lesions may be associated with respiratory infections, they may also be related to nonspecific factors such as sunshine, menstruation and emotional stress.

Meningo-encephalitis. Herpes simplex virus is a relatively common cause of meningo-encephalitis. It may occur during the primary infection or due to the activation of a virus lying dormant after an earlier infection. It develops in apparently normal children and it can occur in the absence of skin lesions. The illness may be very severe and the mortality rate is high. Frontal and temporal lobe abnormalities are found, on the electroencephalogram and a brain scan may demonstrate a 'space-occupying' lesion. A rising titre of antibody in the blood or cerebrospinal fluid confirms the diagnosis. Treatment with acyclovir, if given early, is of some benefit but the improvement in survival with active treatment has not been accompanied by a reduction in the very high rate of chronic neurological handicap.

GLANDULAR FEVER

In developed countries glandular fever, infectious mononucleosis, occurs most often in adolescents and young adults, but is not uncommon in children. Infection is usually sporadic, though epidemics can occur in schools or residential homes. The Epstein-Barr virus is the cause of the infection and is excreted in nasopharyngeal secretions. Close contact is necessary for infection to be transmitted.

The onset of glandular fever is usually insidious and occurs after an incubation period of 4 to 14 days. The clinical features are anorexia, malaise and fever and they are usually accompanied by a sore throat and enlarged glands in most affected children. The tonsillitis may be very severe with a thick white exudate covering the tonsils and surrounding areas. Petechiae may be seen on the palate. Cervical lymph nodes are enlarged, and the spleen is often palpable. A macular rash occurs in 10 to 20 per cent of cases, especially if ampicillin has been given. Hepatitis, often with jaundice is common, but other complications such an pneumonitis and neurological disturbances are rare.

The diagnosis is supported by the presence of atypical mononuclear cells in the blood film. These large cells have an irregular nucleus and pale-staining cytoplasm containing vacuoles, and may account for 10 to 25 per cent of the total white cell count. The test for heterophil antibodies is positive in about 60 per cent of patients in the first week of illness. These antibodies agglutinate sheep red blood cells and are not absorbed by guinea pig kidney cells. Horse red blood cells are also agglutinated and this is the basis of the monospot test. EB virus IgM is present in the early stages of the illness and is indicative of a recent infection. Liver function tests are abnormal in over half of the patients.

Glandular fever is a self-limiting disease for which there is no specific treatment. The lymphadenopathy and splenomegaly may persist for weeks or months, and there may be a long period of debility. The differential diagnosis when tonsillitis is severe includes streptococcal tonsillitis and diphtheria; when lymphadenopathy is prominent it includes leukaemia, toxoplasmosis and cytomegalovirus infection; and when jaundice or a rash are present, infectious hepatitis, measles or rubella may be suspected. The diagnosis is not difficult if the clinical features are characteristic and the appropriate laboratory tests are obtained.

KAWASAKI DISEASE (MUCOCUTANEOUS LYMPH NODE SYNDROME)

First described in Japan, this condition has now been reported from many other countries. The majority of patients are under 5 years of age and present with an acute febrile illness associated with conjunctivitis, pharyngitis and a generalised polymorphous rash. The hands and feet are typically red and oedematous, with peeling of the fingers and toes as the child recovers. Cervical lymph nodes are usually enlarged. Arthritis, urethritis and hepatitis may occur. The fever persists for 1–2 weeks and then settles. A neutrophil leucocytosis, very high ESR and raised platelet counts are found but no organisms have been cultured and auto-antibodies are negative. The most important complication is cardiac involvement with clinical evidence of myocarditis or conduction defects in 20 per cent (especially infants), and death in 1–2 per cent. Coronary artery aneurysms may develop and are detectable by echocardiography, but fortunately slowly resolve in the majority. Post mortem studies show a widespread vasculitis always affecting the coronary arteries.

No infective agent has been isolated and there is no evidence of person-to-person transmission, even in apparent epidemics. Treatment with aspirin in full anti-inflammatory dosage is recommended in the acute stage, and it is reasonable to continue with a small dose to reduce platelet aggregation for some weeks.

ERYTHEMA INFECTIOSUM (5TH DISEASE)

This condition, caused by human parvovirus B19, is characterised by an erythematous maculopapular rash which often begins on the face giving a typical 'slapped cheek' appearance. The rash spreads to the trunk and limbs with central fading of the eruption giving a lacy or reticular appearance. It lasts about a week. There are usually no other symptoms, though arthralgia of the small joints may occur.

ROSEOLA INFANTUM (EXANTHEMA SUBITUM)

This is thought to be caused by human herpes virus 6. The patient is usually under 2 years of age. He develops a high fever, often without appearing particularly ill, though convulsions may occur. Examination reveals only a mild pharyngitis and lymphadenopathy. After 3 or 4 days the temperature drops suddenly to normal and a macular rash appears which lasts for a few hours or a day or 2. The child then makes an uneventful and rapid recovery.

HAND, FOOT AND MOUTH DISEASE

This is caused by a Coxsackie virus. It is common among young children and tends to occur in epidemics. Vesicular leions appear on the palms of the hands or fingers, the soles of the feet and in the mouth. There may be a low grade fever. Mild cases will go undetected.

HEPATITIS A (INFECTIOUS JAUNDICE)

The hepatitis A virus is an enterovirus spread by the faeco-oral route. The illness is normally mild in children. The child may be generally unwell with headache, nausea, vomiting and abdominal pain; they will often be starting to improve when the jaundice and dark urine appear; this may last for a week or 2 before resolving. It is rare for children to develop fulminating hepatitis. Many children do not develop the jaundice and in this situation the diagnosis is difficult. The infection often spreads round the family or to other children in a nursery or school. In these situations the level of hygiene needs to be checked.

POLIOMYELITIS

The introduction of successful immunisation against poliomyelitis has been one of the greatest success stories of modern medicine. A dreadful disease has been eliminated in many countries and there are hopes that it can be erradicated worldwide by the year 2000.

In most people, the poliomyelitis virus produces a mild illness with fever, sore throat, headache and vomiting, lasting up to 3 days. In about one third of affected children this is followed by improvement for 1 to 7 days and then a recurrence of more severe symptoms with pain and stiffness in the neck, back and legs. As in other types of viral meningitis, the cerebrospinal fluid contains increased lymphocytes and protein. Paralysis may develop in association with muscle pain and tenderness. This is due to anterior horn cell damage, is usually asymmetrical, and varies considerably in extent, in the severe forms causing respiratory failure and bulbar paralysis. Once the fever subsides, the spread of weakness and paralysis is halted and there is then a slow improvement over a period of about 18 months. After this time any residual paralysis is likely to be permanent.

The clinical course of poliomyelitis

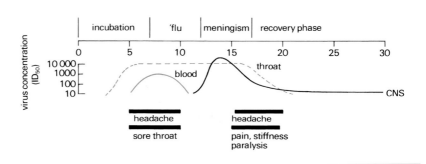

DIPHTHERIA

Diphtheria is now very rare in countries where immunisation is practised. It is caused by one of three strains of *Corynebacterium diphtheriae*. The infection is usually in the throat and is spread by droplets from infected individuals or healthy carriers. The incubation period is 2 to 7 days. The child presents with a sore throat and inflamed tonsils. The pharyngeal exudate may spread with epithelial destruction and membrane formation leading to upper airway obstruction. Exotoxin released by the bacterium may cause myocarditis (second week) and neuritis with paralysis (third to seventh week).

The vaccine, a modified exotoxin, gives a very high level of protection. Treatment of the disease itself requires diphtheria antitoxin to counteract its effects and erythromycin to eradicate the organisms.

PERTUSSIS (WHOOPING COUGH)

Bordetella pertussis is the cause of a prolonged respiratory illness which is particularly dangerous in infancy. After a 7-day incubation period, there is a 'catarrhal' stage lasting 1 to 2 weeks, during which the child is unwell, with signs of upper respiratory tract infection. A cough develops which becomes increasingly severe and paroxysmal. Spasms of coughing may be followed by an inspiratory 'whoop', especially in older children. Vomiting may occur, and the child can become cyanosed or apnoeic during coughing spasms and be left exhausted afterwards. Between spasms there may be no obvious respiratory difficulty and the lungs are clear on examination. This phase lasts 4 to 6 weeks, and the cough gradually improves over another 2 to 3 weeks. The causative organism is cultured in early cases from a nasopharyngeal swab using Bordet-Gengou medium, but is difficult to isolate once the cough is established. A striking lymphocytosis supports the diagnosis.

The most common complication is bronchopneumonia which is especially common in infants and accounts for most of the deaths. Bronchiectasis used to be a well-recognised sequela but is now very uncommon. Convulsions may occur due to asphyxia from severe spasms, intracranial bleeding or encephalopathy. Subconjunctival haemorrhages and facial petechiae due to raised venous pressure during spasms may be alarming but resolve spontaneously.

The treatment of pertussis is largely symptomatic and careful nursing is required. Oxygen, suction and tube-feeding may be necessary. Erythromycin given in the catarrhal stage may abort or modify the illness but the result is often disappointing. Its use in infant contacts is justifiable. No drugs prevent the spasms once the disease is established.

Immunisation against pertussis became the subject of considerable controversy in the mid 1970s, following well-publicised reports of neurological damage associated with reactions to the triple vaccine. The frequency of such reactions and the incidence of natural pertussis and its complications were not known and varying figures were reported. The debate led to a considerable fall in uptake of pertussis immunisation in the UK to 31 per cent in 1978 and as a consequence there was a bad epidemic in 1978–80. It became clear that pertussis is still a serious disease especially in infants. There were at least 30 deaths in England and Wales. At the same time the efficacy of the vaccine in protecting against pertussis, which had been questioned, was clearly demonstrated.

Whooping cough notifications and the effect of vaccination rates

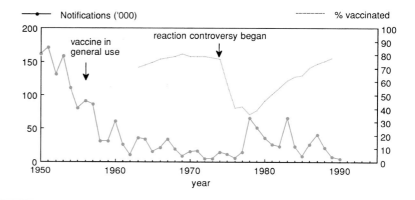

Attempts have been made to establish the risk of encephalopathy following pertussis vaccine, but there is no conclusive evidence of a link. On the other hand the risks from pertussis illness are well established. Immunisation rates have risen again in recent years with a resulting fall in the number of cases. As very little maternal antibody crosses the placenta, the protection of young infants depends on the state of immunity of their older siblings.

SCARLET FEVER

Group A haemolytic streptococci are responsible for a variety of problems in children, especially tonsillitis. Sequelae such as rheumatic fever and acute glomerulonephritis are important, but have become rare in western societies. Scarlet fever results from infection with a strain of the organism which produces an erythrogenic toxin.

After an incubation period of 2 to 4 days, the child develops tonsillitis, fever, headache and malaise. The rash develops within 12 hours of the onset and rapidly becomes generalised. It consists of a fine punctate erythema which blanches on pressure. The face is spared, but the cheeks are flushed so that the child is indeed 'scarlet', apart from the area around the mouth. The tongue has a thick white coating through which the inflamed papillae project, the 'white strawberry tongue'. By day 4 or 5 the tongue peels, leaving a 'red strawberry' appearance. The skin rash fades after a few days, or sooner if penicillin is given, followed by desquamation, especially on the hands and feet. This may persist for some time and is useful in making a retrospective diagnosis. Scarlet fever may also follow infection of wounds or burns.

Treatment with penicillin leads to a rapid recovery, but a 10 day course is necessary to eradicate the streptococcal infection.

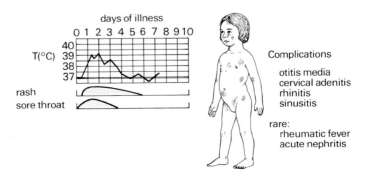

Scarlet fever: incubation period 2 to 4 days

days of illness

0 1 2 3 4 5 6 7 8 9 10

T(°C) 40 39 38 37

rash

sore throat

Complications

otitis media
cervical adenitis
rhinitis
sinusitis

rare:
rheumatic fever
acute nephritis

TUBERCULOSIS

Tuberculosis is no longer the 'captain of the Kings of Death' in Europe, but remains a major problem in many developing countries. The incidence of TB in Europe fell steadily as a result of better social conditions and nutrition, and with the advent of effective chemotherapy. Most children with the disease are now identified because they are contacts of infected adults, who may be asymptomatic. In the UK children of Asian families are at special risk of infection from recent adult immigrants. They account for 40 per cent of the 488 children reported with TB in 1983 in England and Wales.

The incidence is declining in all groups, at an average annual rate of 19 per cent for Indian children, 17 per cent for Pakistanis and 5 per cent for whites since 1978/9. Only 4 per cent of Welsh schoolchildren were found to be tuberculin positive on routine testing in 1980, indicating that they had had a primary infection or BCG vaccination.

Primary infection

Mycobacterium tuberculosis is spread by droplets, and primary infection may occur in the lung, skin or gut. One outbreak in Nottingham occurred in tooth sockets following dental extractions by a dentist with pulmonary TB. Sensitivity to tuberculin develops 4–8 weeks after infection, as shown by a positive Mantoux or Heaf test. Tuberculin tests may be negative if there is severe malnutrition or overwhelming infection. Hypersensitivity reactions such as erythema nodosum (red shiny lumps on the shins) or phlyctenular conjunctivitis occur in a few instances. Only about 1 in 20 of those infected develop disease.

Primary tuberculosis

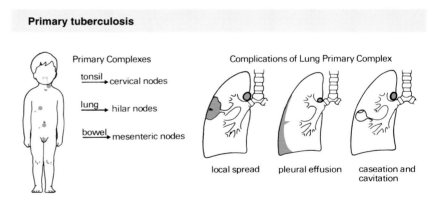

In these, the local infection spreads locally and to the lymph nodes; together these constitute the primary complex. Most such lesions heal slowly by fibrosis and may calcify, the process taking 12–18 months. Complications may arise from the local progression of the primary complex, especially in the lungs. An area of bronchopneumonia develops, or enlargement of the hilar nodes leads to bronchial obstruction, sometimes with rupture of the node into a bronchus. Pleural effusions occur in older children as a hypersensitivity reaction. Empyema, caseation and cavitation are seen more often in malnourished children from developing countries. Unless the lesion cavitates into a bronchus, children with primary TB do not cough up sputum and are not infectious. They may have no cough at all, but a general malaise and vague ill health. Adult pulmonary TB, characterised by cavitation results either from new infection or a breakdown of the primary complex. Tubercle bacilli can persist in a dormant form and cause disease many years later.

Lung complications of tuberculosis

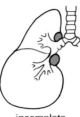 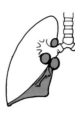 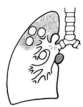

incomplete obstruction— overinflation

complete obstruction— collapse

rupture of node into bronchus— fibrosis and cavities

Gastrointestinal lesions

A primary focus in the tonsillar region may present with cervical adenitis and progress to a 'cold' abscess. This is usually due to human TB but may follow infection with a bovine strain after drinking unpasteurised milk. A similar infection in the small bowel occasionally leads to malabsorption, stricture formation and peritonitis. Cervical adenitis may also occur with infection due to atypical mycobacteria.

Miliary TB and meningitis

Blood stream spread is the most serious complication of primary TB and accounts for at least 70 per cent of childhood deaths due to TB. The risk is greatest in young children especially in developing countries, and almost always occurs within 1 year of infection. The child presents with fever, anorexia and loss of weight. Enlargement of the liver and spleen is common and choroidal tubercles may be seen on examining the fundi. Scattered crepitations may be heard over the lungs, and the chest X-ray shows generalised mottling. There is often associated meningitis, which develops insidiously with gradual progression of lethargy, headache, convulsions and coma. Cranial nerve lesions may develop. A tuberculoma of the brain is much commoner in developing countries than in Europe and presents as a space-occupying lesion.

Miliary TB

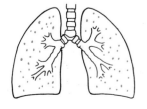

In TB meningitis the CSF is opalescent with increased lymphocytes and protein but low sugar concentrations. A few organisms may be seen on microscopy of the deposit. A culture may take some weeks to grow so treatment should not be delayed. Unfortunately hydrocephalus and other long term neurological damage are common in survivors.

Tuberculosis of the bones and joints can develop as a result of blood stream spread within 3 years of the primary infection. Renal infection may not become apparent for 5 or more years.

Treatment. Active tuberculous infection requires prompt effective chemotherapy. The current recommendation for pulmonary infection is to give isoniazid and rifampicin for 9 months or to give these drugs for 6 months adding pyrazinamide for the first 2 months. For miliary infection or meningitis three drugs should be used for the first 2 months and then continue with isoniazid and rifampicin for 12 or 18 months. Children found to have recently converted their Heaf test from negative to positive should also be treated, mainly to prevent blood stream spread. In this situation isoniazid alone is given for 6 months or isoniazid and rifampicin for 3 months. Older children with a strongly positive tuberculin test and a clear X-ray should be kept under regular supervision and only treated if there is evidence of progression.

Prevention. TB is a notifiable disease. It is essential to trace contacts of newly diagnosed patients and perform a Heaf test and chest X-ray. If the Heaf test is negative, it should be repeated after 6 weeks. If still negative BCG vaccination should be given. The aim of BCG vaccination is to produce a highly modified primary infection with attenuated organisms. It has been shown to give 80 per cent protection against TB and to protect completely against miliary spread.

In parts of the UK BCG immunisation is offered to 11–13 year old children who are Heaf negative; some areas have stopped doing this routinely because they consider that the risks of tuberculous do not justify it. Newborn infants from high risk families (certain ethnic groups and those with a recent history of TB in a close relative) are offered BCG at birth. In countries with a high incidence of TB routine neonatal immunisation is advisable. Initial Heaf testing in neonates is not necessary. Following BCG the Heaf test becomes positive, though not strongly so, and it may revert to negative after some years. Natural infection gives a strongly positive reaction.

BCG is an intradermal injection

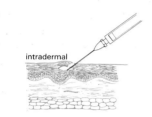

intradermal

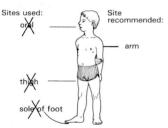

Sites used: oral, thigh, sole of foot

Site recommended: arm

MALARIA

Malaria is endemic in many parts of the world. As a consequence of increase in international travel more children suffering from malaria are seen in non-endemic countries. 'Where have you been?' is now an important question to ask of children presenting with an unexplained high fever.

Characteristically the fever is intermittent and the spleen enlarged, but these signs are not always present. There may be associated vomiting and rigors. The treatment is normally quinine or mefloquine if the species of organism is unknown since *Plasmodium falciparum* may be resistant to chloroquine.

Travellers to countries where malaria is endemic should take appropriate precautions such as physical protection against bites. Chemo-prophylaxis should also be taken starting a week before and continuing 4–6 weeks after return.

HUMAN IMMUNODEFICIENCY VIRUS

This virus has become widespread worldwide in the 1980s. The virus is normally transmitted by sexual contact or by injection of blood or blood products. The most common source of infection in children is by vertical transmission to the infant from its mother. Another significant group of children affected by the virus are those with haemophilia who received blood products before blood was routinely screened.

Children may remain asymptomatic for years, possibly forever. However many go on to develop autoimmune deficiency syndrome (AIDS). By early 1991, 67 cases of AIDS in children had been reported in the UK to the British Paediatric Surveillance Unit, with a further 144 who were HIV positive. About two thirds of these were children born to infected mothers, most of the others had haemophilia, with a few becoming infected via blood transfusions. This is likely to be an underestimate.

The children present with general ill health, failure to thrive and recurrent infection. Mortality is high. Management is of the immune deficiency state. Drugs are being developed which may delay the progress of the illness.

IMMUNISATION

Protection against some of the infectious diseases is available in the form of immunisation which is given at various stages during child-hood. Immunisations for different diseases are scheduled to balance the risks of disease with the child's ability to produce a good immunologi-cal response. Immunisation should not be given if the child is acutely unwell or if a severe reaction has occurred to a previous dose of that vaccine. Live attenuated vaccines (e.g. poliomyelitis, measles, mumps, rubella, BCG) should not be given to children with immune deficiency states, including those on cytotoxic drugs and high doses of corticosteroids, because of the risk of severe generalised infection. Three weeks should elapse between live vaccines to ensure adequate immune responses to the second one.

For the recommended immunisation programme for the UK 1992 see Appendix B.

A vaccine against *Haemophilus influenzae* was introduced in the UK in 1992 and is given in three doses at the same time as the primary course of DPT. Other vaccines are available and used in particular circumstances. Influenza A, hepatitis B, anthrax, rabies, are given to certain high risk groups. Typhoid, cholera, yellow fever, menigococcus C, Japanese B encephalitis and tick borne encephalitis are recommended for travellers to countries where these illnesses are endemic. Other vaccines are being developed and it is likely that more will come into routine use over the next decade.

IMMUNE DEFICIENCY

Contact with infecting organisms is one of the major challenges that face the newborn infant as he establishes an independent existence. Cellular immunity is present at birth, and although the neutrophil count is relatively low the infant is able to respond to bacterial infection with a leucocytosis. Humoral immunity is not well developed in infancy, but the infant is protected initially by maternal IgG antibodies which cross the placenta, and IgA which he receives in colostrum and breast milk. IgM does not cross the placenta, but the infant is capable of producing it in response to infection.

Maternally provided IgG globulins are progressively catabolised so that the infant's circulating immunoglobulins fall to a minimal level at 2 to 3 months. The subsequent rise parallels endogenous production as a result of exposure to environmental antigens. IgM concentrations reach normal adult levels earliest followed by IgG and then IgA.

Sometimes there is a delay in synthesis of immunoglobulins, especially in preterm babies. Low levels of IgA are particularly common and may persist for years. IgA is important in the protection of mucosal barriers and its absence predisposes to recurrent respiratory infection.

Most children with recurrent infections are normal, but immunological investigation should be undertaken when recurrent bacterial or fungal infections occur.

Examples of diseases due to defects in the body defences

Immune deficiency	Pathogens	Disease	Treatment
Humoral	Bacteria, pneumocystis	Agammaglobulinaemia	Gammaglobulin
Cellular	Viruses, tuberculosis, candida	DiGeorge syndrome (absent thymus)	Thymus graft
Stem cell	Bacteria, pneumocystis, viruses, tuberculosis, candida	Combined immune deficiency syndrome	Bone marrow graft
Complement deficiency	Bacteria		Antibiotics
Neutrophil disorders	Bacteria	Chronic granulomatous disease	Antibiotics

There are a number of rare inherited disorders of the immune mechanisms, the immune deficiency syndromes. However, immunological deficiencies may also occur in association with systemic illness, for example transient immunosuppression occurs during viral infections, especially measles, and the resulting susceptibility to infection contributes to malnutrition which in turn impairs defence mechanisms. Susceptibility to infection also occurs in relapsed nephrotic syndrome which limits the available immunoglobulins. Corticosteroid and toxic therapy also reduces immunological competence.

BIBLIOGRAPHY

American Academy of Pediatrics 1986 Report of the Committee on Infectious Diseases ('The Red Book'), 20th edn. American Academy of Pediatrics
Benenson A S 1985 Control of communicable diseases in man, 14th edn. American Public Health Association, Washington
British Paediatric Association 1988 Report of a working party on AIDS in infancy and childhood. British Paediatric Association, London
Christie A B 1987 Infectious diseases, 4th edn. Churchill Livingstone, Edinburgh
Department of Health 1990 Immunisation against infectious disease. HMSO, London
Emond R T D, Rowland H A K 1987 Colour atlas of infectious diseases, 2nd edn. Wolfe Medical, London
Farrar W E, Lambert H P 1984 Infectious diseases. Gower, London
Krugman S, Katz S L, Gershon A A, Wilfert CM 1985 Infectious diseases of children. CV Mosby, St. Louis
Morley D 1973 Paediatric priorities in the developing world. Butterworths, London
Rudd P, Nicoll A 1991 Manual on infections and immunizations in children. Oxford University Press, Oxford
Walker E, Williams G 1985 ABC of health travel, 2nd edn. British Medical Association, London

7 Hazards

Causes of death (1–14 years, 1988)

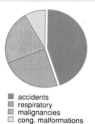

- accidents
- respiratory
- malignancies
- cong. malformations

Accidental deaths (0–14 years)

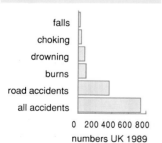

falls
choking
drowning
burns
road accidents
all accidents

0 200 400 600 800
numbers UK 1989

Accidents are by far the commonest cause of death in children over the age of a year. Recently in the UK the number of deaths due to accidents has declined but still approximately 700 children between the ages of 1 and 14 years die each year as a result of an accident. Road accidents are by far the commonest cause of childhood accidental fatalities, followed by choking, drowning and burns. For every child who is killed, many are seriously injured and many more receive minor injuries. Again in the UK about 150 000 children each year have to be admitted to hospital following an accident; this represents nearly a fifth of all paediatric admissions and one child in 80 of the whole child population. As many as one child in six attends a hospital casualty department each year with an injury and a similar number seek advice from their general practitioner. As well as killing and injuring children, accidents are also expensive.

How do accidents in childhood differ from those affecting adults? Three factors are important in any accident: the causative agent or situation, for example a car or a swimming pool; the circumstances in which it took place, for example the degree of parental supervision; and most important of all, the child himself. The type of accident is related to the age, sex, intelligence, social circumstances and personality of the child. Physical and mental development is particularly important. The toddler is fearless and inquisitive, but spends most of his time indoors, so that he is susceptible to falls, burns and self-poisoning. The child who has just started school is impulsive but inexperienced, and therefore likely to be knocked down by a car. The older school child is vigorous and adventurous, he is likely to fall and injure himself while climbing or to drown in a quarry or canal.

An understanding of the cause of accidents may lead to prevention. A young toddler cannot be reasoned with and therefore he must be protected by those around him and by those who design his house and its contents. The young school child can be actively taught about the dangers of traffic, but equally those who design schools, playgrounds and streets must take account of his inexperience. The older child can scarcely be prevented from taking risks and resents adult interference. He must learn to come to terms with himself and the amount of risk he can safely take. Most minor accidents are unavoidable and it is both unrealistic and possibly undesirable to seek ways of avoiding them altogether for they are all part of a child's experience and education. But it is surely the duty of planners and educators to try to reduce the number of serious accidents which cause death or severely damage children to an absolute minimum.

INJURIES

Road traffic accidents

Over half of all accidental deaths are a result of road accidents. As in most accidents, it is predominantly boys who are killed or injured. Most road accidents occur when the child is on foot and is hit by a moving vehicle. In a minority the child is either riding a bicycle or is a passenger in a car. The management consists of dealing with the multiple injuries in order of priority.

Road accident fatalities

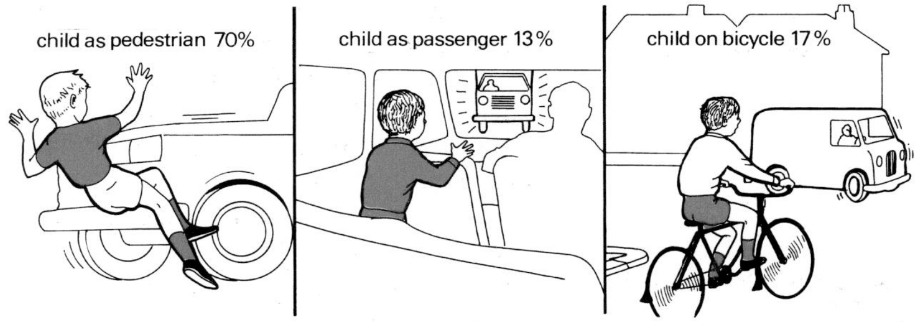

child as pedestrian 70%   child as passenger 13%   child on bicycle 17%

Falls

Children frequently suffer slight head injury as a result of falling out of beds, cots or windows, down stairs or from trees, climbing frames and so forth. While such injuries are not usually fatal, they are a common cause of hospital admission.

Head injury

Injury to the brain is a common cause of death in childhood accidents, and many of the survivors are left with permanent damage. However, of all the children admitted to hospital for observation after head injury, only 5 per cent will prove to have major brain trauma.

Management. Most head injuries are minor. Hospital admission is necessary if the injury was severe or associated with loss or alteration of consciousness. It is also necessary if there is blood or cerebrospinal fluid oozing from the nose or ears, if a scalp wound overlies a fracture, or if a fracture crosses the groove of the middle meningeal artery. A skull fracture is not itself an indication of the severity of injury – many serious brain injuries occur in the absence of a fracture. Pallor and vomiting are very common after minor head injury in young children and result from vagal stimulation. Many children can be allowed home if instructions regarding observations are given to the parents.

Complications. Cerebral oedema is the commonest serious complication of head injury in children, because the soft skull transmits the injury force to the brain rather than absorbing the impact as the harder adult skull does. Pallor, vomiting and impaired consciousness result and may last hours or days. Adequate ventilation is important since a high $PaCO_2$ increases intracranial pressure still further by increasing cerebral blood flow.

Intracranial bleeding is less common. It may be extradural, usually from the middle meningeal artery and therefore rapid in onset, or else subdural from cerebral veins and of slower onset. The head injury observations are intended to make early detection of intracranial bleeding or worsening cerebral oedema possible. Increasing intracranial pressure (ICP) is assessed by a falling level of consciousness as measured on the Glasgow Coma Scale, a falling pulse rate and rising blood pressure, and alteration in size and light reaction of the pupils.

Glasgow coma scale					
Best motor response		Verbal response		Eye opening	
Obeys	6	Orientated	5	Spontaneous	4
Localise	5	Confused conversation	4	To speech	3
Withdraws	4	Inappropriate words	3	To pain	2
Abnormal flexion	3	Incomprehensible	2	Nil	1
Extensor response	2	Nil	1		

A cranial CT scan will show whether the increase in ICP is due to oedema, contusion or haemorrhage (and will identify the origin of the latter). If there is localised bleeding surgery is necessary to decompress the brain, remove the clot and stop the bleeding source. Otherwise raised ICP is treated with cooling, hyperventilation and drugs such as mannitol to reduce brain swelling. Increasingly, ICP is being directly monitored.

Profile of head injuries

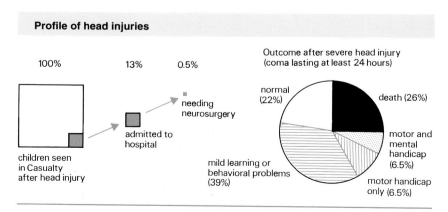

100%   13%   0.5%

Outcome after severe head injury (coma lasting at least 24 hours)

needing neurosurgery

normal (22%)

death (26%)

admitted to hospital

motor and mental handicap (6.5%)

children seen in Casualty after head injury

mild learning or behavioral problems (39%)

motor handicap only (6.5%)

BURNS AND SCALDS

Most accidents involving burns and scalds occur at home, particularly in poorer families. The inquisitive toddler is fascinated by matches and by flames. He knocks over paraffin heaters, goes too close to the open fire and sets light to his clothes, grasps a saucepan of boiling water by the handle and pulls it over himself or pulls a boiling electric kettle by the flex. Burns outside the home involving bonfires and fireworks tend to happen to older children.

The immediate treatment is to relieve the pain, ensure an adequate airway, and then assess the extent of the burns. If more than 10 per cent of the child's surface area is burned, intravenous fluids (plasma and saline) are necessary. If more than 50 per cent of the child's surface area is affected, the chances of survival are poor. Large quantities of fluid, blood and protein are lost from the burned areas and have to be replaced. A careful eye must be kept on the child's urine output and haematocrit. Tetanus toxoid and antibiotics are frequently used. Skin grafting may well be necessary at a later date. Children who have been burned are often also psychologically scarred too.

Supervision of toddlers in the home is the most important aspect of prevention of burns and scalds. The decreasing use of open fires and paraffin heaters, and the increased use of central heating has resulted in a decline in the incidence of burns in children in the last 20 years, but scalds remain common.

Causes of home accidents: fires, hot liquids and cleaning fluids

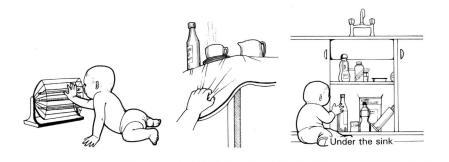

Under the sink

DROWNING

Most drowning accidents occur in inland waters, swimming pools and baths. About a quarter occur in the sea. Again, boys are more commonly involved than girls. Swimming and life saving lessons at school, wearing life-jackets on boats, and supervised pools and beaches are important preventive measures.

Children die during drowning either as a result of laryngeal spasm, when the cause of death is cerebral anoxia (dry drowning), or else water may enter the lungs, rapidly leading to respiratory failure with cardiac arrest (wet drowning). In either situation, the child may respond well to immediate cardiac massage and artificial ventilation once the airway has been cleared. Sometimes, if the water is muddy or polluted, the child may be revived only to die later with progressive pneumonia and pulmonary oedema (secondary drowning).

CHOKING

Over 50 children die each year by choking on foreign bodies or food. An affected child is distressed, making violent respiratory efforts and becoming progressively cyanosed, but making no noise as the obstruction lies at the level of the larynx, wedged between the vocal cords. Death results if the child is unable to remove the obstruction by his efforts. The traditional first aid measure of violent slaps on the back is often unsuccessful, but abdominal compression (the Heimlich manoeuvre) can be life-saving. The rescuer stands behind the child with his clenched hands in the epigastrium – a short sharp squeeze directed inwards and upwards compresses the residual air in the lungs and may dislodge the obstruction.

POISONING

Few children die as a result of poisoning, but many thousands attend hospital each year for treatment. Occasionally a child may intentionally ingest a poison, but in most cases the self-poisoning is accidental. Children may also be poisoned deliberately by their parents or inadvertently by their doctors. Most children who ingest a poison are fearless, inquisitive toddlers attracted by the appearance of tablets, medicines,

Some poisonous berries

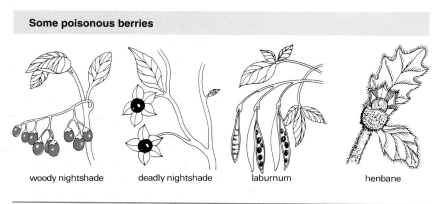

woody nightshade   deadly nightshade   laburnum   henbane

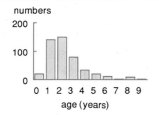

Age of children admitted with poisoning

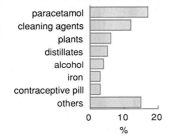

Common 'accidental' poisons (Nottingham admissions 1991)

household and garden substances, berries, seeds or fungi. They will eat almost anything, regardless of taste. It has been shown that a child is particularly likely to ingest a poison when the family is under some sort of stress, presumably because of decreased supervision.

The management of a poisoned child consists of removal of the poison, followed by observation for the expected symptoms and signs. Treatment is generally symptomatic and nonspecific. Vomiting is induced to remove the poison from the stomach by giving syrup of ipecacuanha. Gastric lavage is rarely necessary, but emetic administration is obviously inappropriate for the unconscious child and in such cases the stomach should be emptied by lavage, but only after intubation with a cuffed endotracheal tube. Induced vomiting serves little purpose if more than 4 hours have passed since the ingestion, although there are exceptions, for example in cases of ingested aspirin and atropine, which delay gastric emptying. Vomiting is also to be avoided after ingestion of corrosive substances, or volatile agents such as paraffin or turpentine which are likely to be inhaled and may cause lung damage.

If the side effects of a poison are not known, information can be obtained at any time of day or night from one of the regional poison centres. Children likely to have ingested a toxic agent are admitted to hospital for observation. If respiratory failure develops, mechanical ventilation is necessary. If cardiovascular shock occurs, intravenous plasma or saline should be given.

Aspirin

Aspirin is a respiratory stimulant and a cell poison. When taken in large quantities it produces nausea, vomiting, tinnitus and dehydration. Hyperventilation with deep sighing respirations is a consequence of both metabolic acidosis and respiratory stimulation. Hypoglycaemia, hyperglycaemia and an increased prothrombin time may occur in cases of severe poisoning. Fortunately children do not usually ingest sufficient amounts of aspirin to develop symptoms. If they do, then active steps should be taken to hasten the excretion of aspirin. When blood levels of salicylate are high, excretion should be enhanced by inducing a diuresis and reducing tubular reabsorption of the drug by making the urine alkaline. As with most poisons, there is no specific antidote.

Iron tablets

Iron tablets are frequently swallowed by toddlers because they are likely to be available (for example, iron tablets may be prescribed during pregnancy) and because they look like sweets. A small child can be fatally poisoned by as little as 2 grams of iron. The progress of a poisoned child can be divided into four phases. Firstly, within an hour of the ingestion the child develops severe gastrointestinal symptoms, diarrhoea, vomiting, haematemesis and melaena. These symptoms may gradually subside so that the child seems well. However, some hours later, the serious third phase may develop with iron encephalopathy manifested by coma and fits, liver damage and circulatory collapse. Finally, a child who survives this may develop scarring of the stomach and pylorus as a consequence of local irritation. Iron ingestion is an indication for gastric lavage. The iron chelating agent desferrioxamine is useful. It can be left in the stomach to prevent further absorption of iron and it can be administered parenterally to enhance iron excretion and lessen the severity of the poisoning.

Tricyclic agents

Tricyclic agents such as amitriptyline and imipramine are among the most dangerous drugs consumed by young children. They may be available because one of the parents is taking them for depression or because a child in the family is being treated for bed-wetting. The effects of poisoning include respiratory and cardiovascular depression, as well as cerebral stimulation leading to irritability, excitation, hallucinations and fits, with exaggerated tendon reflexes. They have a marked atropine-like action, with fixed dilated pupils, a dry red skin, sinus tachycardia, urinary retention and paralytic ileus. Finally, their most serious effect is on heart rhythm, resulting in atrial and ventricular tachycardias, fibrillation or heart block. There is no specific antidote, only symptomatic treatment. Diazepam is used for sedation, and antiarrhythmic drugs are occasionally necessary.

Alcohol

Alcohol is a dangerous acute poison in young children who drink it accidentally or older school children who drink it experimentally. The acute encephalopathy is often enhanced by severe hypoglycaemia which is particularly common in children and occasionally causes death. Blood glucose must be carefully monitored at the bedside and IV glucose given if it falls to low levels.

Prevention. Important recent developments have led to a decrease in the incidence of severe accidental poisoning in children. Child-resistant containers have been developed which can only be opened by lining up an arrow on the lid with an arrow on the bottle or by pushing the lid down and twisting it open at the same time. In the UK it is compulsory for all aspirin and paracetamol tablets to be prescribed in this way, and pharmacists are encouraged to dispense other dangerous tablets in this form too. 'Blister packs' are also helpful. It takes the child a long time to eat sufficient tablets to cause symptoms, and he frequently loses interest or is discovered in the act.

Child resistant containers

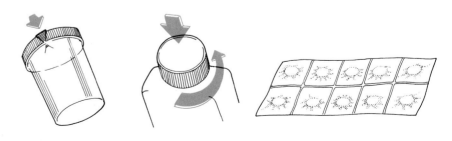

OTHER HAZARDS

The risk of a noxious agent producing permanent damage is highest in the earliest phase of development, embryogenesis. A number of such agents have been identified as being associated with a high incidence of congenital abnormalities. Harmful environmental factors after birth are less easy to identify because so many children are exposed to potential hazards, and the ill effects may be quite subtle, making an association difficult to prove. Two hazards will be considered here, one physical, the other chemical.

Smoking

The harmful effects of smoking on those who actually smoke are well known. Chronic bronchitis, lung cancer and coronary heart disease are three common conditions whose incidence is greatly increased in smokers. Many school children now smoke regularly and are therefore at risk. It is obviously important to try to dissuade children from taking up smoking by appropriate health education in schools. It is also known that the children of smoking parents have a higher incidence of bronchitis and pneumonia; this applies particularly to babies and young children. Presumably the passive inhalation of tobacco smoke by the children at home is the important factor.

Lead

Lead is an environmental element which is undoubtedly harmful. If it is ingested or inhaled in large quantities it can produce a serious illness which may be lethal or result in brain damage. It is probable too, that chronic exposure to environmental lead has a harmful effect on mental development. There are several sources of lead. It used to be present in paint, so that children who chewed painted surfaces were liable to be poisoned. Water in lead pipes may contain sufficient lead to cause poisoning. Lead fumes produced by burning car batteries may produce toxic symptoms. Asian families use lead salts ('surma') in cosmetics applied regularly to the conjunctivae of the child and this may cause poisoning. More recently, there has been concern about atmospheric lead. Lead is present in exhaust fumes from vehicles and blood lead levels are higher in urban children and in those living close to major motorways. It has been suggested that this chronic exposure to moderate amounts of atmospheric lead may produce permanent intellectual impairment.

A child who has ingested lead may show symptoms of encephalopathy, with irritability, drowsiness, convulsions and eventually coma. Papilloedema may be present. Colicky abdominal pain is common and an abdominal X-ray may actually show radio-opaque lead fragments in the gastrointestinal tract. The diagnosis is made on the clinical picture, a history of exposure to a source of lead and investigations. Blood lead levels can be measured and are a guide to severity of poisoning. Lead affects many enzyme systems, but particularly those involved in haem synthesis. Measurement of blood levels of haem precursors forms the basis of a screening test for early lead poisoning which can be carried out in children who are at risk. In chronic poisoning, lead interferes with the growing ends of bones producing the X-ray sign 'lead lines'.

The treatment of a poisoned child is directed at removing lead from the body. This is achieved by using lead-chelating agents which increase lead excretion. In severe cases with encephalopathy, calcium edetate (EDTA) and dimercaprol (British Anti-Lewisite, BAL) are given parenterally. In less severe cases oral D-penicillamine is used. If there are signs of raised intracranial pressure, cerebral oedema can be lessened by intravenous mannitol or dexamethasone. The source of the lead must obviously be identified and removed. Severe lead poisoning carries a high mortality and survivors are often neurologically handicapped.

BIBLIOGRAPHY

Blumer J L, Reed M D 1986 Pediatric toxicology. Pediatric Clinics of North America, vol 33, no. 2. W B Saunders, Philadelphia (Chapters on gastric lavage and all the common poisons)
Dreisbach R H 1983 Handbook of poisoning, 11th edn. Lange, California
Ellenhorn M D, Barceloux D G 1988 Medical toxicology – diagnosis and treatment of human poisoning. Elsevier, New York (A large reference work)
Haddal L M, Winchester J F 1983 Clinical management of poisoning and drug overdosage. WB Saunders, Philadelphia (A large reference work)
Meadow R 1989 ABC of child abuse: poisoning. British Medical Journal 298: 1445–1446
Piomelli S, Rosen J F, Chisholm J J 1984 Management of childhood lead poisoning. Journal of Pediatrics 105: 523–532
Proudfoot A T 1982 Diagnosis and management of acute poisoning. Blackwell Scientific Publications, Oxford
Sharples P M et al 1990 Causes of fatal childhood accidents involving head injury in Northern region, 1979–86. British Medical Journal 301: 1193–7.
Sharples P M et al 1990 Avoidable factors contributing to death of children with head injury. British Medical Journal 300: 87–91.
Vale J A, Meredith T J 1981 Poisoning – diagnosis and treatment. Update Books, London

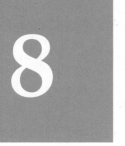

Airways and Lungs

8

Acute respiratory infections and attacks of asthma account for a large number of family practitioner consultations and hospital admissions, especially in pre-school children. Most are viral infections of the upper respiratory tract; respiratory syncytial, rhinovirus influenza, para-influenza and adenoviruses, which on average occur 6–8 times a year in this age group. Children with older siblings who are in day nurseries, or whose parents smoke are at greater risk. Serious lower respiratory tract infections occur mainly in infants. Pneumonia is still an important cause of death in the first year of life.

Respiratory infection may play a part in the sudden infant death syndrome which is also common in the winter months. The symptoms and signs of the precipitating illness are often trivial.

Apart from asthma, chronic lung disease is uncommon in children. Most infections resolve without sequelae, but recurrent respiratory infections in early childhood may be associated with chronic obstructive lung disease in adult life. Some of the survivors of neonatal intensive care have severely damaged lungs which can improve with growth but do predispose them to further problems.

Normal respiratory rates (breaths/min)

newborn	30–60
6 mths	30–45
1–2 yrs	25–35
3–6 yrs	20–30
7 yrs+	20–25

UPPER RESPIRATORY TRACT INFECTIONS

Coryza (common cold)

Nasal discharge and obstruction due to rhinovirus infections is common, and can lead to feeding difficulty in infants. Nasal aspiration or the use of decongestant nose drops for a few days is helpful.

Pharyngitis and tonsillitis

In pharyngitis, nasal symptoms are associated with a sore throat and generalised redness of the pharynx. Again most are due to viruses. Streptococcal tonsillitis is less common and usually presents with fever. A tonsillar exudate and cervical lymphadenopathy are found on examination. It may be complicated by scarlet fever, acute glomerulonephritis and, rarely in the UK, rheumatic fever. Treatment is with penicillin for 10 days. A tonsillar exudate may also be found in glandular fever, sometimes with palatal haemorrhages.

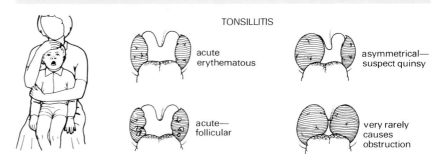

Examination of the throat

TONSILLITIS

acute
erythematous

asymmetrical—
suspect quinsy

acute—
follicular

very rarely
causes
obstruction

Tonsillectomy may be considered for children who have very frequent episodes of tonsillitis, or who have had a peritonsillar abscess (quinsy). Very large tonsils and adenoids may cause airway obstruction with sleep apnoea and, rarely, pulmonary hypertension.

Otitis media

Acute infection of the middle ear causes fever, pain and sometimes discharge. Infants present with irritability, crying and vomiting and are unable to localise their discomfort. The ears should always be examined carefully, and the diagnostic red bulging tympanic membrane sought. Otitis media may be viral or bacterial, and antibiotic therapy should be given unless the signs are minor. Paracetamol, to relieve pain and fever, and nasal decongestants help. Acute mastoiditis is now uncommon but should be suspected if there is pain, swelling and redness behind the ear.

Recurrent otitis media may be associated with blockage of the Eustachian tube due to enlarged adenoids, and adenoidectomy may resolve the problem.

Chronic exudative otitis media ('glue ear') is common. Fluid in the middle ear causes a variable hearing loss which may be unsuspected for prolonged periods and lead to problems at school. Drainage and the insertion of grommets may be required.

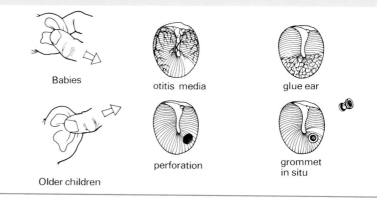

Pulling the ear to straighten the auditory canal and four possible findings

Babies

otitis media

glue ear

perforation

grommet
in situ

Older children

Sinusitis

Maxillary sinusitis can complicate upper respiratory infection, but the frontal sinuses are not developed in young children. Sinusitis causes fever, pain and local tenderness. Recurrent or persistent infection sometimes leads to a postnasal drip and cough.

UPPER AIRWAY OBSTRUCTION

Acute upper airway obstruction is usually due to laryngotracheo-bronchitis (croup). An inhaled foreign body and epiglottitis are less common and other causes are rare.

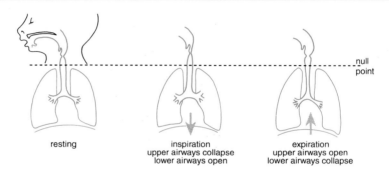

Airways collapse

resting

inspiration
upper airways collapse
lower airways open

expiration
upper airways open
lower airways collapse

null point

Laryngotracheobronchitis (croup)

Croup tends to occur most often in autumn, and it is usually due to respiratory viral infection, especially para-influenza. A cold is followed by the sudden onset of difficult breathing with stridor. Airway obstruction is often more severe in infants, in whom the natural tendency for the airway to collapse in inspiration adds to the stridor and degree of obstruction. Anxiety makes matters worse. Intercostal and subcostal recession indicate the increased work of breathing, and the child should be watched carefully for evidence of hypoxia (rising heart and respiratory rates, restlessness, cyanosis). Intubation or tracheostomy is occasionally needed, but most cases settle in a warm relaxed atmosphere.

In older children airway obstruction is less likely to occur but there will be a sore throat, barking cough and loss of voice. The infection tends to spread down the respiratory tract leading to cough and wheeze.

Epiglottitis

In this condition, severe airway obstruction may develop very rapidly due to oedema and inflammation of the epiglottis and surrounding structures. It is due to infection with *Haemophilus influenzae* type B and is associated with septicaemia. The child will be very unwell, febrile and drooling saliva, with marked difficulty in breathing and a variable degree of stridor. The neck is often held extended and the child is most comfortable sitting up. This position should not be altered and the throat

Clinical features of epiglottitis

- flushed
- unable to talk
- unable to swallow
- drooling
- inspiratory stridor

should not be examined, as efforts to do so may lead to complete obstruction and cardiorespiratory arrest. Wait until an anaesthetist is present to intubate the child. Almost all children with epiglottitis require intubation for 1–3 days. The typical 'cherry red' epiglottis can be observed at the time of intubation. If a skilled anaesthetist is not available, tracheostomy may be a safer option. Antibiotic therapy (ampicillin, chloramphenicol or a cephalosporin) is given and the child should then make a quick recovery.

Persistent stridor

Stridor at birth results from congenital abnormalities of the airway or structures surrounding it. The commonest problem is laryngomalacia ('floppy epiglottis') which improves steadily through the first year though the stridor will become worse with colds and excitement. Persistent stridor with evidence of airway obstruction requires further investigation including laryngoscopy. Pressure on the trachea from a vascular ring or mediastinal tumour is demonstrated by X-ray screening and barium swallow. Recurrent bouts of croup should raise the suspicion of asthma.

Findings at laryngoscopy

     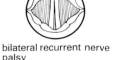

| laryngomalacia | subglottis stenosis | congenital web | juvenile papillomatosis | rt. recurrent nerve palsy | bilateral recurrent nerve palsy |

LOWER RESPIRATORY TRACT INFECTIONS

Acute bronchitis

Upper respiratory tract infections can spread down the airway to involve the bronchial mucosa. The child develops a troublesome cough, sometimes with sputum production. Most children are not severely ill and the condition is self limiting. It is usually due to a viral infection. There may be associated wheezing which responds to bronchodilator therapy, but otherwise a simple cough linctus suffices for treatment. If the cough is spasmodic, with or without vomiting or whooping, and persists for weeks, pertussis is the likely diagnosis.

Acute bronchiolitis

This can be a severe illness, it occurs every winter and results in many infants being admitted to hospital. Ninety per cent are due to respiratory syncytial virus and the remainder to other respiratory viruses. The infection spreads rapidly to the bronchioles, causing mucosal damage and airway obstruction. The infant, usually 2–10 months old, develops a cough and rapid breathing often with audible wheeze. Difficulty in feeding often leads to hospital admission. The infant is usually afebrile

Chest X-ray findings in bronchiolitis: depressed diaphragm, horizontal ribs and streaky hilar shadows

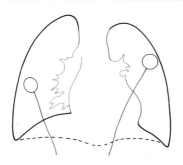
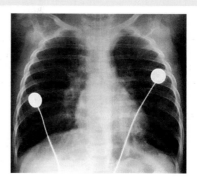

but has a high respiratory rate with intercostal and subcostal recession. The chest appears over-inflated, and the liver is pushed down.

On auscultation, there is generalised wheeze and extensive crepitations. The chest X-ray confirms over-inflation of the lungs and there are often patchy areas of collapse. Respiratory syncytial virus infection is confirmed by immunofluorescence of nasopharyngeal secretions.

The infants require good nursing care with minimal handling and frequent observation because episodes of apnoea or bradycardia may occur. Oxygen saturation should be measured regularly using a cutaneous probe, and oxygen given by head box or nasal cannula to maintain a satisfactory level. Tube feeding is often required, and rarely artificial ventilation is necessary. Antibiotic treatment is not indicated unless there is evidence of secondary bacterial infection, which is rare. Steroids and bronchodilators are ineffective. Ribavirin may be given by inhalation using a small particle aerosol generator and has some beneficial effect, but in view of the good outcome for most infants with bronchiolitis and the expense and difficulty of this treatment, its use currently is restricted to infants with serious underlying problems, such as bronchopulmonary dysplasia or congenital heart disease, in whom the mortality rate is much higher. In normal infants the mortality is 1–2 per cent and the illness lasts about 10 days. A high proportion will go on to have recurrent episodes of wheeze with colds over the next few years.

Derbyshire chair

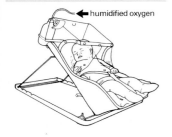

humidified oxygen

Pneumonia

Consolidation of the lung parenchyma may be due to viral or bacterial infection, or both. Bacterial infection is more common in developing countries, where pneumonia is an important cause of infant deaths. The child presents with fever and upper respiratory symptoms progressing to rapid breathing and cough, with a variable degree of systemic upset. Signs of consolidation, apart from a raised respiratory rate, are difficult to detect in infants though localised crackles are heard as the disease progresses.

A chest X-ray will show the extent of the consolidation. Identification of the causative organism is often difficult, but culture of sputum or

Surface markings of the lobes of the lung; a reminder

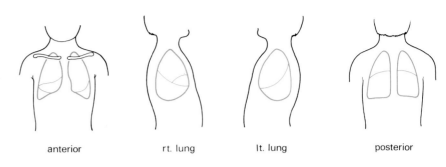

anterior   rt. lung   lt. lung   posterior

Causes of pneumonia

Viral
RSV – Main cause in infants
Influenza A, B – Common
Para influenza 1, 3 – Common
Adenovirus – Uncommon

Bacterial
Strep. pneumoniae – Common,
all ages
Mycoplasma pneumoniae
Common, especially 5–14 yrs
Staph. aureus – Uncommon
Haemophilus influenzae –
Uncommon in UK
Group B streptococcus –
Newborn
Gram negative organisms –
Uncommon, secondary
invaders

nasopharyngeal aspirate and blood culture should be undertaken, as well as immunofluorescence for respiratory syncytial virus. Antibiotic treatment is based on the likely pathogens and the age of the child.

Viral pneumonia. Primary viral infections can spread down the respiratory tract into the lungs and should be expected in any child, particularly in the first year of life, in whom a respiratory illness has resulted in marked constitutional effects and/or circulatory failure. Influenza, para-influenza, adenoviruses and RSV are among those most commonly implicated. Clinical examination gives little clue to the patchy shadowing that may be seen on a chest X-ray. Although the infection may be thought to be due to a virus, broad spectrum antibiotics are given.

Streptococcal pneumonia. This is the commonest cause of bacterial pneumonia, especially in younger children. It produces an acute illness with fever, chest pain and rapid respiration often with grunting. The child may complain of pain in the abdomen or shoulder, depending on the site of infection. Lobar or segmental consolidation is apparent on examination and confirmed by X-ray. A pleural effusion may be present. Treatment with penicillin leads to rapid improvement and there is complete clearing of the radiological changes in 3–4 weeks.

Haemophilus influenza type B pneumonia. In the world this is reported to be the second most common cause of bacterial pneumonia. The chest X-ray usually shows the scattered pattern of bronchopneumonia rather than a lobar shadow. Most respond to oral amoxicillin.

Mycoplasma. This infection tends to have a rather insidious onset and subacute course. Wheezing is common, and the X-ray changes are often more extensive than would be expected from the clinical findings. The diagnosis is confirmed by demonstrating a specific antibody response. The illness lasts some weeks, and antibiotic treatment probably makes little difference though erythromycin may be of some benefit.

Staphylococcal pneumonia. This form of pneumonia has become uncommon but should be considered in young children who are severely ill. There is usually a high fever and septicaemia, with segmental or lobar consolidation which may be complicated by empyema or pneumothorax requiring drainage. Appropriate antibiotic therapy and supportive management is required. As the consolidation resolves, pneumatocoeles become apparent radiologically and resolve slowly over some months.

Features seen on chest X-ray with lung infection

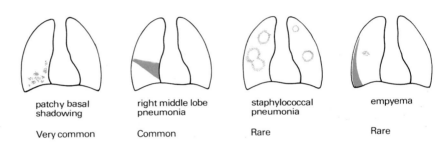

patchy basal shadowing	right middle lobe pneumonia	staphylococcal pneumonia	empyema
Very common	Common	Rare	Rare

If pneumonia is atypical or slow to clear, other pathogens, especially TB, and the possibility of an underlying abnormality should be considered.

Recurrent or persistent lower respiratory infection is a common problem in the winter months. Cough is often due to associated asthma, or to retained secretions sometimes with segmental collapse. An inhaled foreign body, aspiration of gastric contents or underlying disease such as cystic fibrosis should be considered. Congenital abnormalities of the airway or lungs are rare.

Bronchiectasis

Persistent infection leads to damage and dilatation of the bronchi, with chronic cough and sputum. This may occur as a consequence of pneumonia, pertussis or measles especially in malnourished children, but has become very uncommon in the UK. Most cases of bronchiectasis in childhood are now due to cystic fibrosis, and a small number are secondary to ciliary dyskinesia or immune deficiency states.

CYSTIC FIBROSIS

Cystic fibrosis (CF) is the commonest cause of chronic suppurative lung disease in children in the UK, and also the commonest cause of pancreatic insufficiency. It occurs in about 1 in 2500 births and is inherited as an autosomal recessive condition, 1 in 25 of the population being carriers. The gene has been identified on chromosome 7. Seventy per cent of north European patients have the ΔF508 mutation and are either homozygous or heterozygous with one of the many other mutations which have been identified. Apart from the small group of patients who have no clinical pancreatic insufficiency and who do not carry ΔF508, there is poor correlation between genetic and clinical state. The gene has been shown to code for a large protein which is situated in the apical membrane of secretory epithelial cells and controls the transport of sodium and chloride, and hence water, across the cell. This leads to the typical high salt content of the sweat, which is due to failure of reabsorption of sodium and chloride, and to the thick secretions produced by the epithelial cells in some organs. This causes pancreatic duct obstruction with gradual pancreatic fibrosis and biliary cirrhosis and obstruction of the vas deferens. In the lungs, thick mucus obstructs the small airways and predisposes to infection.

Presentation

Presenting symptoms in 100 Nottingham patients		
	<1 yr	> 1 yr
Meconium ileus	23	–
Sibling affected	7	6
Diarrhoea and FTT	10	0
Respiratory	0	14
Respiratory and GI	17	14
Total	**60**	**40**

The majority of patients present in infancy with diarrhoea and failure to thrive, often with recurrent or persistent respiratory problems in addition, but the severity of the initial symptoms is variable. About 20 per cent present with meconium ileus, a form of neonatal bowel obstruction due to thick meconium. Some heath services are now screening newborn infants for CF using the immunoreactive trypsin test on the blood spot taken for screening for PKU and hypothyroidism. If the level is raised it is repeated at 4 weeks, and if still high then the infant is referred for further investigation. The blood spot can also be used for genetic studies which may lead to rapid confirmation of the diagnosis (see Chapter 2).

Diagnosis

The diagnosis of cystic fibrosis is confirmed by the demonstration of raised levels (>60 mmol) of sodium and chloride in the sweat. Over 100 mg sweat must be obtained and the test must be positive on at least two occasions. In addition, supporting evidence for the diagnosis is sought. Pancreatic insufficiency is associated with fat globules in the stool on microscopy and very low or absent levels of stool chymotrypsin. There are no specific respiratory symptoms or signs.

Management

Lungs. The lungs are normal at birth, but the child later develops a tendency to frequent and prolonged infections with a cough which is often accompanied by a wheeze. As the disease progresses, sputum is produced and the cough becomes chronic. Clubbing develops early and in severe cases there may be chest deformity and growth retardation. The rate of progression of lung disease is very variable. Chest X-rays are usually normal in small children, but they may show evidence of air trapping and some increase in line shadows. Later generalised bronchial wall thickening and dilatation occurs with mottled shadows due to infection or sputum retention.

The sputum typically cultures Haemophilus species, *Staphylococcus aureus* and/or *Pseudomonas aeruginosa*. Pulmonary function tests confirm airflow obstruction and increased lung volumes with an eventual fall in vital capacity and oxygen saturation as respiratory failure

Chest X-ray in advanced cystic fibrosis showing patchy collapse and consolidation, cystic shadows, linear shadows and overinflation

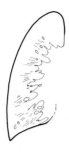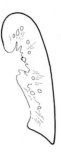

Bilateral:
patchy collapse consolidation
cystic shadows
linear shadows
overinflation

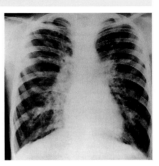

develops. Many patients have abnormal liver function tests, and a few develop portal hypertension which may lead to haematemesis. Abdominal pain associated with a right iliac fossa mass ('meconium ileus equivalent' or distal intestinal obstruction syndrome) may occur in older patients.

The aim is to drain secretions, prevent infection where possible and treat it promptly and effectively. Parents are taught how to perform postural drainage regularly and older children learn self-physiotherapy techniques. Exercise should be encouraged. Antibiotic therapy should be based on the results of regular sputum or cough swab cultures and given in high dosage for prolonged periods when infection occurs. Once *Pseudomonas aeruginosa* is well established it cannot be eradicated, and as IV antibiotic therapy is usually required it is only practical to treat intermittently though nebulised antibiotics may be used long term with some benefit. Bronchodilators and mucolytics are useful for some patients. Immunisation against measles and influenza is recommended, as viral infections are also very important.

Cystic fibrosis: complications

Respiratory	Other
Bronchiectasis	Abdominal pain (DIOS)
Wheezing	Biliary cirrhosis
Haemoptysis	Portal hypertension
Pneumothorax	Gall stones
Nasal polyps	Diabetes mellitus
Sinusitis	Growth failure
Allergic aspergillosis	Delayed puberty
Lobar collapse	Male infertility
Cor pulmonale	Rectal prolapse

Malabsorption. Pancreatic enzyme supplements have to be taken with all meals and snacks but may not control the malabsorption completely. The children should have a high energy, high protein diet and do not need to restrict fat. Dietary supplements may be required at times of illness and for older children with anorexia. All patients should have supplements of vitamins A, D and E. Extra salt is needed in hot weather or if the child is febrile. A few older patients develop diabetes and require insulin.

General care

With regular treatment, growth should be normal at least until 9 or 10 years. Puberty may be delayed and growth poor in older patients with severe lung disease. The outlook for cystic fibrosis has improved greatly, and many children have years of virtually normal life attending normal schools and taking part in activities. The need for regular treatment and constant anxiety causes a great deal of family stress, and many teenage patients have difficulty accepting the situation and complying with treatment. Current median life expectancy is about 25 years, but for infants born in the 1990s it is estimated to be around 40 years, irrespective of any advances in treatment which may become available. Heart/lung transplantation has greatly improved the quality of life and survival of some patients but is limited by the shortage of donors.

ASTHMA

Asthma is characterised by an episodic cough and wheeze associated with a variable air flow obstruction which responds to bronchodilator therapy. The incidence of asthma is at least 10 per cent in primary school children and much higher in the pre-school age group in whom diagnosis can be difficult. Asthma appears to be becoming more frequent and probably also more severe. It is a very common cause of hospital admission and missed school and causes much distress to parents and children.

Asthma triggers

Viral respiratory infections
Allergens:
- house dust mite
- grass pollens
- pets

Exercise
Excitement and upset
Nonspecific irritants:
- cigarette smoke
- pollution
- sprays

The atopic tendency is inherited in a dominant manner, but different members of the family may have asthma, eczema, hayfever and other allergic problems in varying combinations and degrees of severity. Inhalation of an allergen leads to a type 1 allergic response and the release of histamine and other mediators resulting in muscle spasm, mucosal oedema and mucus production, and all contribute to airways obstruction. Asthmatics have a variable degree of bronchial hyper-reactivity, and develop airway obstruction with exercise, cold air and nonspecific irritants such as fog and cigarette smoke. Viral respiratory tract infections are the major trigger of attacks in younger children. Acute attacks are characterised by shortness of breath, wheezing and intercostal recession and limitation of activity.

Diagnosis

In older children, evidence of airflow obstruction can be obtained by measuring peak expiratory flow rate or FEV, during an attack or by exercise, and demonstrating an improvement after an inhaled bronchodilator is given.

Peak expiratory flow rates measured by a Wright's Peak Flow Meter

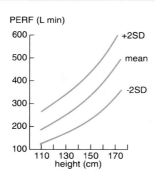

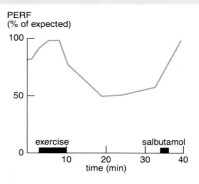

Normal values are related to height rather than age. The serial measurements are those of a child with exercise-induced bronchospasm who responded to salbutamol

In younger children, diagnosis rests on persistent or recurrent cough and/or wheeze and the clinical response to treatment. Between attacks most children are well, there are no signs to be found on examination and lung function is normal. Skin tests for common allergens confirm that the child is atopic and may help to identify important allergens for the individual, such as animals.

Allergens

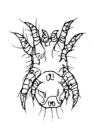

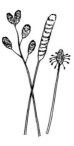

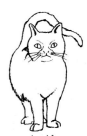

D. pteronyssimus   pollens   animal fur

Management

Asthma is a very variable condition and the pattern often changes as children grow older, so treatment needs to be reviewed regularly and adjusted as necessary. The aim is to control the symptoms so that the child can live a normal active life, using a minimum of drug therapy. Parents and children need to learn a good deal about asthma and its treatment, and to have an appropriate plan of action for dealing with acute attacks as it is these that create most anxiety.

Allergen avoidance is advised, though efforts to eliminate the house dust mite from bedrooms have been disappointing so far. Young children with troublesome asthma should not have pets, especially cats, in the house and parents are advised not to smoke.

The main drugs used in asthma

Bronchodilators 'Relievers'
e.g.   Salbutamol
        Terbutaline

Prophylactic 'Preventers'
e.g.   Sodium cromoglycate
        Beclomethasone
        Budesonide

Drug therapy. All patients are treated by inhalation if it is at all possible, by a method appropriate for their age. Most children will manage a dry powder inhaler or a metered dose inhaler with a spacer device from about 3 years of age with appropriate tuition. Very few can use a metered dose inhaler properly alone under the age of 10. Children under 3 may cooperate with a spacer and facemask or require a nebuliser. Delayed release oral preparations are useful for nocturnal symptoms.

All patients should have a bronchodilator available at all times to use for episodes of cough and wheeze and before exercise. This may be all the treatment required by children with mild episodic asthma. If symptoms are frequent and persistent, regular preventative treatment is recommended though there are often major problems with compliance. Sodium cromoglycate is very effective and entirely safe and should be tried first. If, after 4–6 weeks of regular treatment, the child has not improved or if initial good control is not maintained, treatment is changed to an inhaled steroid, budesonide or beclomethasone. The dose is then adjusted as necessary to maintain control of symptoms at the lowest possible dose. Oral steroids should be avoided for long term treatment in view of their side effects, especially growth retardation, but are entirely safe in occasional short courses.

Asthma

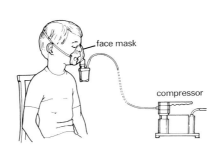

face mask

compressor

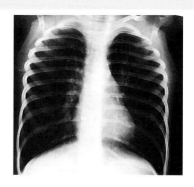

Acute attacks

The introduction some years ago of nebulised bronchodilator therapy has revolutionlised the management of acute attacks of asthma, and many families now have nebulisers at home. In the absence of a nebuliser, the child should be given 5–10 puffs of salbutamol or terbutaline from a metered dose inhaler using a spacer or a paper cup as a face mask.

High dose bronchodilator therapy may resolve the attack, but if the child does not respond, or the improvement is not maintained, oral prednisolone should be given without delay. A single high dose may be adequate if given early but a more severe and prolonged attack needs further treatment. The progress of an attack should be carefully observed and peak expiratory flow rate measured regularly if possible, as clinical assessment can be unreliable. If improvement is not rapid, hospital admission should be considered.

Death in asthma is due to hypoxia causing an acute cardiorespiratory arrest. Respiratory failure due to exhaustion occurs rarely. All children with severe attacks should be given oxygen and monitored closely. IV fluids, aminophylline and hydrocortisone may be required but artificial ventilation is rarely necessary.

Prognosis

Most children with asthma improve as they grow older. Pre-school children who wheeze only with colds are likely to lose their symptoms by 5–8 years. In general the more severe the asthma, the older the age at which it is likely to improve. Asthma may recur in adult life, and teenagers should be advised to avoid smoking and potential allergens at work.

REFERENCES

Chernick V (ed) 1990 Kendig's disorders of the respiratory tract in children, 5th edn. W B Saunders, Philadelphia

Goodchild M, Dodge J 1985 Cystic fibrosis — Manual of diagnosis and management, 2nd edn. Bailliere Tindall, London

Phelan P D, Landan L I, Olinsky A (eds) 1990 Respiratory illness in children, 3rd edn. Blackwell Scientific Publications, Oxford

Warner J O et al 1989 Management of asthma — a consensus statement. Archives of Diseases in Childhood 64: 1065–79

Warner J O et at 1992 Asthma: a follow up statement from an international paediatric asthma consensus group. Archives of Diseases in Childhood 67: 240–248

Heart

Now that rheumatic fever is rare, congenital abnormalities have become the main cause of heart disease in children. Acquired heart disease still occurs but it is not common; congenital heart defects, however, occur in approximately seven to eight infants per thousand live births and heart disease thus forms the commonest single group of serious congenital abnormalities. Less than a quarter of affected children will die in the first year of life, the majority within the first month. These children have severe cardiac abnormalities which, in many cases, are complex and inoperable. However, the number of children with severe lesions who are now surviving beyond the first year is increasing, a tribute to the skill and ingenuity of cardiac surgeons. Ten to 15 per cent of children with congenital heart disease have more than one cardiac abnormality. Ten to 15 per cent have an associated non-cardiac abnormality; the skeletal, gastrointestinal and genito-urinary systems are the most commonly involved. There are nine common congenital heart lesions which together make up 90 per cent of all cases. The remaining 10 per cent consist of numerous rarer, more complex anomalies.

Aetiology

As with most congenital defects, the precise aetiology is unknown but both genetic and environmental factors have been identified. Family studies suggest that the mode of inheritance is polygenic, although occasionally single gene mutations occur. If a mother has a child with a congenital heart defect, the chances of a second child being affected are about three times higher than if her child had no heart defect. Children with chromosomal abnormalities have a greatly increased incidence of congenital heart disease; nearly half of all children with Down syndrome have a cardiac lesion. Maternal rubella in the first trimester of pregnancy, maternal diabetes and drugs in pregnancy (like thalidomide, alcohol, phenytoin) are environmental factors associated with an increased incidence of congenital heart disease.

Antenatal detection

Severe congenital heart disease can be detected at 16–18 weeks gestation by fetal echocardiography. Increasingly, this is being used as a screening test for severe heart abnormalities but it is particularly useful in the case of families where a previous baby has had a heart abnormality.

Presentation

Congenital heart disease usually presents in one of the three following ways.

Heart murmur. This is the commonest mode of presentation. Most murmurs are detected in the first year of life, either on routine examination in the newborn period or in the child health clinics. A minority are not discovered until the child starts school or on coincidental examination.

Heart failure. A number of lesions will cause heart failure, commonly in the first year of life. The symptoms and signs are similar to those found in an adult. The baby becomes breathless, particularly after the exertion of feeding or crying. He may have difficulty completing feeds and as a consequence fails to thrive. Sweating is often a prominent symptom. On examination, the baby has a rapid respiratory rate and a rapid pulse rate. Heart enlargement is usually present and can be detected clinically; a thrill or murmur may be present and there is often a gallop rhythm due to a third heart sound. Invariably, the liver is enlarged due to venous congestion. Oedema of the dependant parts of the body is rarely seen. Fine moist sounds of pulmonary oedema are less easily heard in babies than in adults. If frank pulmonary oedema is present, the baby may be centrally cyanosed and the cyanosis will disappear when oxygen is given.

Cyanosis ('blue baby'). If the heart defect results in unsaturated venous blood by-passing the lungs, central cyanosis will be present and is not corrected while breathing 100 per cent oxygen. This lack of response to oxygen helps to distinguish cyanosis due to heart disease from cyanosis due to severe lung disease, especially in the newborn period when this distinction can be difficult. Long-standing central cyanosis results in clubbing of the fingers and toes and secondary polycythaemia. A child with cyanotic congenital heart disease often has a reduced exercise tolerance and fails to grow normally.

Heart failure in infancy

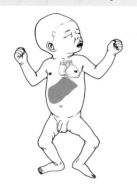

Symptoms
breathlessness on exertion (especially feeding and crying)
sweating
failure to thrive

Signs
rapid breathing
rapid heart rate
enlarged heart
murmur
enlarged liver

Investigations

Investigations must be carried out urgently in symptomatic infants. A chest X-ray and electrocardiogram are essential investigations in the assessment of a child with suspected heart disease. Echocardiography using ultrasound is a non-invasive investigation which gives detailed information about the anatomy of the heart and great vessels. The additional use of Doppler ultrasound provides haemodynamic information. Almost all lesions which cause heart failure or cyanosis in infancy, and many of those which produce a murmur, can be confidently diagnosed by echocardiography. Cardiac catheterisation is an invasive investigation, only performed in specialist units; it enables the pressures and saturations within the cardiac chambers to be measured and, with angiocardiography following injection of radio-opaque dye, permits precise anatomical and physiological diagnosis. It is particularly useful for estimating the severity of a lesion, and judging the need for surgery in asymptomatic patients.

The innocent murmur

Many babies and children have heart murmurs without any structural abnormality of the heart. Indeed, in one reported series, a cardiologist detected a heart murmur in the majority of healthy school children on routine examination! Such murmurs are termed innocent, or functional. They are diagnosed as being innocent on the basis of their characteristics and are associated with a normal chest X-ray, cardiac ultrasound and ECG. If a murmur is obviously innocent, no follow-up is necessary. If there is uncertainty an expert opinion should be sought as soon as possible, before the seeds of cardiac neurosis are sown. There are three types of innocent murmur:

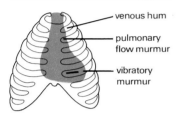

Innocent murmurs

venous hum

pulmonary flow murmur

vibratory murmur

Venous hum. This is a blowing, continuous murmur heard at the base of the heart, often just below the clavicles. It varies both with respiration and the position of the head, and disappears when the child lies down. It is due to blood flow through the systemic great veins and is sometimes confused with a patent ductus arteriosus.

Pulmonary flow murmur. This is a soft, systolic ejection murmur heard in the pulmonary area (the second left intercostal space). It is due to rapid flow of blood across a normal pulmonary valve and is especially prominent when the cardiac output is high, for example after exercise, in febrile children or in cases of anaemia.

Vibratory murmur. This is a short, buzzing murmur heard in systole at the left sternal edge or at the apex of the heart. It is variable and changes with position.

If a murmur is pansystolic, diastolic, loud or long, associated with a thrill or with cardiac symptoms, it is not innocent.

Congenital heart disease can conveniently be classified into two groups: (1) acyanotic due to either a left to right shunt or obstructive lesion, and (2) cyanotic with either increased or diminished pulmonary flow.

ACYANOTIC LESIONS WITH A LEFT TO RIGHT SHUNT

A common type of congenital heart defect is a hole between the two sides of the heart, at the level of either the atria, the ventricles or the great arteries. In fetal life, pulmonary blood flow is small and the pressures in the right ventricle and pulmonary artery are high. With the onset of regular respirations, the pulmonary vascular resistance falls, with a consequent fall in the pressures on the right side of the heart. Since the pressure on the left side of the heart now exceeds that on the right side, blood will start to flow from the left side to the right side through the hole. The fall in pulmonary vascular resistance occurs rapidly in the first few days after birth and then more slowly over the next few weeks, so that by the age of about 3 months the left to right flow of blood reaches a maximum. There is therefore an additional circulation of blood from the left side of the heart to the right side, thence to the lungs and back to the left side of the heart again. This is termed a shunt. If the hole is small, the shunt may be trivial, but if it is large, it may represent the majority of the cardiac output, so that the blood flow through the pulmonary artery may be several times greater than the flow through the aorta. A large shunt imposes an added burden on the heart, with consequent hypertrophy, dilatation and sometimes failure. Because of the high pulmonary vascular resistance immediately after birth, frequently a murmur is not heard and in babies with a simple left to right shunt, heart failure is uncommon in the first few weeks of life.

A left to right shunt, if appreciable, will give rise to a number of consistent findings, regardless of the site of the hole. Clinical examination may show an enlarged heart with hypertrophy of one or both ventricles. Signs of ventricular hypertrophy will be present on the electrocardiogram. A chest radiograph will reveal an enlarged heart with a prominent pulmonary artery and an increase in vascular markings (pulmonary plethora) due to the high pulmonary blood flow.

ATRIAL SEPTAL DEFECT (OSTIUM SECUNDUM)

Atrial septal defect

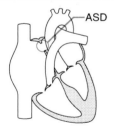

In the majority of atrial septal defects, the hole is in the atrial septum in the region of the fossa ovalis, the site of the foramen ovale: this is the ostium secundum defect. Because the right ventricle is less muscular and easier to fill with blood than the left ventricle, blood will flow from the left atrium to the right atrium through the defect, thence to the right ventricle and the lungs. The right side of the heart therefore takes the whole of the added burden of the shunt.

Natural history. Symptoms are rare in infancy and uncommon in childhood, even if the shunt is large. However in the third or fourth decade, heart failure, pulmonary hypertension or atrial arrhythmias may occur.

Clinical features. Because symptoms are unusual in childhood, most children with atrial septal defects present with a heart murmur. The murmur is often quite soft and frequently not detected until the child is at school. If symptoms do occur, they are of breathlessness or tiredness on exertion, or recurrent chest infections.

Examination. The child is well, pink and has normal pulses. The right ventricle may be easily felt. There is a systolic murmur at the second left interspace. This is due not to flow of blood across the defect, but to a high flow of blood across a normal pulmonary valve. If the shunt is large, a mid-diastolic tricuspid flow murmur may be heard too. The

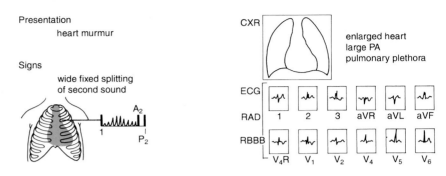

Presentation, examination and investigation of atrial septal defect

aortic and pulmonary components of the second sound are widely separated because the excessive filling of the right ventricle delays closure of the pulmonary valve. Furthermore, the time interval between these two sounds does not vary with respiration ('fixed splitting') because the two atria function as a single unit and respiration affects them both equally.

Investigations. The chest X-ray shows cardiomegaly with prominent atrium and pulmonary artery, and pulmonary plethora. The electrocardiogram shows right axis deviation, right ventricular hypertrophy and in most cases right bundle branch block. The diagnosis is confirmed by echocardiography.

Treatment. If the defect is moderate or large, closure is advisable, using cardiopulmonary bypass. Repair is by simple suture or by insertion of a patch of pericardium.

ATRIAL SEPTAL DEFECT (OSTIUM PRIMUM)

Although less common than secundum defects, ostium primum defects are more serious. The hole is situated low down in the atrial septum and represents a failure of development of the septum primum in fetal life. The defect is just above the atrioventricular valves, and usually extends to the insertion of the anterior leaflet of the mitral valve, so that the latter is cleft and frequently incompetent. An ostium primum atrial septal defect represents the mild end of the spectrum of developmental abnormalities involving the central portion of the heart, endocardial cushion defects. In the most severe form, the defect extends from the atrial septum, through the origin of both atrioventricular valves into the ventricular septum. This is described as an atrioventricular canal defect and gives rise to a large left to right shunt and both mitral and tricuspid incompetence. The endocardial cushion defects are particularly common in children with Down syndrome.

Clinical features. Heart failure commonly develops in infancy and childhood and there is a high mortality without surgery. The development of severe pulmonary hypertension is common, especially in Down syndrome. There are commonly signs of heart failure with marked cardiac enlargement. The child is often breathless at rest, with deformities of the lower ribs (Harrison's sulci). He is pink, with normal pulses. Clinically, the heart is large with increased activity of both ventricles. In addition to the auscultatory signs of an atrial septal defect there may be an apical pansystolic murmur signifying mitral regurgitation.

Investigations. The chest X-ray shows marked cardiomegaly, prominent pulmonary arteries and pulmonary plethora. The electrocardiogram is frequently diagnostic, showing left axis deviation and right bundle branch block. Catheterisation is required to assess the size of the shunt and the degree of mitral incompetence.

Treatment. Early surgery is usually advised for children with ostium primum defects. The defect is closed and the cleft mitral valve repaired. It is a more difficult and risky operation than that for a secundum defect.

VENTRICULAR SEPTAL DEFECT

Ventricular septal defect

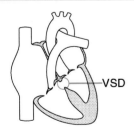

This is the commonest of all congenital heart lesions. Usually a single defect is found in the membranous portion of the ventricular septum, adjacent to the tricuspid valve, or below the aortic valve. Less commonly, single or multiple defects are found in the muscular part of the septum. In 25 to 30 per cent of affected children other heart defects are also present.

Natural history. There are four possibilities:

1. The hole may close spontaneously. This occurs in perhaps as many as 50 per cent of cases, usually in early childhood but sometimes in later childhood, adolescence or adult life.
2. The hole may remain the same size. Since the heart is growing throughout childhood, the defect becomes relatively smaller.
3. Stenosis of the outflow tract of the right ventricle (the infundibulum), may occur. This raises the pressure in the right ventricle and steadily reduces the size of the left to right shunt. Eventually the shunt may reverse and the child will become cyanosed. The child in effect develops Fallot's tetralogy.
4. Progressive pulmonary hypertension may develop. If the left to right shunt is large, the torrential pulmonary blood flow irreversibly damages the smaller pulmonary vessels, giving rise to pulmonary

hypertension. This makes he defect inoperable and considerably reduces the child's life span.

Clinical presentation depends on the size of the defect and whether pulmonary hypertension is present.

Small ventricular septal defect ('maladie de Roger')

Since the shunt through the defect is small, the child is symptom-free and the heart murmur is often picked up on routine examination. The child is well, pink and has normal pulses, and the heart is not enlarged. Frequently there is a thrill at the lower left sternal border. On auscultation a harsh, pansystolic murmur is heard at the same site due to flow of blood through the defect. The heart sounds are normal.

Investigations. The chest X-ray and electrocardiogram are usually normal. Catheterisation is unnecessary.

Treatment. There is a risk of bacterial endocarditis and antibiotic prophylaxis is therefore necessary at the time of dental extractions, etc.

Moderate ventricular septal defect

Symptoms usually occur in infancy, with breathlessness on feeding and crying, failure to thrive and recurrent chest infections. As the child gets older, the symptoms tend to improve and may disappear altogether, because of actual or relative closure of the defect.

Examination. The baby is breathless at rest but is pink, with normal pulses. The heart is enlarged clinically with prominent activity of both ventricles. There is a systolic thrill at the lower left sternal border. On auscultation there is a loud, harsh pansystolic murmur, maximal at this site but heard all over the chest. There is frequently an apical mid-diastolic murmur, caused by an increased flow of blood across a normal mitral valve. The second heart sound is noticeably split and the pulmonary component may be louder than normal.

Investigations. The chest X-ray shows cardiomegaly, prominent pulmonary arteries and pulmonary plethora. The electrocardiogram shows biventricular hypertrophy, since both ventricles are involved in the shunt. Cardiac catheterisation should be carried out if the child does not improve with age or if there is evidence of pulmonary hypertension.

Treatment. If symptoms are prominent, diuretics should be given. Surgery should be avoided because of the tendency to spontaneous improvement. Exceptions are continuing symptoms and the development of pulmonary hypertension.

Large ventricular septal defect

When the pulmonary vascular resistance falls to its lowest level at about three months of age, the shunt through a large defect is great and results in heart failure. Symptoms of breathlessness on feeding usually start earlier than this and sweating is very common. Affected babies may be

Clinical features of ventricular septal defect

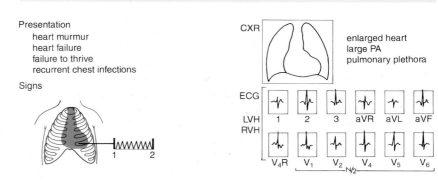

Presentation
    heart murmur
    heart failure
    failure to thrive
    recurrent chest infections

Signs

CXR — enlarged heart, large PA, pulmonary plethora

ECG — LVH, RVH — 1 2 3 aVR aVL aVF — V₄R V₁ V₂ V₄ V₅ V₆

severely ill with congestive cardiac failure, and they have an increased tendency to chest infections which often precipitates episodes of failure.

Examination. The baby is usually underweight, breathless and ill. If there is frank pulmonary oedema, cyanosis will be present. The heart is large clinically with increased ventricular activity and a systolic thrill. Signs of heart failure will be present. On auscultation, there is a harsh systolic murmur which is caused by increased flow across the pulmonary valve. A pulmonary systolic ejection and a mitral mid-diastolic flow murmur are usually heard and the pulmonary second sound is loud.

Investigation. The chest X-ray shows very marked cardiomegaly, large pulmonary arteries and pulmonary plethora. The electrocardiogram shows biventricular hypertrophy. Echocardiography will display the defect but catheterisation is necessary to measure the size of the shunt and the pulmonary artery pressure.

Treatment. The initial treatment is medical. The infant in heart failure is nursed in a semi-sitting position. Diuretics (usually frusemide or a thiazide) are given, together with potassium supplements or a potassium sparing diuretic such as spironolactone. The success of treatment can be gauged by regular weighing and by recording the size of the liver. As the heart failure responds to treatment there will be a rapid weight loss and a progressive decrease in liver size. If the baby does not respond to treatment, surgical closure is necessary. This is best done as a single stage operation, using cardiopulmonary bypass. Such an operation in an ill baby requires the highest medical and surgical skills. An alternative method of surgical treatment is to place a constricting band around the base of the pulmonary artery, thus reducing the size of the shunt. A second operation is required to remove the band and close the defect.

PATENT DUCTUS ARTERIOSUS

Patent ductus arteriosus

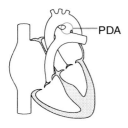
PDA

This is a common congenital heart lesion, either singly or in combination with other heart defects. It is particularly common in girls, in children whose mothers had rubella in early pregnancy and in babies who are born prematurely. In fetal life the ductus arteriosus, which is a large vessel with a muscular wall, diverts blood from the right ventricle and pulmonary artery into the aorta. Within the first 24 hours after birth, it closes in response to oxygenated blood. Spontaneous closure of a ductus arteriosus which remains patent after the first few days of life is unlikely, the only exception is the premature baby in whom closure of the ductus may still occur at any time in the first 3 months of life. As the pulmonary vascular resistance falls after birth, a left to right shunt of blood from the aorta to the pulmonary artery occurs through the ductus (the opposite direction to the flow in fetal life).

Small ductus

The child is symptom free and a heart murmur is detected routinely or coincidentally. He is pink with normal pulses. On auscultation there is a loud, continuous murmur heard best below the left clavicle. The murmur extends through systole into diastole because the pressure in the pulmonary artery is lower than that in the aorta throughout the whole cardiac cycle. It has a rough 'machinery' quality.

Investigations. Chest X-ray and electrocardiogram are normal. Echocardiography with Doppler demonstrates the duct.

Treatment. Surgical ligation is recommended because of the risk of bacterial endocarditis. The operation itself carries a very low risk.

Large ductus

The severity of symptoms is related to the size of the shunt. The child may be underweight with a reduced exercise tolerance and increased tendency to chest infections. At the other end of the spectrum, severe heart failure may develop in infancy. On examination the child is often small and thin. An increased respiratory rate is common. There is no

Clinical features of a patent ductus arteriosus

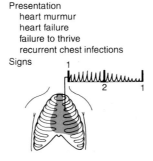

Presentation
  heart murmur
  heart failure
  failure to thrive
  recurrent chest infections
Signs

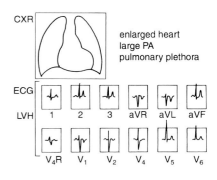

CXR
enlarged heart
large PA
pulmonary plethora

ECG
LVH

cyanosis, but the pulses are easily felt, being full and collapsing in nature. The diastolic blood pressure is low and pulse pressure is wide. The heart is enlarged clinically with a prominent left ventricle and there is a systolic thrill in the pulmonary area. On auscultation, there is a harsh systolic murmur which may extend through the second sound into early diastole. The length of the murmur depends on the pulmonary artery pressure. This is high in large shunts so that blood only flows from left to right during systole. The pulmonary second sound is loud. A mitral (mid-diastolic) flow murmur may be heard.

Investigations. The chest X-ray shows the typical features of a left-to-right shunt. The electrocardiogram shows left ventricular hypertrophy. The diagnosis is confirmed by echocardiography.

Natural history. If the duct is small, the only risk to the patient is from bacterial endocarditis, or more accurately, endoarteritis. This is appreciable. If the duct is larger, heart failure may occur in infancy, or may occur for the first time in adult life. Pulmonary hypertension and shunt reversal can occur.

Treatment. If heart failure is present, medical treatment is necessary. Surgery should be carried out as soon as the child's condition allows.

PULMONARY HYPERTENSION

A large left to right shunt with a high pulmonary blood flow may produce an elevation of pulmonary artery pressure simply because of the increased flow (hyperdynamic pulmonary hypertension). Following surgical closure of the defect, the pulmonary artery pressure returns to normal. Persisting high pulmonary blood flow may result in permanent damage to the smaller pulmonary vessels with consequent narrowing and irreversible pulmonary hypertension. If the defect is closed under these circumstances, the pulmonary artery pressure remains elevated. When the pulmonary artery pressure reaches systemic levels the left to right shunt ceases and may actually reverse.

Clinical features. The child becomes mildly cyanosed, with clubbed fingers and toes, but otherwise may appear remarkably well. However, exercise tolerance is usually considerably reduced. On examination, the right ventricle is prominent and heaving, and the pulmonary second sound is palpable. On auscultation there is usually a systolic ejection murmur in the pulmonary area due to blood flow through the huge pulmonary artery, not through the shunt, and sometimes an early diastolic murmur signifying pulmonary incompetence. The pulmonary component of the second sound is very loud.

Investigations. A chest X-ray shows an enlarged heart with a prominent right atrium. The pulmonary artery is greatly increased in size but its smaller branches are not seen. The electrocardiogram shows right axis deviation, right atrial hypertrophy and right ventricular hypertrophy. Cardiac catheterisation is needed to demonstrate the site of the shunt and to measure the pulmonary artery pressure.

The development of severe, irreversible pulmonary hypertension as a result of a large left to right shunt is called the Eisenmenger syndrome. Although it was originally described in association with a ventricular septal defect (Eisenmenger complex), it may occur with a left to right shunt at any site. It is particularly likely to occur in cases of large ventricular septal defects, atrioventricular canal defects and transposition of the great arteries where there is a large shunt. No surgical correction is possible and the life expectancy of affected children is considerably reduced. Heart–lung transplantation may be an option for these patients.

OBSTRUCTIVE LESIONS

The commonest examples are aortic stenosis, coarctation of the aorta and pulmonary stenosis. The chamber of the heart proximal to the obstruction hypertrophies in an attempt to overcome it. If the obstruction is severe, heart failure may result.

AORTIC STENOSIS

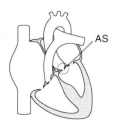
Aortic stenosis

AS

This is a common congenital heart lesion which may occur in isolation or in combination with other heart defects. In the majority of cases the aortic valve itself is narrowed by congenital deformity. The deformed valve may be bicuspid instead of tricuspid and the cusps are frequently fused at the edges. The degree of stenosis may worsen as the child gets older, with thickening and calcification of the cusps. A bicuspid aortic valve may open normally in childhood, but becomes thickened and narrowed in adult life. If the aortic valve is particularly narrowed and rigid, a degree of aortic incompetence is common too.

Occasionally, aortic obstruction may be above or below the aortic valve. In supravalvular stenosis, the ascending aorta above the valve is narrowed. This is often associated with an unusual facial appearance, mental handicap and hypercalcaemia in infancy (William syndrome). In subvalvular aortic stenosis, there may be a fibrous diaphragm below the valve obstructing the flow of blood from left ventricle to aorta, or there may be excessive hypertrophy of the left ventricle and interventricular septum which obstructs the outflow tract of the left ventricle during systole, that is, a hypertrophic obstructive cardiomyopathy.

Clinical features. Severe aortic stenosis results in heart failure in infancy results. In most other instances a heart murmur is detected routinely. A minority of older children with severe aortic stenosis may feel faint or dizzy on exertion, and lose consciousness. This is an indication for urgent treatment. Bacterial endocarditis is a complication of aortic stenosis of any degree.

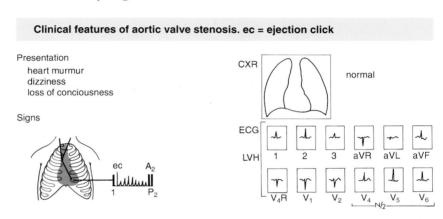

Clinical features of aortic valve stenosis. ec = ejection click

Presentation
  heart murmur
  dizziness
  loss of conciousness

Signs

CXR — normal

ECG — LVH

Examination. The child appears well and is pink. The pulses are often small in volume, and of the slow rising, plateau type. The systolic blood pressure may be low. On palpation, the left ventricle is prominent and a thrill may be palpable at the lower left sternal border, in the suprasternal notch and in the neck over the carotid arteries. On auscultation there is a systolic ejection murmur heard at the apex and lower left sternal edge, which is conducted upwards into the neck. There is usually an ejection click immediately before the murmur. The aortic second sound is soft and delayed. If the stenosis is severe the aortic second sound may actually occur later than the pulmonary component so that there is apparent paradoxical splitting of the second sound with respiration.

Investigations. A chest X-ray may show a prominent left ventricle with post-stenotic dilatation of the ascending aorta. An electrocardiogram shows varying degrees of left ventricular hypertrophy relating to the severity of the stenosis. The aortic valve gradient can be measured by ultrasound.

Treatment. If echocardiography shows a gradient across the aortic valve greater than 40 mmHg, cardiac catheterisation is necessary to confirm the findings. The stenosis can be relieved by balloon valvuloplasty — with a catheter tip passing through the aortic valve from the femoral artery, a balloon is inflated to widen the stenosed valve. If this is un-successful or the aortic stenosis is severe, an open aortic valvotomy is necessary. Residual stenosis and incompetence are common, but aortic valve replacement is avoided where possible until children have stopped growing. Aortic stenosis is the one congenital heart lesion in which strenuous activity should be avoided because of the risk of sudden death. Prevention of bacterial endocarditis is important.

COARCTATION OF THE AORTA

Coarctation of aorta

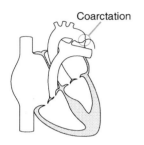

This is a localised narrowing of the descending aorta, close to the site of the ductus arteriosus and usually distal to the left subclavian artery. Arterial blood bypasses the obstruction reaching the lower part of the body through collateral vessels which become greatly enlarged. The left ventricle hypertrophies to overcome the obstruction and heart failure may result. The systolic blood pressure in the upper part of the body is usually elevated.

Clinical presentation. If the narrowing is severe, heart failure may occur in the first few days or weeks of life. In most cases, however, the diagnosis is made on routine or coincidental examination, either because a murmur is heard, or the femoral pulses cannot be felt or because of the discovery of hypertension. Occasionally, a child or adult may present with a complication such as a subarachnoid haemorrhage from rupture of an intracranial aneurysm or bacterial endarteritis.

Examination. The child is well and pink. The brachial and radial pulses are normal but the femoral pulses are either absent or weak and delayed. There is usually systemic hypertension and the left ventricle may be prominent. On auscultation, a systolic ejection murmur is usually heard over the left side of the chest, especially at the back. Collateral arteries are often palpable over the scapulae.

Investigations. A chest X-ray may show a prominent left ventricle. In older children rib notching may be seen where the enlarged intercostal arteries have eroded the under side of the ribs. An electrocardiogram may show left ventricular hypertrophy.

Clinical features of coartation of the aorta

Presentation
  heart murmur
  absent femoral pulses
  hypertension

Signs

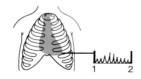

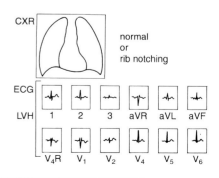

Treatment. Surgery is recommended in all but the mildest cases and should be carried out soon after the diagnosis is made. The narrowed segment of aorta is resected and the two ends sewn together. In infants, the proximal portion of the left subclavian artery can be used to repair the aorta after excision of the narrowing. Earlier surgery is more effective in permanently treating the hypertension but as the child grows there is a risk that relative narrowing at the site of the coarctation will occur again, requiring further surgery.

HYPOPLASTIC LEFT HEART

In this condition, the left ventricle is underdeveloped, frequently with hypoplasia or atresia of the mitral valve, aortic valve and arch of the aorta. The ductus arteriosus is patent and blood therefore by-passes the left-sided obstruction. Affected babies present in the first few days after birth with severe progressive heart failure. They are pale and shocked, with very weak pulses. Unfortunately it is a relatively common condition for which there is no treatment apart from symptom relief. Diagnosis is made by echocardiography, sometimes in fetal life, and death occurs in early infancy.

PULMONARY STENOSIS

Pulmonary stenosis

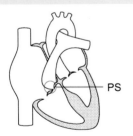

PS

In this condition the pulmonary valve is congenitally deformed, thickened and narrowed. The right ventricle hypertrophies in an attempt to overcome the obstruction. The muscular outflow tract of the right ventricle, the infundibulum, also hypertrophies and this may increase the degree of obstruction.

Clinical presentation. If the stenosis is severe, the infant presents with right sided heart failure. There may be cyanosis from a right to left shunt of blood through the foramen ovale. In mild and moderate cases a heart murmur is heard on routine examination. Symptoms are rare in childhood. However, in cases of moderate stenosis, dysfunction of the right ventricle and arrhythmias are liable to occur in adult life.

Examination. In mild to moderate cases the child is well, pink, and has normal pulses. Right atrial hypertrophy produces a large 'a' wave in the jugular venous pulse. The right ventricle is heaving and a systolic thrill is palpable in the pulmonary area. On auscultation, there is usually an ejection click followed by a systolic ejection murmur caused by blood flowing across the narrowed valve. The murmur is heard in the upper part of the left chest anteriorly and is conducted to the back. The

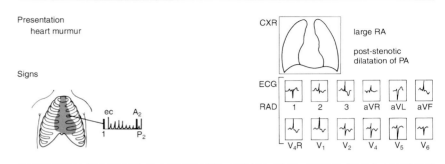

Clinical features of pulmonary valve stenosis

Presentation
  heart murmur

Signs

ec A₂

CXR large RA

post-stenotic
dilatation of PA

ECG

RAD 1 2 3 aVR aVL aVF

V₄R V₁ V₂ V₄ V₅ V₆

pulmonary component of the second sound becomes softer and more delayed as the stenosis increases.

Investigations. A chest X-ray shows post-stenotic dilatation of the pulmonary artery. An enlarged right atrium and right ventricle are seen in severe cases. An electrocardiogram shows varying degrees of right axis deviation, right atrial hypertrophy and right ventricular hypertrophy, according to the severity of the stenosis. The pulmonary valve gradient is measured by Doppler ultrasound.

Treatment. If the Doppler gradient across the valve exceeds 40–50 mmHg cardiac catheterisation with balloon valvuloplasty is carried out. This is highly successful — the narrowing is reduced by 75 per cent or more and does not usually recur.

CYANOTIC HEART DISEASE

A minority of babies or children with congenital heart disease are centrally cyanosed because unsaturated blood is bypassing the lungs. An affected child may be quite well at rest, even though he may be very blue. However, when the body's demand for oxygen increases during exercise, he becomes very easily tired and breathless. Even though the arterial oxygen saturation may be very low, the child's intelligence is usually normal. Secondary polycythaemia follows chronic hypoxia. This is to the child's advantage at first since it increases the actual amount of oxygen that can be transported in the blood. However, when the packed cell volume exceeds a certain limit, the viscosity of the blood increases with a resultant tendency to thrombosis, particularly in cerebral vessels. Embolism from thrombosis and haemorrhage from consumption coagulopathy are also well recognised complications of cyanotic heart disease.

Cyanotic heart disease can be subdivided into two types. In the first type the lungs are under-perfused as blood shunts from right to left by-passing the lungs. Fallot tetralogy is the commonest example. In the second type, the lungs are normally filled or even over-perfused with blood, but cyanosis results because there is inadequate mixing of the systemic and pulmonary circulations. Transposition of the great arteries is the commonest example.

FALLOT TETRALOGY

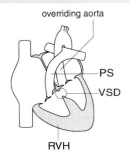

Fallot tetralogy

overriding aorta

PS

VSD

RVH

The two essential features of this condition are a large ventricular septal defect, usually sited high up in the membranous part of the septum beneath the aortic valve, and stenosis of the pulmonary valve or infundibulum. There is therefore resistance to the flow of blood through the pulmonary valve with a consequent shunt of blood from the right to left ventricle and thence to the aorta. In fact, since the septal defect is just below the aortic valve, the aorta appears to override the right ventricle and the shunt is directly from the right ventricle to the aorta. Pulmonary or infundibular stenosis leads to right ventricular hypertrophy. The overriding of the aorta and right ventricular hypertrophy, in combination with the ventricular septal defect and pulmonary stenosis, make up the tetralogy originally described by Fallot. The main pulmonary artery is small and in the most severe cases may not be patent (pulmonary atresia with a ventricular septal defect).

Clinical features. Affected children are usually pink in the newborn period, although a heart murmur due to blood flow through a narrow infundibulum or pulmonary valve may be detected. Cyanosis develops and increases over the next few weeks or months. Sometimes the baby may be quite pink when at rest, only becoming cyanosed with the exertion of crying or feeding. Sometimes cyanotic 'attacks' or 'spells' occur. An affected baby is relatively well most of the time but is prone to attacks during which he becomes extremely cyanosed and pale often with loss of consciousness. Such spells result from reduced systemic vascular resistance, increasing the right to left shunt and preventing blood from reaching the lungs. As the children become older, cyanosis at rest becomes more obvious, exercise tolerance is reduced and the typical squatting may occur. The latter is a manoeuvre to gain symptomatic relief after exercise in which the child squats down on his haunches with his knees up to his chest. It traps unsaturated venous blood in the legs preventing it from returning to the heart and also raises aortic pressure by obstructing the femoral arteries, with consequent reduction in size of the right to left shunt.

Heart failure is extremely rare in Fallot tetralogy but the thromboembolic complications of polycythaemia, bacterial endocarditis and cerebral abscess may occur.

Examination. The affected child may be cyanosed at rest with clubbing of the fingers and toes. The heart is not enlarged clinically but the right

Clinical features of Fallot tetralogy

Presentation
  cyanosis
  poor exercise tolerance
  squatting

Signs

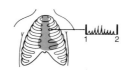

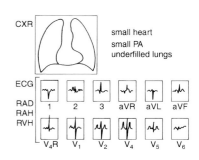

CXR — small heart, small PA, underfilled lungs

ECG — RAD, RAH, RVH

ventricle is easily felt and there may be a systolic thrill in the pulmonary area. On auscultation, there is a systolic ejection murmur in the pulmonary area and a single second heart sound. No murmur arises from blood flow through the septal defect because the pressures in the two ventricles are similar.

Investigations. The chest X-ray shows a normal size heart with the apex above the left diaphragm but the left heart border is concave because the main pulmonary artery is small and the heart is said to look like a boot. The lung fields are oligaemic. The electrocardiogram shows right axis deviation, right atrial hypertrophy and right ventricular hypertrophy. The diagnosis is made by echocardiography.

Treatment. This is surgical in all cases. Symptomatic infants require a palliative shunt to improve their symptoms until they are old enough for a total correction. A shunt operation is the creation of a communication between the pulmonary and systemic circulation (an artificial ductus arteriosus). The most commonly performed type is the modified Blalock procedure where a tube of Goretex is used to connect the subclavian and the pulmonary arteries on either the left or right side. After the age of a year, a total correction is carried out using cardiopulmonary bypass — the hole is closed and the pulmonary valve and infundibulum are widened. Results of surgery are excellent.

TRANSPOSITION OF THE GREAT ARTERIES

In this heart lesion, the aorta and pulmonary artery are 'transposed' so that the aorta arises from the right ventricle and the pulmonary artery from the left ventricle. This means that there are two isolated circulations, pulmonary and systemic, working in parallel. Obviously this would not be compatible with life were it not for the fact that there must be some mixing between the two circulations. In fetal life, the baby is in no difficulty because the pulmonary blood flow is very

Transposition

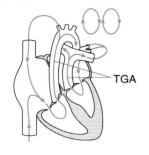

TGA

small. After birth however, as the ductus arteriosus and foramen ovale begin to close, progressive cyanosis develops. The severity of the symptoms depends on the degree of mixing of the two circulations through these fetal channels. In some cases, a large ventricular septal defect or a large patent ductus arteriosus may be present, in which case there is a high pulmonary blood low and only slight cyanosis. In the simple form however, progressive cyanosis develops in the first hours or days after birth. Without treatment, few children survive the first year of life.

Clinical features. Progressive cyanosis develops within the first few hours or days of life. The affected baby becomes increasingly blue and acidotic. Breathlessness and heart failure may follow.

Examination. Cyanosis is the major physical sign and persists even if the baby is given 100 per cent oxygen. There are usually no heart murmurs but the second sound is loud because the transposed aorta lies anteriorly, close to the chest wall.

Investigations. The chest X-ray is often typical. The heart is slightly enlarged and is said to look like an egg lying on its side. The vascular pedicle of the heart is narrow because the aorta and pulmonary artery lie one in front of the other. The lung fields are normally filled or plethoric. Diagnosis is made by echocardiography.

Clinical features of transposition of the great arteries

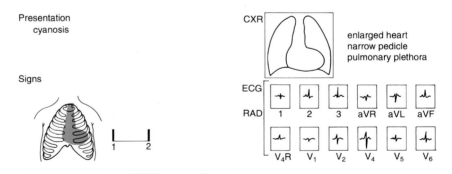

Treatment. A shunt between the systemic and pulmonary circuits is urgently needed. It is created by means of a balloon atrial septostomy (Rashkind procedure). A special double lumen catheter is passed via the inferior vena cava, right atrium and foramen ovale into the left atrium. A balloon near the catheter tip is inflated with contrast medium and catheter and balloon are then pulled sharply back through the atrial septum, tearing it and creating a large septal defect. This allows mixing of blood and improves the cyanosis.

The definitive corrective operation is an anatomical repair, in which the pulmonary artery and aorta are switched to their rightful ventricles. It is usually carried out in the first week or two of life.

CARDIAC ARRHYTHMIAS

Children often have cardiac arrhythmias which are of no clinical significance; sinus arrhythmia is the most common example. A number, however, have symptoms which are a direct result of an abnormality of heart rhythm.

Paroxysmal supra-ventricular tachycardia

This is a regular, rapid rhythm at the rate of 240 to 300 beats per minute. It is due to impulses originating in the atrioventricular node re-entering the atria via an accessory pathway and thus exciting the atrioventricular node prematurely. Since the heart rate is so rapid, diastolic filling of the ventricles is impaired and cardiac failure arises. The younger the patient, the less well is the rapid heart rate tolerated and the earlier heart failure develops. The tachycardia is paroxysmal and frequently recurs. About a quarter of the children with this disorder have an underlying cardiac defect, either congenital or acquired.

Clinical features. Paroxysmal tachycardia may be noted *in utero* or occur at any time in infancy, childhood or adult life. As the heart rate suddenly becomes rapid, the baby may go pale, start to breathe quickly and vomit. After a few hours, symptoms of heart failure occur and death may result if no treatment is given. Older children can usually recognise the onset of the tachycardia, and describe palpitations. Paroxysms may occur spontaneously or be precipitated by illness. Return to sinus rhythm produces a diuresis.

Examination. The child looks pale but may be otherwise well. A baby is more likely to show obvious signs of heart failure. The pulse is very rapid, regular and weak. It does not gradually slow when carotid sinus or eyeball pressure is applied.

The ECG of supraventricular tachycardia

supraventricular tachycardia
(rate 280/min)

sinus rhythm
(rate 140/min)

Investigations. The electrocardiogram shows a heart rate in excess of 240 beats per minute. The P waves may be present, abnormal, or absent, and the QRS complexes are normal. Between paroxysms, the electrocardiogram shows normal sinus rhythm. A number of children show the Wolff-Parkinson-White syndrome, an electrocardiographic abnormality comprising a short P-R interval and slurring of the beginning of the QRS complex.

Treatment. In some cases an attack can be terminated by vagal stimulation. In an infant this is best achieved by eliciting the diving reflex — the infant's face is immersed for a few seconds in ice cold water. In a child, straining (the valsalva manoeuvre), carotid sinus massage or eyeball pressure can be tried. If this fails, then anti-arrhythmic drugs are used; adenosine or flecainide in an infant, verapamil in an older child. Digitalisation is often effective but slow. In an emergency DC shock may be necessary. Recurrent attacks can be prevented or suppressed by regular digoxin or a beta–adrenoreceptor blocking drug.

Complete heart block

Complete heart block with atrioventricular dissociation may occur in otherwise normal children or in children with underlying congenital or acquired heart disease. It is usually congenital and is sometimes suspected before birth. The ventricular rate of contraction is in the region of 50 per minute and may increase with exercise. Many affected children lead normal, healthy lives and remain symptom-free. A minority have classical Stokes–Adams attacks in which they fall to the ground and lose consciousness. They need an artificial pacemaker.

SUBACUTE BACTERIAL ENDOCARDITIS

This is a well recognised complication of congenital as well as rheumatic heart disease. The risk is highest with those lesions which result in a turbulent jet of blood, such as a ventricular septal defect, coarctation, patent ductus and aortic stenosis. The endocardium becomes infected in the presence of a bacteraemia which may occur during dental treatment or cardiac surgery. As in adults, *Streptococcus viridans* is the commonest infecting organism.

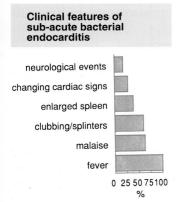

Clinical features of sub-acute bacterial endocarditis

neurological events
changing cardiac signs
enlarged spleen
clubbing/splinters
malaise
fever

0 25 50 75 100
%

Clinical features. Fever, malaise and anorexia are usually the presenting symptoms. Peripheral signs include clubbing of the nails and splinter haemorrhages. The spleen may be palpable and the physical signs of the heart defect can change rapidly as the endocarditis damages the heart valves.

Investigations. The diagnosis is made on one or more positive blood cultures. Microscopic haematuria is common, and the white count and ESR are usually raised.

Treatment. Bacteriocidal antibiotics are given parenterally in large dose for a period of 6 weeks. The combination of benzylpenicillin and gentamicin is particularly useful for *Strep viridans* but frequent monitoring of serum levels for killing activity against the organism is necessary.

Prevention. Any child known to have a congenital heart lesion, no matter how trivial, needs antibiotic prophylaxis with dental treatment and should carry a card to show to his dentist. The card states that the child has congenital heart disease and that in the event of dental treatment (extraction, fillings or scaling) antibiotics should be given. The usual practice is to give oral amoxycillin as a single large dose 1 hour before the treatment. Similar prophylaxis is also necessary before surgery involving the middle ear, tonsils or adenoids.

RHEUMATIC FEVER

There has been a dramatic decline in this disease which used to cause much illness in children and permanent valvular damage in adults in the Western world. It remains common, however, in the Middle East and Africa. The decline of the disease is probably the result of diminished virulence of the β-haemolytic streptococcus, the introduction of antibiotics and improved social conditions. Rheumatic fever may represent an abnormal immunological response to the β-haemolytic streptococcus, an organism commonly responsible for sore throats and tonsillitis. It is thought that the body confuses its own antigens with those of the organism, thereby causing an autoimmune reaction.

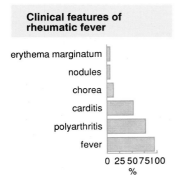

Clinical features of rheumatic fever

Clinical features. One to 3 weeks after a throat infection, the child (usually of school age) develops a fever, malaise and an acute migratory polyarthritis involving the medium-sized joints (knees, ankles, wrists, and elbows). Carditis is common, involving all the layers of the heart. Pericarditis produces a friction rub or a pericardial effusion. Myocarditis produces a tachycardia, cardiac enlargement and arrhythmias. Endocarditis causes systolic and diastolic murmurs. Skin rashes, especially erythema marginatum, and subcutaneous nodules over the occiput or extensor surfaces of the elbows, wrists and fingers are less common. Chorea is a neurological manifestation of rheumatic fever which is rarely associated with carditis.

Investigation. There is usually evidence of a recent streptococcal infection (raised ASO titre and/or positive throat swab) with a raised white count and ESR. The P-R interval is commonly increased in the presence of carditis, often above 0.2 seconds.

Treatment. Penicillin is given to eradicate the streptococcus and high doses of aspirin lower the fever and relieve the arthritis. Steroids shorten the illness but do not reduce the incidence of permanent cardiac damage from the carditis — they are used in particularly severe cases of rheumatic fever. Rheumatic fever tends to recur and carditis is common in subsequent attacks if it occurred in the initial illness. Such recurrent episodes of carditis produce severe rheumatic valvular disease and should be prevented by penicillin prophylaxis for life. On the other hand, children who have no carditis with their initial rheumatic fever have a reduced risk of further relapses and a very low chance of carditis in future episodes.

HYPERTENSION

Unfortunately blood pressure measurement is often overlooked when assessing a child's problems. This attitude arises from the difficulties of

Normal blood pressure in childhood

Age (years)	Mean mmHg Systolic	Diastolic
0–2	95	55
3–6	100	65
7–10	105	70
11–15	115	70

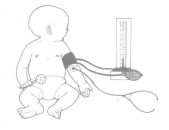

making accurate measurements in a restless young child with equipment which is designed for adults and also because the yield of abnormal readings is very low. With attention to correct technique using suitable cuff sizes and making repeated attempts in a relaxed atmosphere, reliable measurements can be made using a mercury sphygmomanometer. In infants and young children the Doppler method is more reliable. Blood pressure increases with age, height and weight although it should be remembered that the fat arm may give an artificially high reading. Too narrow a cuff in a normal arm also causes this error. There is no precise definition of hypertension in childhood and although the figure 130/85 mmHg is often used, this overlooks those children who fall in the top 5 per cent of the blood pressure distribution for age. A proportion of these high rankers, particularly those with a family history of hypertension, become the adult population at risk from symptomatic hypertension, ischaemic heart disease and cerebrovascular disease. It must be emphasised that no child should be regarded as having an abnormal blood pressure until this has been confirmed on several occasions.

Surveys in several countries have demonstrated that the majority of children with mild asymptomatic hypertension fall into the primary or essential category. In contrast 70 to 90 per cent of those with severe symptomatic hypertension have some underlying cause, most commonly renal parenchymal disease. Greater attention to blood pressure measurement will bring these underlying problems to attention more promptly and may avoid life threatening complications. Hypertension may manifest itself as persistent headache, dizziness, disturbed vision, unexplained irritability, convulsions, and other neurological signs. Naturally, blood pressure should always be measured in the presence of cardiac and renal disorders. Paroxysmal episodes of palpitation and sweating raise the possibility of a phaeochromocytoma.

HYPERLIPOPROTEINAEMIA

The morbidity and mortality arising from atherosclerosis has reached such epidemic proportions in industrial societies that paediatricians can no longer evade their responsibilities in this direction. Fatty streaks are already present in the aortas of children aged 10 to 11 years and the coronary arteries start to show involvement in the early twenties. Both genetic and environmental factors contribute towards atheroma. Currently there is great interest in preventive measures. Some measures, such as antismoking campaigns, the prevention of obesity and the provision of facilities for regular physical exercise are well validated although not always easy to implement; others such as the widescale modification of diet in infants and young children must be approached with caution.

Hyperlipidaemia, and in particular hypercholesterolaemia, has been linked to the development of atheroma. The majority of serum choles-terol is transported as β-lipoprotein, a low density lipoprotein.

Hyperbetalipoproteinaemia (familial hypercholesterolaemia). This is an autosomal dominant condition in which homozygote individuals have a severe disease. They develop tuberous and tendon xanthomata in early childhood and die of ischaemic heart disease in the second or third decade. The heterozygote condition is relatively common, affect-ing approximately 1 in 280 in England and Wales. Fifty-one per cent of heterozygote males and 12 per cent of heterozygote females have a heart attack by the age of 50 years. There is therefore a case for detecting this disorder in early life so that dietary and drug treatment can be introduced before ischaemic disease is established. Cholesterol screening is justified in at-risk families but it is less certain whether it has a place in routine child health surveillance programmes. Children with elevated LDL–cholesterol levels need to be referred to specialist clinics for more detailed lipid and apolipoprotein analysis. Diet remains the main component of lipid-lowering strategies. Anion-exchange resins such as cholestyramine are effective in lowering LDL–cholesterol but compliance is a problem. The new class of drugs which blocks cholesterol synthesis, for example simvastatin, is still undergoing trials in children.

Diet and hypercholesterolaemia. The majority of hypercholesterol-aemia in affluent society is not due to a single, genetically-inherited disorder but reflects the impact of a high animal fat diet on a polygenically susceptible population. Within families there is a significant correlation between the serum cholesterol concentrations of children and those of their parents. The family history should include details of the occurrence and age of onset of ischaemic heart disease so that advice can be offered in an attempt to safeguard at-risk children. It is obviously sensible to reduce the fat intake, particularly from dairy products, but there is still insufficient evidence for the radical exclusion of cholesterol. Children tend to acquire the tastes of their parents and habituation to high fat or salt diets or smoking may well contribute to the future toll of athero-sclerosis.

BIBLIOGRAPHY

Anderson R H, Macartney F J, Shinebourne E A, Tynan M (eds) 1987 Paediatric
    cardiology, vols 1 and 2. Churchill Livingstone, Edinburgh
Jordan S C, Scott O 1989 Heart disease in paediatrics, 3rd edn. Butterworths, London

10 Gut

Normal function of the gastrointestinal tract depends on a carefully regulated balance between motility, sphincter tone, exocrine secretion and integrity of the absorptive surfaces. These functions begin to evolve early in fetal life: digestive enzymes and primitive swallowing movements are first detectable in the 12-week fetus and regular flow of amniotic fluid into the gut occurs from 20 weeks; by term this amounts to approximately 500 ml per day or half the total amniotic volume.

Gut function must undergo abrupt adjustment and maturation with birth and the onset of intermittent oral feeding. There is a marked increase in small intestinal mucosal surface area and this is at least partially mediated by gut hormones such as gastrin which are released in response to milk feeds. Digestive enzymes show a varied pattern of maturation, lactase activity being fully developed at term whereas trypsin takes 12 months to reach maximal levels. Although the gut is probably sterile at birth, it is rapidly colonised by bacterial entry through the mouth and anus. A normal microflora contributes to the available supply of vitamin K, folic acid and biotin. Immunological protection is provided to the newborn by secretory IgA antibodies in the maternal milk and by the transplacental passage of IgG antibodies. Endogenous IgA is produced in the first 3 to 4 weeks and is a major component of the barrier against bacteria and other antigens. Infants with immunological deficiencies are liable to develop gastrointestinal symptoms after 3 months of age when the reserve of maternal IgG is exhausted.

ACUTE ABDOMINAL PAIN

In children the 'acute abdomen' is a common and testing problem. Surgical conditions which require prompt diagnosis and treatment have to be distinguished from a large number of medical disorders. Careful general examination and urinalysis is essential.

Acute appendicitis

Appendicitis is the commonest acute surgical emergency of childhood. Three or four children in every 1000 have their appendix removed each year. It can occur at any age but is usually seen in children over 5 years of age.

Causes of acute abdominal pain

Surgical	Medical (relatively common)	Medical (rare but important)
Acute appendicitis	Mesenteric adenitis	Lead poisoning
Intussusception	Constipation	Diabetes
Intestinal obstruction	Gastroenteritis	Sickle cell crisis
Torsion of ovary or testis	Lower lobe pneumonia	Acute porphyria
Hydronephrosis	Acute pyelonephritis	Pancreatitis
Renal calculus	Henoch Schönlein purpura	Primary peritonitis
	Hepatitis	Meningitis

The characteristic triad of clinical features seen in adults, abdominal pain, low grade fever and tenderness with guarding in the right iliac fossa, is seen in the older child but in infants pain may not be a feature; they are more likely to present with a history of a recent respiratory infection followed by anorexia, vomiting, irritability and a high fever. This often leads to diagnostic confusion and delay so that the incidence of perforation with resulting peritonitis or abscess formation is higher in the younger child. The course of the disease in the young child is extremely rapid: a 2-year-old can progress from apparent normality to perforation in 6 hours! There is no place therefore for prolonged observation in the young patient.

Mesenteric adenitis

Vague central or generalised abdominal pain commonly accompanies viral upper respiratory tract infections. It is due to non-specific inflammation in the mesenteric lymph nodes which provokes a mild peritoneal reaction and stimulates painful peristalsis in the terminal ileum. It is usually possible to distinguish mesenteric adenitis from acute appendicitis, but if there is any doubt 4 to 6 hours after the child is first seen, and in all cases where there is persisting local tenderness, the child must be surgically explored.

Features which distinguish appendicitis and mesenteric adenitis

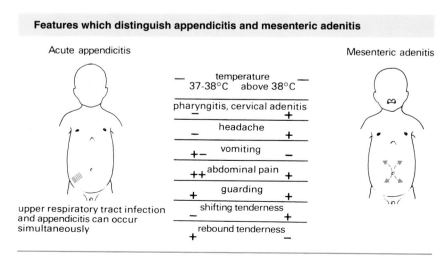

Acute appendicitis

Mesenteric adenitis

	Acute appendicitis		Mesenteric adenitis
temperature	— 37-38°C	above 38°C —	
pharyngitis, cervical adenitis	−	+	
headache	−	+	
vomiting	+−	−	
abdominal pain	++	+	
guarding	+	+	
shifting tenderness	−	+	
rebound tenderness	+	−	

upper respiratory tract infection and appendicitis can occur simultaneously

Primary peritonitis

Primary peritonitis, usually due to pneumococcus, is considerably rarer than peritonitis secondary to appendicitis. Patients with nephrotic syndrome and immune deficiency states are susceptible.

Malrotation

Arrested caecal descent. The midgut loop of the developing embryo elongates by herniating out into the umbilical cord from the sixth to the fourteenth intrauterine weeks. The apex of the loop communicates with the yolk sac by the vitelline duct, and this is the site of a possible Meckel diverticulum. While still in the extra-embryonic coelom a counter clockwise rotation of 270° round the superior mesenteric artery occurs. At about 14 weeks the gut starts to return to the abdominal cavity, the proximal jejunum leading and lying in the left upper abdomen. The caecum is the last portion of the gut to re-enter the abdomen and it initially lies in the subhepatic position. This state of affairs is the most common abnormality seen clinically and to be accurate it should be called arrested caecal descent, not malrotation. It can cause neonatal duodenal obstruction due to Ladd bands, and partial recurrent volvulus in the older child due to the narrow mesenteric attachment between caecum and the duodenojejunal flexure. Often it is asymptomatic but causes severe technical difficulty if the patient develops acute appendicitis.

Maldescent and malrotation

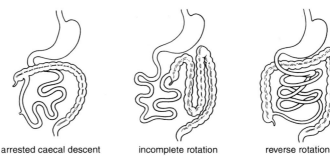

arrested caecal descent   incomplete rotation   reverse rotation

Incomplete rotation. The second anomaly causing clinical problems is correctly called incomplete rotation of the gut, and again is not malrotation. Here rotation in the extraembryonic coelom only amounts to 90° counterclockwise, and the colon and caecum return first to the abdomen and occupy the left side. The small bowel fills the right side. The whole small bowel is suspended by an extremely narrow 1 cm mesenteric attachment between duodenojejunal flexure and caecum, and volvulus in the early days of life is extremely likely. Total small bowel infarction can result.

True malrotation can occur when embryonic rotation is 90° clockwise instead of 270° counterclockwise but this is rare. The duodenum will be anterior to the transverse colon. Clinical problems are unusual.

Meckel diverticulum

This diverticulum is a remnant of the vitellointestinal duct. It arises from the antimesenteric border of the terminal ileum and usually gives no trouble, but very rarely it may become inflamed and then the symptoms and signs mimic acute appendicitis. More commonly the diverticulum causes an intussusception or a volvulus. It may also contain ectopic gastric mucosa in which peptic ulceration can produce haemorrhage or perforation. A technetium scan may help to identify ectopic mucosa.

Intussusception

Intussusception is an invagination of bowel into an adjacent lower segment. The usual origin is the terminal ileum or ileo-caecal valve resulting in an ileocolic intussusception. Although uncommon (2: 1000 live births), it is the most frequent cause of intestinal obstruction in the first 2 years of life.

It presents as paroxysmal pain sometimes with reflex vomiting and a sausage shaped mass is palpable in the right upper abdomen. If there is delay in diagnosis the child will develop fever, a distended abdomen and will pass bloodstained mucus rectally. The diagnosis is usually based on clinical suspicion supported by a plain abdominal X-ray showing a mass and an absent gas pattern over the caecum and ascending colon.

If the history is for less than 24 hours and there are no signs of fever, tenderness or blood rectally, it is appropriate to perform a barium enema both to confirm the diagnosis and to reduce the intussusception by hydrostatic pressure. Hydrostatic reduction has a success rate of approximately 75 per cent, the remaining children require immediate surgery. Surgery has the advantage of establishing underlying causes such as a Meckel diverticulum but such a cause is found in only 5 to 7 per cent. Recurrence is more frequent following barium enema reduction. A barium enema is useful in the diagnosis of chronic recurrent non-obstructive intussusception.

Intussusception: barium enema

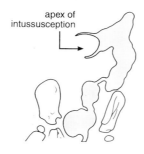

apex of intussusception

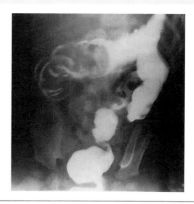

RECURRENT ABDOMINAL PAIN

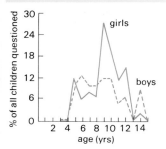

Age of 200 children with recurrent abdominal pain (Apley 1975)

This is a common problem affecting at least 10 per cent of school children. Although no organic cause is found in over 90 per cent, it is essential to identify those with an organic condition promptly. This enables specific management of the problem and confident counselling of children with functional disorders. The majority of children are adequately evaluated on the basis of a careful history and examination. The periodicity of the complaint, the absence of coexistent symptoms and intervening good health reinforce the innocence of the problem. Only a minority justify investigation beyond a blood count and a urinalysis; troublesome cases can be seen during attacks and may warrant additional investigations such as an abdominal ultrasound scan and upper gastrointestinal endoscopy.

Childhood migraine. Children who go on to have classical migraine commonly present with recurrent episodes of prolonged midline abdominal pain associated with nausea or vasomotor symptoms. A positive family history of migraine is an important clue.

Renal tract infection must be excluded by urine culture and microscopy. Loin pain in the absence of urinary abnormality may still be an indication for urinary tract ultrasound examination in case of hydronephrosis due to pelviureteric junction obstruction.

Peptic ulcers are now being diagnosed more often in children, partly as a consequence of the wider application of endoscopy. Sleep disturbance due to nocturnal epigastric pain is a useful clue and may be reinforced by a family history of peptic ulceration. *Helicobacter pylori*, a curved Gram negative micro-aerophilic bacterium, is a cause of gastritis and duodenal ulceration in children as well as adults. The recognition of this organism's role in the aetiology of peptic ulceration has shifted treatment strategy away from H_2-receptor antagonists in favour of schemes

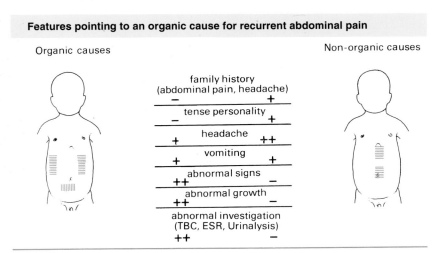

Features pointing to an organic cause for recurrent abdominal pain

Organic causes		Non-organic causes
	family history (abdominal pain, headache)	
−		+
	tense personality	
−		+
	headache	
+		++
	vomiting	
+		+
	abnormal signs	
++		−
	abnormal growth	
++		−
	abnormal investigation (TBC, ESR, Urinalysis)	
++		−

to eradicate *H. pylori*. The place of drug combinations such as colloidal bismuth subcitrate, metronidazole and amoxicillin has still to be evaluated in the young.

Chronic recurrent pancreatitis. Although rare, it may be suggested by a family history and by central abdominal pain radiating through to the back. Clinical suspicion is confirmed by finding calcification of the pancreas on abdominal X-ray.

GASTROENTERITIS

Diarrhoeal illness, frequently superimposed on malnutrition, extracts a terrifying toll from the world's children: at a conservative estimate 10 to 15 million deaths annually. WHO has committed itself to 'Health for All by the Year 2000', major targets being universal availability of safe water supplies and simple but life saving oral rehydration treatment. In the developed world gastroenteritis is common and usually mild but should not be underestimated particularly in vulnerable settings such as neonatal units.

Bacterial gastroenteritis

Bacteria interfere with mucosal integrity by direct invasion, by toxin release, or by adherence to and disruption of the enterocyte brush border. Groups of *E. coli* operate by all three mechanisms, the genetic determinants of virulence being carried in chromosomes or in plasmids. Gene probes are being developed to facilitate the laboratory identification of pathogenic *E. coli*.

Fever is common in bacterial gastroenteritis and in particular in Shigella infection where pyrexial convulsions and marked meningism may precede overt enteric symptoms. Food poisoning may arise due to the ingestion of the exotoxin produced by coagulase positive staphylococcus.

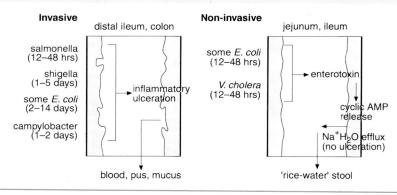

Bacterial gastroenteritis may be due either to invasive or non-invasive organisms

Viral gastroenteritis

In developed countries viral infection is responsible for 50 to 60 per cent of acute gastroenteritis in children under the age of 5 years. Rotavirus, a double stranded RNA virus, is the main agent responsible for winter epidemics of gastroenteritis. There are several different strains of Rotavirus, and of other agents for example Astroviruses, Caliciviruses, and this is an obstacle to the development of effective vaccines. Vomiting may be the only obvious presenting feature as diarrhoea may not occur for several hours and even then a watery stool is liable to be confused with urine in the wet napkins. Colicky abdominal pain with ill-defined tenderness and exaggerated bowel sounds is common. It is important to remember that vomiting and diarrhoea may be the presenting symptoms of surgical conditions, for example appendicitis, Hirschsprung disease and intussusception. They also result from non-gastrointestinal disorders such as upper respiratory tract infections, urine infections and meningitis.

Dehydration

The water loss associated with gastroenteritis places a relatively greater stress on the young infant for he has a higher percentage of body water (80 per cent at term and 60 per cent at 12 months), a higher metabolic rate and a larger surface area to volume ratio. The assessment of dehydration relies upon a series of clinical signs which reflect changes in body, tissues and circulatory status. The tissue changes are more easily recognised in thin than in overweight infants. A recent reliable weight is the best guide to body fluid loss. The clinical estimate indicates the percentage of the expected body weight which needs to be replaced, so that 10 per cent dehydration in a 5 kg infant indicates a replacement volume of 500 ml. It is also necessary to assess the type of dehydration: hypotonic, isotonic or hypertonic (also termed hypernatraemic when the serum sodium is above 150 mmol/l).

Features which differentiate isotonic and hypertonic dehydration

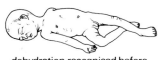

lethargic ; hypotonic ; depressed fontanelle : sunken eyes ; loss of skin turgor

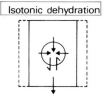

dehydration recognised before circulatory failure

Isotonic dehydration

Na⁺ and H₂0 loss in proportion

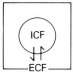

Normal

ICF

ECF

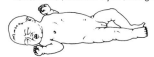

irritable ; hypertonic ; normal or full fontanelle ; normal eyes ; doughy skin

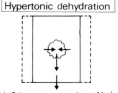

circulatory failure due to masking of dehydration

Hypertonic dehydration

H_2O loss greater than Na^+

Clinical assessment of dehydration

Sign	5% dehydration	10% dehydration
Skin	Loss of turgor	Mottled, Poor capillary return
Fontanelle	Depressed	Deeply depressed
Eyes	Sunken	Deeply sunken
Peripheral pulses	Normal	Tachycardia, poor volume
Mental state	Lethargic	Prostration, coma

Mild dehydration

Mild dehydration (*under 5 per cent*) can be treated in the home by a regimen of clear fluids for at least 24 hours, followed by the gradual reintroduction of a normal diet. There is now a range of formulations available based on the principle that oral rehydration therapy is considerably more efficient when glucose or sucrose is added to an electrolyte solution. In impoverished cultures effective rehydration solutions can be created using cheap local ingredients, for example salt and boiled rice water. It is essential to advise families how to use these solutions appropriately and to avoid unnecessarily prolonged use which places the child at risk of malnutrition.

Oral rehydration therapy

Formulation	UK mmol/L	WHO mmol/L
Na	30–50	90
K	20	20
Cl	30–50	80
citrate	10	10
glucose	200	100
	for use in UK to replace mild faecal electrolyte loss, reduced risk of hypernatraemia	for use in developing world to replace substantial faecal electrolyte loss, to be used in addition to water and milk

Maintenance requirements

Age (months)	H$_2$O (ml/kg)	Na (mmol/kg)	K (mmol/kg)
0-6	150	2.5	2.5
6-12	120	2.5	2.5
12-24	100	2.5	2.5
Over 24	80	2.0	2.0

Moderate to severe dehydration

Moderate to severe dehydration (*over 5 per cent*) requires intravenous therapy and this is especially urgent when there are signs of peripheral circulatory failure. Appropriate management demands an understanding of normal maintenance requirements as well as an assessment of the deficit. Acidosis may accompany dehydration and if severe is treated by providing about half the calculated deficit as sodium bicarbonate:

deficit (mmol) = weight (kg) $\times$ 0.3 $\times$ (24 − observed plasma bicarbonate mmol/l). Antibiotics are not indicated unless systemic spread of bacterial infection is likely. Anti-diarrhoeal agents should be avoided as they have a slow transit time and encourage the persistence of an abnormal bowel flora.

Principles of intravenous therapy

Total fluid requirements

maintenance	0.2 saline in 4.3% glucose plus KCl
+	
deficit	Normal saline plus KCl
+	
ongoing loss	Normal saline plus KCl

Scheme

$0-\frac{1}{2}$ hours	Treat shock immediately	Plasma or Normal saline 20 ml/kg
$\frac{1}{2}-4$ hours	Initial replacement	0.5 Normal or normal saline 10 ml/kg/h (awaiting serum electrolyte results)
4–24 hours	Continuing replacement	
	(a) Serum Na under 150 mmol/l	0.2 Normal saline in 4.3% glucose plus KCl 30–40 mmol/l plan correction in 24 hours
	(b) Serum Na above 150 mmol/l	0.2 Normal saline in 4.3% glucose plus KCl 30–40 mmol/l restrict fluid to 150 ml/kg in first 24 hours and plan total correction over 48 hours

Solutions	Na	K	(mmol/l) Ca	Cl	Lactate
Normal saline (0.9%)	150	—	—	150	—
0.5 N saline in 5% Dextrose	77	—	—	77	—
0.18% N saline in 4.0% Dextrose	30	—	—	30	—
Ringer's lactate solution (Hartmann's solution)	130	5	4	112	27

Complications

Post-gastroenteritis diarrhoea is relatively common in young infants. A short period of lactose-free milk may be required. Refractory cases require careful evaluation. Protracted diarrhoea may be due to secondary lactose intolerance, secondary cow's milk intolerance or bacterial overgrowth. The infant may suffer convulsions for a number of reasons including associated fever, hypo or hypernatraemia, hypoglycaemia or hypocalcaemia. Cerebral damage may follow hypotension or vascular thrombosis. Fluid overload can cause pulmonary oedema particularly if there is oliguria due to pre-renal failure or renal failure due to renal vein thrombosis or medullary necrosis.

MALABSORPTION

Enzymatic degradation of the major nutrients occurs within the gut lumen, at the microvilli and in the cytoplasm of the columnar epithelial cells. Disorders in the lumen may be due to failure of exocrine secretion, for example pancreatic insufficiency in cystic fibrosis, or disrupted bile salt circulation as in cholestatic liver disease. The mucosa may suffer non-specific epithelial damage in a variety of conditions, including coeliac disease and post-gastroenteritis. Other more specific inherited disorders interfere with individual pathways in the epithelium, for example primary congenital alactasia and familial chloride diarrhoea. Malabsorption may also occur due to obstruction of lymphatics in the intestinal wall as in congenital lymphangectasia.

Investigation of malabsorption is relatively complex and must not be initiated until it has been established that the child is failing to gain weight on a normal diet, does not have other systemic diseases and is being cared for in an adequate environment. Stool microscopy may reveal abundant fat globules. Quantitative measures of faecal fat are now largely redundant. Relevant investigations include a sweat test to exclude cystic fibrosis, and abdominal X-rays to rule out malrotation and other structural abnormalities. Intestinal endoscopy and biopsy are useful procedures in suitably selected patients.

Coeliac disease

Coeliac disease is the permanent inability to tolerate dietary wheat or rye gluten. Exposure to gluten results in morphological and functional abnormality of the proximal small intestine which can be reversed by exclusion of gluten. The incidence is about 1 in 2000 in the UK and as high as 1 in 300 in west Ireland. The susceptibility to coeliac disease is inherited but disease manifestation probably depends on early dietary and environmental factors. Breast feeding and delayed gluten exposure appear to be protective. There is a suggestion that human adenovirus 12 infection may trigger the disease. The adenovirus contains an amino acid sequence similar to a region of the gliadin molecule, a component of gluten, and may provoke immune cross-reactivity.

The majority of children with coeliac disease present before the age of two years. The weight record may show progressive growth failure dating from the introduction of gluten-containing solids. In a few, overt malabsorption may not occur for many years, and diagnosis only comes to light after recognition of late growth failure and delayed puberty. Positive IgA gliadin antibodies provide a useful if not entirely specific screening test for coeliac disease. A duodenal or jejunal biopsy is essential for definitive diagnosis, and is generally performed on two occasions

The clinical features of gluten enteropathy

failure to thrive
vomiting
diarrhoea
irritability
anorexia
anaemia
hypotonia
abdominal distension
wasted buttocks
rickets
delayed bone age
short stature
delayed puberty

Normal and abnormal jejunal mucosa

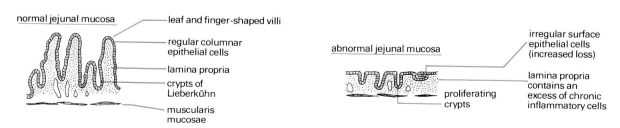

normal jejunal mucosa
— leaf and finger-shaped villi
— regular columnar epithelial cells
— lamina propria
— crypts of Lieberkühn
— muscularis mucosae

abnormal jejunal mucosa
— irregular surface epithelial cells (increased loss)
— lamina propria contains an excess of chronic inflammatory cells
— proliferating crypts

while the child is exposed to gluten before concluding that there is justification for a lifelong restricted diet. There are other causes of temporarily abnormal small intestinal mucosa including post-gastroenteritis and cow's milk protein intolerance. Children with coeliac disease usually show a prompt response when placed on a gluten free diet; parents certainly appreciate the improved mood. Gluten exposure may or may not result in early return of symptoms. Planned challenge prior to confirmatory biopsy may have to be continued for several months before mucosal changes occur. Dietary compliance becomes an increasing problem in adolescence, particularly in those who have few symptoms. There is still some dispute as to whether chronic gluten exposure and mucosal inflammation increases the likelihood of small intestinal lymphoma.

Sugar intolerance

Sugar intolerance results from failure to absorb particular sugars, most commonly lactose. The osmotic load of the undigested sugar results in explosive watery diarrhoea and the intraluminal fermentation produces an excess of lactic acid and carbon dioxide. The fluid stools are acid (pH less than 5.5) and contain reducing substances.

Lactose intolerance

Secondary lactose intolerence is common after gastroenteritis. It contributes to loose stools but is usually short-lived and does not result in significant malabsorption or necessitate major dietary adjustment. Severe or recurrent gastroenteritis, especially in malnourished infants, can damage the small intestinal mucosa and cause symptomatic lactase deficiency. Coeliac disease and cytotoxic therapy are other examples of gut insults that lead to secondary lactase deficiency. A diet has then to be designed which excludes lactose and replaces it with glucose or glucose polymers which are more readily absorbed. An attempt should be made to distinguish lactose intolerance from cow's milk protein intolerance although both conditions are treated by selecting a lactose-free soya milk.

Lactose intolerance also occurs in premature infants, as a rare inherited disorder in Caucasians (autosomal recessive), and as a frequent finding in non-Caucasians after early childhood (autosomal dominant).

Others

Sucrase–isomaltase deficiency can occur after severe mucosal damage or be inherited in an autosomal recessive mode.

Galactose–glucose malabsorption is extremely rare, and results in severe persistent diarrhoea from birth.

CHRONIC DIARRHOEA

Chronic non-specific diarrhoea

Persistent diarrhoea in a thriving child is a very common complaint. The most frequent explanation is an exaggerated gastrocolic reflex repeatedly provoked by frequent snacks and cold drinks. Simple measures such as restricting fluid intake to meal times obviates the need for antidiarrhoeal preparations of dubious therapeutic value.

Cow's milk protein intolerance

This is a mainly clinical diagnosis which is made when either acute or chronic symptoms appear to be related to cow's milk ingestion. Acute reactions after small amounts of milk include vomiting, diarrhoea, urticaria, stridor and bronchospasm, and when this happens the association with milk intake is fairly readily established. It is more difficult to confirm that chronic effects such as failure to thrive, rectal bleeding, anaemia and hepatosplenomegaly are due to a reaction to milk protein. Immunological studies indicate a variety of mechanisms. Susceptible infants may have enhanced absorption of antigenic quantities of lacto-globulin in early infancy and this may in turn be related to transient IgA deficiency or follow gastroenteritis. Jejunal biopsy shows variable villous flattening. The disorder is usually temporary and can be managed by dietary adjustments. Protein is given in the form of casein hydrolysate, chicken meat or soy protein.

Other food intolerance

Children may have clearly documented hypersensitivity to one or more foods, for example eggs and fish. More difficult are the claimed associations between a wide range of food substances and problems such as behavioural disturbance, headaches and even convulsions. While it is appropriate to conduct sensibly structured dietary trials, the doctor must ensure that the child is not exposed to unfounded, bizarre or deficient diets. Allergy to egg is not a contraindication to immunisation unless the child has had an anaphylactic reaction following food containing egg.

Acrodermatitis enteropathica

This is a rare autosomal recessive disorder linked to a defect of zinc metabolism. The infants develop severe diarrhoea and failure to thrive with a characteristic rash over the mucocutaneous junctions and pressure areas. There is also alopecia and nail dystrophy. The onset is delayed if the child is breast fed. Without appropriate therapy it is a fatal condition, and until the recognition of the value of zinc supplements the disease was controlled by the use of diodoquin.

Crohn disease

This is uncommon in children but the incidence appears to have increased over the last 30 years. The cause is unknown although both Crohn disease and ulcerative colitis occur more often within families than would be expected by chance. Lack of breast feeding and a higher frequency of diarrhoeal illnesses in infancy appear to be predisposing factors. Presenting features include recurrent abdominal pain, anorexia, growth failure, fever, diarrhoea, oral and perianal ulcers, and arthritis. Diagnosis is often delayed by confusion of the symptoms with functional complaints. Crohn disease should be considered in adolescents with suspected anorexia nervosa. Measurement of an acute phase reactant such as C-reactive protein or ESR help to screen for the disease.

The granulomatous involvement of the gut may be diffuse so that both upper and lower endoscopy with biopsy, as well as contrast studies of the bowel, play a part in assessment. The resulting malnutrition leads not only to growth failure but also aggravates the disease process. Energetic nutritional programmes based on elemental diets correct the growth failure and induce remission of active disease. This nutritional approach is at least as effective as corticosteroids, and avoids the hazard of iatrogenic growth impairment. There is a place for surgical resection of localised disease which either causes anatomical problems such as obstruction or which accounts for persisting growth failure.

Ulcerative colitis

Ulcerative colitis presents with diarrhoea containing visible blood and mucus. It is important to exclude an infectious cause for an initial presentation of colitis. The early episodes of ulcerative colitis may be intermittent and short-lived. Others produce more systemic upset with abdominal pain, weight loss, arthritis, and liver disturbance. Skin manifestations include erythema nodosum and pyoderma gangrenosum.

Colonoscopy with multiple mucosal biopsy is an invaluable tool for confirming the disease and assessing its extent. Although the disease may be limited to a proctosigmoiditis at outset, approximately 60 per cent of children will go on to have more extensive involvement of the colon.

Acute attacks of proctosigmoiditis are treated with topical corticosteroid preparations; enemas, foam or suppositories. More extensive disease requires oral or systemic corticosteroids with careful supervision because of the risks of fulminant colitis. Sulphasalazine or similar drugs are valuable for treating mild symptomatic disease and sustaining remission. Extensive refractory colitis may be an indication for immunosuppressant therapy with azathioprine or cyclosporin. The disruption of repeated episodes, poor nutrition, anaemia and drug side-effects may be such that colectomy is justified. There is also the cumulative risk of mucosal dysplasia and neoplasia. When colectomy is indicated, the procedure of choice is restorative proctocolectomy with ileal reservoir.

Food allergy colitis

Milk protein allergy can provoke colitis in infants and cause frankly blood-stained diarrhoea.

INTESTINAL PARASITES

In the developing world these provide a further threat to children's health and result in malabsorption, anaemia and chronic diarrhoea.

Giardia lamblia

Giardiasis is caused by ingestion of food or water contaminated by the cysts of this flagellate protozoan. It is endemic in most countries and prevalence is high in young and malnourished children. Host factors are important in determining whether the trophozoite form adheres to small intestinal mucosa and disrupts structure and absorptive function.

The clinical spectrum of infection ranges from asymptomatic cyst carriage to severe diarrhoea and malabsorption. Diagnosis can be confirmed by microscopy of stool, jejunal juice or intestinal biopsy. Metronidazole is the treatment of choice but treatment failure is common.

Enterobius (threadworm)

Enterobius is a frequent cause of perianal and vulval pruritis. The mobile thread-like worms are easily recognised on separating the buttocks of the sleeping child. They are difficult to eradicate and justify treatment only when symptomatic. The entire family must be treated with, for example, piperazine. Hygiene measures are also necessary to break the cycle of self-infection.

Ascaris lumbricoides

Roundworm infection follows ingestion of the eggs. The larvae migrate via the portal system to the lungs where they ascend the bronchial tree to re-enter the gut. Heavy infestation may result in pneumonitis and eosinophilia during the larval phase. Gut symptoms are rare but include pain, obstruction and appendicitis. Piperazine treats the adult phase.

Ankylostoma (hookworm)

Hookworm is a major cause of iron deficiency in hot, humid climates. Bephenium hydroxynaphthoate is an effective treatment.

Threadworm, roundworm, hookworm and toxocara

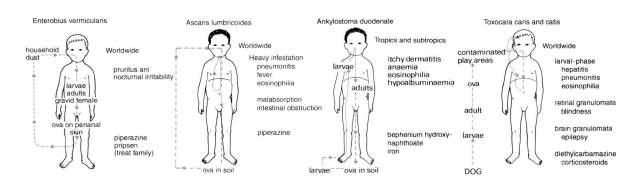

Toxocara canis and catis

Toxocara canis and catis may have their migratory larval phase in children who are in close contact with animal excreta. Infection produces eosinophilia, hepatomegaly and bronchospasm. The larvae may encapsulate in the eye producing retinal granulomata, or in the brain acting as potential epileptogenic foci.

Taenia

Taenia saginata (beef tapeworm) and Taenia solium (pork tapeworm). The adult worms inhabit the intestinal canal of man. It is also possible for man to be infected by the larval phase of T. solium as a result of consumption of inadequately cooked pork. The larvae or cysticerci may encapsulate and calcify in the tissues. The adult tapeworms may be killed by niclosamide.

CONSTIPATION

Constipation is a frequent complaint in all age groups and reflects a common obsession with regular bowel function. It is valid to differentiate the problem of infrequent hard stools from the less worrying complaint of infrequent normal stools. Healthy infants show a considerable variation in the pattern of bowel frequency depending on their diet, and indeed mother's diet if breast fed. They may also show alarming colour changes and vigorous abdominal contractions during defaecation which may be interpreted by mother as straining. Genuine hard stools may result from an inadequate milk intake, hunger stools, or from over strength artificial feeds where the free water is diverted to facilitate renal solute excretion. The change from an artificial milk formula or breast milk to cow's milk is accompanied by production of smaller, harder and less frequent stools. Their passage may require more effort and resulting anal irritation may provoke withholding, and a pattern of behaviour which can evolve into troublesome constipation. Constipation may accompany more generalised disorders but it is seldom the chief complaint. Hypothyroidism, idiopathic hypercalcaemia and neuro-muscular problems fall into this category.

In older children, acute constipation is a common accompaniment of febrile illnesses and the resulting hard stools may cause an anal tear which in turn initiates the cycle of faecal retention and chronic constipation. The prompt use of gentle laxatives and abundant fluids facilitates healing of the traumatised anal margin and helps the child to regain confidence in his toilet activities. It is sad that so many of these children are allowed to develop chronic constipation with all its attendant problems. These include abdominal pain, anorexia, vomiting, failure to thrive, and a predisposition to urinary tract infections. The accumulation of hard stool in the rectal ampulla leads to an acquired megacolon. The distension of the rectum results in relaxation of the internal sphincter so that the child must continually call on the external sphincter and the levator ani, which are voluntary muscle groups, in order to resist stool passage. Eventually this effort fails and the external sphincter is no longer able to prevent constant leakage of faecal matter. The soiling is often the

Chronic constipation

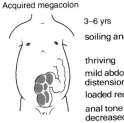

Acquired megacolon

3–6 yrs

soiling and constipation

thriving

mild abdominal distension

loaded rectum

anal tone decreased

soiling

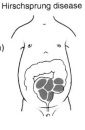

Hirschsprung disease

neonate	60–70%
later	30–40%

constipation (occasionally diarrhoea)

failure to thrive

gross abdominal distension

empty rectum

anal tone normal or increased

no soiling

dominant complaint and the families become desperate in their attempts to cope with this unsocial problem. Examination confirms the presence of the indentable faecal mass, the perianal soiling and the firm stool just within the internal sphincter.

Treatment requires an enthusiastic but relatively simple approach. The main objectives are to dislodge the faecal mass, overcome withholding behaviour and promote a regular bowel habit. Success revolves around the child regaining confidence in being capable of painless easy defaecation. A short course of a powerful liquid laxative is an effective means of dislodging the faecal mass. More refractory cases may require a brief course of enemas but the oral approach is more satisfactory for both child and therapist. This is followed by a programme of copious fluids, a high roughage diet and Senokot at a dosage sufficient to amplify the gastrocolic reflex. The child must learn to take advantage of the latter by spending 5 to 10 minutes on the toilet after breakfast and the evening meal. It is worth checking that the child has firm foot support so that he can obtain the optimal mechanical advantage while sitting on the toilet. The use of laxatives may cause the soiling to be worse during the initial period of treatment and parents must be warned about this. In most children, the physical and emotional problems improve in parallel with the recovery of normal bowel function. In a minority there are more profound behavioural problems which warrant a careful psychiatric evaluation.

Although chronic constipation can usually be overcome by this regimen, in some children the possibility of short segment Hirschsprung disease arises. If the problem persists in spite of anal dilatation under general anaesthetic, re-evaluation is necessary.

Hirschsprung disease

Hirschsprung disease must be considered if constipation presents in infancy. The incidence is 1 in 4500 live births. It accounts for about 10 per cent of neonatal intestinal obstruction, but it may also present in the older child. It results from failure of migration of ganglion cells to the submucosal and myenteric plexuses of the large bowel. The aganglionic segment, which remains tonically contracted and aperistaltic, invariably involves the internal sphincter. Sometimes there is a very short segment, but 80 per cent involve the recto-sigmoid colon and 15 per cent extend to the more proximal colon. In one large series 85 per cent developed difficulties in the first month of life and 95 per cent by the end of the first year.

The typical infant fails to pass meconium within the first 24 hours of life, develops progressive abdominal distension, refuses to feed and finally has bilious vomiting. A severe form of enterocolitis with perforation and septicaemia may complicate this picture and has a high mortality rate. The older child suffers with intermittent bouts of intestinal obstruction from faecal impaction, failure to thrive, hypochromic anaemia and hypoproteinaemia. Soiling is extremely unusual but not unknown in Hirschsprung disease. On examination, the upper abdomen is distended with gas as well as faeces, the costal margin is flared and the umbilicus is displaced downward. Characteristically, the anal canal and rectum are free of faeces and may feel narrow and grip the finger. The diagnosis may be confirmed by barium enema of an unprepared colon, rectal biopsy and ano-rectal manometry. The latter demonstrates an absence of the normal reflex inhibition of the internal anal sphincter on rectal distension. Surgical treatment often entails an initial colostomy to relieve the obstruction. The subsequent definitive operation is designed to bypass the aganglionic segment and bring the normal bowel down to the anus.

Surgical approaches to Hirschsprung disease

Swenson

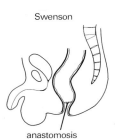

anastomosis

Duhamel

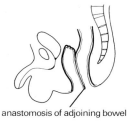

anastomosis of adjoining bowel

Soave

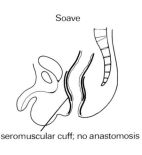

seromuscular cuff; no anastomosis

LIVER DISEASE

Hepatomegaly

Liver disease presents with hepatomegaly, jaundice, metabolic disturbance or haemorrhagic problems either singly or in combination. The normal liver has a soft, smooth, non-tender edge 1 to 2 cm below the costal margin. An enlarged liver may be a transient finding accompanying acute disorders like infectious hepatitis or glandular fever, or it may be long-standing, requiring detailed investigation.

Persistent neonatal jaundice

Jaundice persisting beyond the second week is abnormal and in considering the possible cause, a distinction must be made between conjugated and unconjugated hyperbilirubinaemia.

Breast milk jaundice. Breast milk jaundice is a relatively uncommon problem, and may be due to a complex steroid in the milk which inhibits hepatic glucuronyl transferase. It is seldom necessary to advise against breast feeding in this condition as it resolves spontaneously. It is often confused with jaundice due to fluid deprivation.

Prolonged neonatal jaundice

Crigler-Najjar syndrome. Crigler-Najjar syndrome is a rare, autosomal recessive condition in which hepatic glucuronyl transferase is deficient or absent. The most severe form causes neonatal kernicterus and is

Causes of persistent neonatal jaundice

Unconjugated hyperbilirubinaemia	Conjugated hyperbilirubinaemia

Infection, e.g. urinary tract
Hypothyroidism
Haemolytic anaemia
High gastrointestinal obstruction
Breast-milk jaundice
Transient familial hyperbilirubinaemia
Crigler-Najjar syndrome
	(a) Neonatal hepatitis syndrome
	    Congenital infection, e.g. rubella,
	    cytomegalovirus, toxoplasmosis
	    Metabolic
	    α_1-antitrypsin deficiency
	    Galactosaemia
	    Tyrosinosis
	    Cystic fibrosis
	    Storage disorders
	(b) Duct obstruction or obliteration
	    Extrahepatic biliary atresia
	    Intrahepatic biliary hypoplasia
	    Choledochal cyst

incompatible with life. A milder variety may respond to long term phototherapy.

Neonatal hepatitis. Neonatal hepatitis is not a discrete entity but is the end result of a range of injurious processes which produce a similar histological picture, hepatocellular necrosis and inflammatory cell infiltrates in the portal tracts and lobules. Infants with conjugated hyperbilirubinaemia must be investigated for the known infective, genetic and metabolic causes, and it has to be appreciated that neonatal hepatitis is part of a spectrum of hepatic injury which overlaps with biliary atresia.

Biliary atresia. Biliary atresia is an acquired condition of early post-natal life in which a previously patent biliary tree becomes sclerosed. Without surgical intervention to re-establish bile drainage, cirrhosis and a fatal outcome are inevitable. It affects approximately 1 in 14 000 infants and is the single most common cause of childhood liver related death in the UK. The cause of the inflammatory process remains unknown. All infants with persistent jaundice must have their stool colour checked; pale stools suggest obstructive jaundice. The child may be thriving and without conspicuous hepatomegaly but can still be at risk of developing biliary cirrhosis unless prompt diagnosis and surgery is provided. Diagnosis is based on finding conjugated hyperbilirubinaemia, elevated transaminases, an absent gall bladder on ultrasound imaging, and a supportive needle liver biopsy. Tests to exclude the recognised causes of neonatal hepatitis are also performed but it is important that a decision regarding surgery is reached promptly and preferably before age 60 days. Bile drainage is created by anastomosing the porta hepatis to a Roux-en-Y loop of jejunum, a hepatic portoenterostomy or Kasai procedure. 60–70 per cent of those operated on before 60 days become jaundice-free, this figure falls to 25–35 per cent if surgery is later. Long-term survival depends on the status of liver fibrosis and cirrhosis. An increasing proportion are having good quality survival into adult life. Others develop portal hypertension or progressive liver failure. Liver transplantation is now a realistic option for children who fail to benefit from initial surgery.

Alpha$_1$-antitrypsin deficiency is an important cause of neonatal heptatitis. The deficiency is associated with PiZ or Pi nul phenotypes of protease inhibitor. It is unclear why deficiency in some families manifests as liver disease while in others it predisposes to emphysema in early adult life. There is a spectrum of severity of liver involvement from subclinical hepatitis through to severe cholestasis and cirrhosis. As yet there is no specific treatment but attempts are underway to genetically engineer replacement therapy. Genetic counselling must advise heterozygote parents of a 25 per cent risk of recurrence. Gene probing directed at a fragment of chromosome 14 is available.

Infectious hepatitis

Hepatitis A (incubation 15 to 50 days). Hepatitis A infection is the commonest cause of jaundice in older children. It spreads by the oral route and is usually mild or subclinical. Anorexia, fever, vomiting and abdominal pain may precede the jaundice. Elevation of serum transaminase levels is the first biochemical abnormality and they remain raised for up to three weeks in most cases. Passive immunisation with pooled immunoglobulin provides protection and may be indicated for family and other close contacts. Hepatitis A-specific IgM is the best single marker of recent infection.

Hepatitis B (incubation 50 to 180 days). Hepatitis B is uncommon in European children, but infection and chronic carrier status are frequent in developing countries. Vertical transmission from carrier mothers to newborn babies is a major route of spread, and contributes to a new generation of chronic carriers. Infected infants are seldom symptomatic but are vulnerable to cirrhosis and hepatocellular carcinoma. Programmes to protect infants with combined passive and active immunisation schedules are now established.

Non-A, non-B hepatitis. This diagnostic category is being further defined as new immunological markers are identified. Hepatitis C is transmitted by blood products and provokes chronic liver disease. Infectious mononucleosis and cytomegalovirus also cause acute hepatitis.

Reye syndrome

Reye syndrome is a relatively rare but important disorder characterised by acutely disturbed liver and brain function. The liver involvement is not an inflammatory process as in acute hepatitis, but is a disruption of mitochondrial integrity and function which results in metabolic problems, notably hypoglycaemia and hyperammonaemia. Liver biopsy reveals a diffuse microvesicular fatty infiltration. Cerebral function is also disturbed and there is a threat of progressive cerebral oedema with altered consciousness and convulsions. Reye syndrome is a convenient term for this pattern of illness, but it probably represents a variety of interreactions between genetic susceptibility and environmental insults. Patients may have inherited disorders of mitochondrial function, for example errors of the urea-cycle, or fatty acid transport and oxidation.

Various viral illnesses have been identified as triggers. Epidemiological and experimental evidence has also incriminated aspirin as a causative factor, and hence the decision to withdraw product licences for salicylates in children.

Particular attention must be paid to children who present with refractory vomiting, reduced consciousness and convulsions. Low blood glucose, elevated plasma ammonia, high liver transaminases and prolonged coagulation raise the possibility of Reye syndrome or allied metabolic disorders. Management must be within an intensive care setting with facilities for ventilation and control of raised intracranial pressure. Effectively managed, Reye syndrome is a self-limiting condition but there is a high mortality and many survivors are handicapped.

Chronic hepatitis

Chronic liver inflammation is caused by a wide range of congenital disorders and environmental insults. We have already dealt with important early disorders such as congenital infection and alpha-1–antitrypsin deficiency. In a world-wide context hepatitis B and possibly C generate a vast amount of chronic liver disease. In older children other causes include autoimmune chronic active hepatitis, sclerosing cholangitis usually associated with chronic inflammatory bowel disease, Wilson disease, drugs, and biliary obstruction. The chronic inflammation carries the threat of progressive fibrosis, disruption of liver architecture and cirrhosis. The progress of the liver damage may be highlighted by chronic jaundice or ill-health, but it can also be an insidious process which only comes to light when the child presents with bleeding problems, splenomegaly, ascites or growth failure.

Autoimmune chronic hepatitis

This is predominantly a disease of older children and young adults with females accounting for over 70 per cent. Genetic susceptibility is linked to HLA antigens B8 DR3, but the environmental trigger that causes a cellular immune reaction against liver cell specific antigens has yet to be established. It may present as an apparent acute hepatitis, or more gradually with intermittent fever, acneiform rashes, colitis, arthritis and hepatosplenomegaly. Elevated liver transaminases and hyper-gammaglobulinaemia are characteristic, and autoantibodies are usually positive. The prothrombin time is usually prolonged. Formal diagnosis hinges on the liver biopsy which shows widening of the portal tracts with chronic inflammatory cell infiltrate, and destruction of the limiting plate at the junction of portal tracts and parenchyma together with hepatocyte necrosis. Immunosuppressant therapy is indicated in order to relieve symptoms and to delay the progression to cirrhosis. Recommended regimens incorporate prednisolone and azathioprine, with repeat liver biopsy to determine whether remission has been achieved. Long-term follow-up is necessary as there is a high risk or relapse.

Wilson disease

Wilson disease (hepatolenticular degeneration) is a rare, autosomal recessive disorder of copper metabolism which can readily escape prompt diagnosis. The classically described features of copper deposition at the peripheries of the cornea (Kayser–Fleischer rings), neurological problems, and a low caeruloplasmin may be absent in the young. Children can present with either acute or chronic hepatitis, deteriorating school performance, haemolytic anaemia, proteinuria or arthralgia. Liver problems typically present before neurological complaints, and unfortunately acute liver failure or cirrhosis may determine the prognosis. Wilson disease needs to be considered in any child with otherwise unexplained acute or chronic hepatitis. Investigations include plasma caeruloplasmin measurement, liver biopsy with copper estimation, and studies of urinary copper excretion. Diagnosis before irreversible tissue damage allows for a good response to treatment with penicillamine which promotes urinary clearance of copper ions. Liver transplantation is an option for patients who present too late to benefit from chelation therapy. Genetic counselling and screening of siblings is essential.

Childhood cirrhosis

Cirrhosis may evolve as the end stage of recognised liver disease, or may already be established at first presentation with portal hypertension or liver failure. The liver failure may lead to sudden deterioration, or may be more gradual with growth impairment, intermittent ascites and a coagulation disorder. Children can tolerate cirrhosis for years, sustaining adequate growth and a nearly normal lifestyle. Investigations should be aimed at identifying the underlying cause but this cannot be defined in a substantial proportion of cases. The degree of liver dysfunction needs to be assessed so that steps can be taken to correct reversible problems such as malnutrition, vitamin deficiency, ascites and electrolyte imbalance. Attention to these factors can considerably delay the final liver decompensation. Liver transplantation is now a realistic option for the management of these children with one year survival in the region of 70 to 80 per cent and promising long-term results. The difficulty is recognising when a child's quality of life has deteriorated to the extent that justifies this major step and the ensuing dependence on immunosuppressant therapy.

Causes and clinical features of cirrhosis in childhood

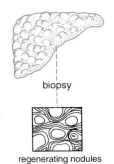

CAUSES

Genetic (metabolic/storage) cirrhosis
e.g. α₁-antitrypsin deficiency
    Wilson disease
    galactosaemia
    cystic fibrosis

Post-necrotic cirrhosis
e.g. neonatal hepatitis
    chronic aggressive hepatitis
    drugs, toxins, poisons
    venous congestion

Biliary cirrhosis
e.g. extrahepatic biliary atresia
    intrahepatic biliary hypoplasia
    choledochal cyst

biopsy

regenerating nodules
broad bands of fibrosis

CLINICAL FEATURES

Portal hypertension
    oesophageal varices
    splenomegaly
    hypersplenism
    ascites

Hepatic failure
    failure to thrive
    fatigue, anorexia
    spider naevi
    finger clubbing
    liver palms

Portal hypertension

This usually presents as intestinal bleeding and splenomegaly, but the spleen may not be palpable immediately after a severe haemorrhage.

The majority of cases are due to thrombosis of the portal vein; either idiopathic or secondary to sepsis of the umbilical vein and portal system in infancy. Hepatic cirrhosis and congenital hepatic fibrosis may also cause portal hypertension. The exact cause needs to be established by selective angiography of the coeliac axis and by a liver biopsy. If portal vein thrombosis is diagnosed, the long-term management should be as conservative as possible as splenorenal shunts are technically difficult and seldom successful before the age of 10 years. There is a tendency for bleeding from the oesophageal varices to improve with age.

Congenital hepatic fibrosis   Congenital hepatic fibrosis may be either sporadic or familial and is diagnosed by liver biopsy which shows marked portal fibrosis but retention of the normal hepatic lobular architecture. It may be associated with polycystic disease of the kidneys.

Causes of hepatomegaly and clinical signs which may aid diagnosis

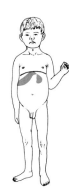

Causes

- Systemic infection
  infectious hepatitis
  glandular fever
- Primary liver disease
  chronic hepatitis
  polycystic disease
  hepatocellular carcinoma
- Other neoplasia
  leukaemia
  reticulosis
  nephroblastoma
  neuroblastoma
- Metabolic storage
  glycogenoses
  lipidoses
  mucopolysaccharidoses
- Cardiac

Signs

mental retardation
  mucopolysaccharidoses

Kayser-Fleischer rings:
  Wilson disease

spider naevi:
liver palms:
finger clubbing
  chronic liver failure

splenomegaly
collateral veins
ascites
  portal hypertension

bone lesions
  lipidoses

LIVER ENZYME DEFICIENCIES

Glycogen storage diseases   Enzyme deficiencies with their resulting disorders have been recognised for each of the steps in the pathways of glycogen synthesis and degradation. They enter into the differential diagnosis of recurrent hypoglycaemia, hepatomegaly, muscle weakness with cramps, and congestive cardiac failure.

Type I: Glucose-6-phosphatase deficiency is a serious disorder, usually presenting in infancy, and manifest by hepatomegaly, hypoglycaemia and a metabolic acidosis. The enzyme deficiency prevents the normal glycaemic response to intramuscular glucagon and can be confirmed by liver biopsy. Frequent glucose feeds and restriction of galactose and fructose intake are helpful in treatment.

Type III: Debranching enzyme deficiency and type VI: liver phosphorylase deficiency present in a similar although milder fashion and can be diagnosed by measurement of leucocyte enzyme levels.

Type II: Acid maltase deficiency (Pompe disease) results in excessive glycogen deposition in both liver and muscle, with cardiac muscle especially involved. The majority of affected infants present soon after birth with poor feeding, weakness, tachypnoea and cardiac failure. Muscle or leucocyte enzyme analysis confirms the diagnosis but treatment is supportive only and the child will survive only for a matter of months.

Galactosaemia

Galactosaemia is a very rare, recessively inherited disorder but its importance lies in the disastrous consequences of its being overlooked. It results from deficiency of the enzyme, galactose-l-phosphate uridyl transferase, which is essential for galactose metabolism. Affected infants are normal at birth but shortly after the commencement of milk feeds the majority develop jaundice, vomiting, diarrhoea, and fail to thrive. If the disorder remains unrecognised liver disease, cataracts and mental retardation will result. The urine contains galactose and is characteristically Clinitest positive but Clinistix negative, the latter being specific for glucose. Specific enzymatic techniques confirm the diagnosis and establish the necessity of a lactose-free diet.

Hereditary fructose intolerance

This is another rare enzyme deficiency in which prompt recognition can prevent the onset of life-threatening complications. The low activity of aldolase B not only results in the accumulation of fructose-l-phosphate but also causes a secondary inhibition of hepatic pathways responsible for maintaining normoglycaemia. In susceptible children, fructose-containing foods provoke abdominal pain, nausea, vomiting and symptoms of hypoglycaemia. In the longer term hepatomegaly, growth failure and liver failure occur. A detailed dietary history reveals normal health until the introduction of sucrose into the diet, and suspicion may be substantiated by a fructose tolerance test or by liver enzyme analysis. Therapy involves the elimination of all fructose containing items from the diet.

Benign fructosuria

Benign or essential fructosuria is an asymptomatic deficiency of the enzyme fructokinase.

BIBLIOGRAPHY

Milla P J, Muller D P R 1988 Harries' paediatric gastroenterology. Churchill Livingstone, Edinburgh
Mowat A P 1987 Liver disorders in childhood, 2nd edn. Butterworths, London
Tripp J H, Candy D C A 1985 Manual of paediatric gastroenterology. Churchill Livingstone, Edinburgh

Urinary Tract and Testes

Renal function undergoes a major transition with the onset of extra-uterine life and the demands of water conservation and electrolyte homeostasis. Although nephron formation is complete before birth the newborn kidney contains less than 20 per cent of its adult cellular component, and the total renal blood flow is reduced due to higher renal vascular resistance. The glomerular filtration rate at term averages 20 ml per minute per 1.73 m^2 with adult values only being reached in the second year of life. The functional limitations of the newborn kidney are reflected in higher blood urea and phosphate levels, and a lower plasma bicarbonate concentration.

The higher metabolic rate of the infant in relation to body weight, greater insensible water losses and the inability to control oral intake, increase the susceptibility of young patients to dehydration and metabolic abnormalities. Acute renal failure with acidosis, uraemia and hyperkalaemia can develop very rapidly in the young infant.

RENAL FUNCTION TESTS

Urinalysis. A multiple urine test strip can be employed and it is preferable to examine a fresh morning sample of urine.

Proteinuria. This can signify renal disease but transient proteinuria is also common during febrile illnesses or after exercise. Heavy proteinuria with oedema suggests nephrotic syndrome.

Postural or orthostatic proteinuria is suggested by the absence of significant proteinuria on a first morning specimen compared to one tested after the child has been ambulant. Measurements of proteinuria on 24 hour urine collections have now been replaced by measuring protein to creatinine ratios on spot urine samples (normal ratio <20 mg/mmol).

Haematuria. Microscopic haematuria may also be a transient finding but macroscopic haematuria always requires further investigation. The commonest cause is urinary tract infection. Microscopy of fresh urine

Urinary output (ml/day)	
infant	250–600
child	500–1000
adolescent	500–1500
adult	500–2000

should always be performed to confirm the presence of red blood cells rather than a false positive test due to free haemoglobin, myoglobin, beeturia, drugs or confectionary dyes.

Glycosuria and aminoaciduria. Glycosuria and aminoaciduria may be secondary to elevated serum levels or may be the result of tubular defects.

Urine pH and osmolality. Normal urine pH is between 5 and 7 and is affected by dietary intake. Formal acidification tests may be required if renal tubular acidosis is suspected. A first morning urine sample after fasting overnight provides a useful screening test of renal concentrating ability with normal values being above 800 mOsm per kg (specific gravity above 1.020).

Nitrite and leucocyte tests. Many test strips now incorporate nitrite detection which can indicate the presence of urinary infection when nitrate is reduced to nitrite. Leucocytes may also indicate infection but false positive and negative tests do occur.

Microscopy. This may give useful information especially in the presence of proteinuria or haematuria. Fresh urine should also be used when examining for casts. Red blood cell casts suggest glomerulonephritis. The presence of increased white blood cells, above 5 per high powered field, or motile bacteria suggest urinary tract infection. The latter needs confirmation by urine culture.

Blood tests. These will include full blood count, electrolytes including bicarbonate, urea, creatinine, calcium, phosphate, alkaline phosphatase and albumin. Urea levels can be effected by dehydration, protein meals and drug therapy so plasma creatinine levels are favoured for monitoring renal function. However, it should be remembered that the plasma creatinine can remain within the normal range until the glomerular filtration rate is less than 50 per cent of normal.

Glomerular filtration rate (GFR). Derived from 24 hour urine volume and measurement of plasma creatinine, this is very liable to error in young children because of difficulty of collection techniques. The approximate GFR can be derived from the plasma creatinine using the equation: GFR/1.73 m^2 surface area = 38 × height (cm)/plasma creatinine (μmol/l). The rate of fall in the blood concentration of injected isotope, chromium-51 EDTA or ^{99}Tc-DTPA is used for more precise measurement.

Radiological investigations. Ultrasound is now the investigation of choice for urinary tract problems with the intravenous urogram (IVU) being reserved for when further details of the urinary tract are required. The micturating cystourethrogram (MCUG) is still required to exclude reflux or lower urinary tract obstruction. Increasing use is made of radionuclide investigations such as DMSA (to define scars from

Urine microscopy

red blood cells   white blood cells

hyaline casts   epithelial cells

crystals   bacteria

vesicoureteric reflux and differential function) or ^{99}Tc-DTPA (to define obstruction and as an indirect method for following reflux).

URINARY TRACT MALFORMATIONS

These are relatively common but most are functionally insignificant, for example duplex systems. A small proportion are lethal and may have important genetic implications. The increased use of ultrasound in pregnancy has resulted in renal malformations being diagnosed more frequently *in utero*. Fortunately most abnormalities are unilateral. Intervention techniques to relieve fetal obstructive uropathy are under investigation but initial results have been disappointing.

Renal agenesis. This results in oligohydramnios and compression of the fetus, Potter syndrome. Other urinary tract malformations such as polycystic kidneys or obstructive lesions may also cause oligohydramnios. The degree of the associated pulmonary hypoplasia is critical to early survival.

Unilateral renal hypoplasia and dysplasia. This may be an incidental finding but a large multicystic dysplastic kidney may present as an abdominal mass in a newborn infant. Differentiation from hydronephrosis is important. The function of the apparently normal contralateral kidney must be carefully assessed as part of the evaluation.

Polycystic kidneys. Infantile polycystic disease results in grossly enlarged spongy kidneys and cystic changes in the liver and other viscera. The bilateral kidney enlargement is conspicuous at birth or in early infancy. There are several varieties with an autosomal recessive inheritance. The adult form, with autosomal dominant inheritance, can also present in early life although most survive to be young adults and are therefore capable of transmitting the abnormal gene.

Potter syndrome

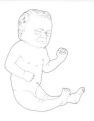

epicanthic folds
broad flattened nose
floppy, flow set ears
receding chin
pulmonary hypoplasia
urogenial system defects
leg deformities

Renal tract anomalies causing obstruction

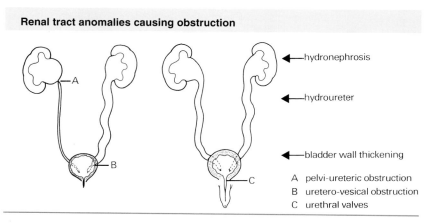

hydronephrosis
hydroureter
bladder wall thickening

A   pelvi-ureteric obstruction
B   uretero-vesical obstruction
C   urethral valves

Serous cysts. These are very common in adults and have to be distinguished from cancers, but they are rare in childhood. They appear to be an acquired condition.

Obstructive malformations These produce unilateral or bilateral hydronephrosis.

Pelviureteric junction (PUJ) obstruction. PUJ obstruction is the commonest cause of hydronephrosis and may be produced by intrinsic stenosis, functional obstruction or compression from an aberrant artery or bands. Treatment for PUJ obstruction is by pyeloplasty.

Vesicoureteric junction (VUJ) obstruction produces megaureters. Treatment is by reimplantation of the ureter which often requires tapering at its lower end.

Horseshoe kidney

Horseshoe kidneys. Horseshoe kidneys produce a characteristic IVU picture — the upper poles are further from the midline than the lower poles. Hydronephrosis due to PUJ obstruction may occur.

Ureteric duplication. The bifid ureter is more common than complete duplication. Usually there is a strong family history of this abnormality. When the ureters enter the bladder separately the ureter draining the upper renal moiety is situated in a lower position or maybe ectopic. Since it has a longer intravesical course it is liable to become obstructed resulting in hydronephrosis of the upper pole. The ureter draining the lower moiety has a short intravesical course and is therefore prone to vesico-ureteric reflux resulting in chronic pyelonephritis of the lower pole.

Ureteric duplications

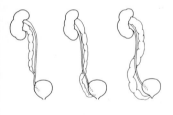

Ureterocoele. Ureterocoele is an expanded end of either a normally situated ureter or one which enters the bladder ectopically. It affects girls more than boys and the abnormality may appear as a filling defect of the bladder. Occasionally it can prolapse through the bladder neck and may appear as a mass in the vagina.

Urethral valves

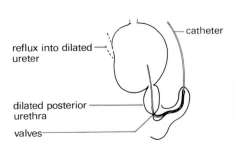
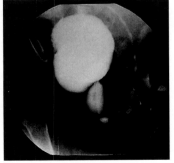

Posterior urethral valves. Posterior urethral valves are the commonest cause of lower urinary tract obstruction in the male child. The diagnosis may be made on antenatal ultrasound or postnatally on routine examination of a healthy neonate who has a distended bladder with a poor urinary stream. Otherwise infants may present with a urinary infection and septicaemia, or overflow incontinence in later years. The kidneys show secondary bilateral hydronephrosis due to obstruction and/or vesicoureteric reflux. Diagnosis is by MCUG and treatment is by ablation of valves via endoscopy. Temporary diversion is rarely necessary. Chronic renal failure can develop at any age and reflects the degree of renal dysplasia and residual renal mass.

Bladder exstrophy. This results from failure of midline fusion of the infra-umbilical midline structures. Males are affected more commonly than females. Clinically, the bladder mucosa is present as a small contracted circular plaque in the low abdomen, the umbilicus is abnormally low, the penis up-turned and epispadic, the pubic bones unfused and the lower limbs therefore apparently externally rotated. In girls the genital tract is normal although vaginal stenosis may need surgery in early adult life. Bladder and especially bladder neck reconstruction is extremely difficult and many children are treated by urinary diversion.

Urachal remnants may persist producing blind tracts or cysts in the lower abdominal wall. Complete patency between the bladder and umbilicus is exceptionally rare.

Prune belly syndrome. This occurs almost exclusively in males and is a triad of deficiency of abdominal muscles, complex genito-urinary malformation and bilateral undescended testes. Pulmonary hypoplasia may prove fatal in the newborn period but other less affected children can survive with appropriate therapy.

URINARY TRACT INFECTIONS

This is a common and important paediatric problem because it is a significant cause of morbidity in childhood. Association with vesicoureteric reflux may lead to renal damage (reflux nephropathy) which can give rise to hypertension and end stage renal disease in late childhood or adult life. Approximately 2–3 per cent of girls and less than 1 per cent of boys are at risk of asymptomatic urine infections throughout childhood. Proven bacterial infections warrant further investigation and this needs to be more comprehensive in pre-school children who are most at risk of developing renal scars.

The younger the child the more non-specific the symptoms. In the newborn prolonged jaundice, excessive weight loss or a septicaemic episode may be secondary to urinary tract infection. The young child may also present with poor weight gain, irritability, fever, vomiting and diarrhoea. In any septicaemic infant suprapubic aspiration of the urine should be considered a routine part of the infection screen, along with blood cultures and lumbar puncture. Otherwise every effort should be made to obtain a proper clean catch urine. Positive urine cultures based on bag specimens are often misleading.

Organisms derived from bowel flora are the commonest infecting agents. Some individuals are more prone to urinary tract infections than others and this may be associated with abnormal Gram negative bacterial colonisation of the introitus and periurethral areas. Studies showing increased adherence to uroepithelial cells by pyelonephritogenic bacteria may allow improved preventative measures in the future.

Management. Management of acute infection includes copious fluids, mild analgesia if required, and antibacterial therapy; septicaemia or acute pyelonephritis merits intravenous ampicillin, gentamicin or a cephalosporin. Oral therapy for less severe cases includes trimethoprim, amoxycillin, nalidixic acid, nitrofurantoin or a cephalosporin. A 7 to 10 day course of chemotherapy is usually sufficient and a sterile urine should be obtained following treatment. Prophylaxis with bedtime administration of antibiotics is generally continued until investigations are complete.

All proven urinary tract infections require radiological evaluation. Initially this is an ultrasound which is often combined with a plain abdominal X-ray to show details of the spine and exclude renal calculi. Children under 2 years of age are investigated further with an MCUG to rule out vesicoureteric reflux with which renal scarring and damage may be associated. The MCUG is only performed in older children if pyelonephritis is strongly suspected, or if there is a history of repeated urinary tract infections or renal problems in relatives. Reflux can be a familial problem. It is therefore justified to screen other family members (usually by ultrasound alone) when gross reflux is present in one child. If moderate to severe reflux is detected then any associated scarring of the kidneys can be documented by DMSA scanning.

Grades of vesicoureteric reflux during micturating cystogram

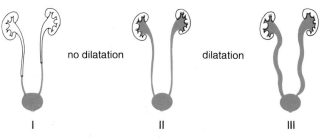

no dilatation   dilatation

I   II   III

no or little risk of renal damage   increased risk of renal damage

The presence of vesicoureteric reflux warrants continuous prophylaxis with antimicrobial agents such as trimethoprim (2 mg/kg/single dose) or nitrofurantoin (2 mg/kg/single dose). Previously many of these children were subjected to surgery for reimplantation of the ureters, but since reflux will cease spontaneously in a large number of children maintained on prophylactic therapy alone, surgery is now generally restricted to cases of urinary obstruction, or to children with 'breakthrough' urinary infections while on prophylaxis.

Drugs commonly used in the treatment of urinary tract infection

Drug	Dose	Comments	Side effects
Trimethoprim	4 mg/kg/day	Useful in prophylaxis. Good compliance	Rashes, vomiting
Amoxycillin	20 mg/kg/day	Less useful in prophylaxis	Rashes, diarrhoea
Nitrofurantoin	3.5 mg/kg/day	Useful in prophylaxis	Nausea, vomiting
Nalidixic acid	50 mg/kg/day	Useful in boys with proteus infection	Rashes
Cephradine	50 mg/kg/day	Less useful in prophylaxis	Allergic reactions
Gentamicin	2 mg/kg/day	Parenteral use only	Nephrotoxic, ototoxic

It is important to emphasise general preventive measures in all children with urinary tract infection. These include a regular bowel habit, adequate fluids, proper voiding techniques and double micturition, good hygiene and the avoidance of irritants such as bubble baths and nylon underwear.

Older children may complain of an urethral syndrome with frequency and dysuria and no bacteriological confirmation of urine infection. Viral infections may play a role but acute vulvitis or balanitis may be associated with poor hygiene, perineal candidiasis or contact sensitivity to nylon pants.

Sexual abuse should also be borne in mind in a child with recurrent urinary tract symptoms, especially with genital signs.

Screening. Extensive surveys have attempted to monitor the impact of detection, investigation and treatment of asymptomatic bacteriuria in schoolgirls aged 5 to 12 years. The results suggest that such screening is not worthwhile and that kidney damage associated with infection generally occurs before 5 years. Screening the preschool child is time consuming and the yield of treatable abnormalities is small.

HAEMATURIA

Haematuria may occur as an isolated symptom or may be accompanied by signs of a systemic disorder, for example Henoch Schönlein purpura or acute glomerulonephritis. It may be associated with renal colic due to clot, calculus, or obstructive malformation, or a loin mass, for example Wilms tumour or hydronephrosis. Red cell casts and significant proteinuria establish glomerular lesions while pyuria and bacteriuria point to infection, the latter being the commonest cause for haematuria in childhood. An abdominal ultrasound or IVU is indicated if renal tract pathology is suspected. Cystoscopy is seldom required unless the blood staining is prominent at the start or finish of the stream. Renal biopsy is reserved for children whose haematuria is persistent, and accompanied by significant proteinuria, hypertension or impaired renal function. Fictitious haematuria may be part of the syndrome of Munchhausen by proxy where blood is added to the child's urine by a close relative.

Causes of haematuria with examples

Infection	bacteria, viruses, tuberculosis, schistosomiasis
Trauma	
Glomerulonephritis	post-streptococcal, mesangial IgA nephropathy
Calculus	
Congenital abnormality	hydronephrosis due to pelviureteric obstruction
Tumour	Wilms tumour
Vascular	arteritis, infarction
Bleeding disorder	
Drug induced	cyclophosphamide
Exercise induced	
Fictitious	

Recurrent or persistent haematuria. Recurrent macroscopic haematuria exacerbated by upper respiratory tract infections suggests IgA nephropathy or Berger disease. Some healthy children with persistent microscopic haematuria and similar findings in other family members fall into the category of benign familial haematuria. A positive family history of nephritis in association with sensorineural nerve deafness suggests Alport syndrome which is X-linked, and boys with this condition tend to be affected more severely than girls. Longer term follow up of patients with recurrent haematuria suggests that there may be more morbidity than previously suspected.

Acute haemorrhagic cystitis. This may occur with viral infection, notably adenovirus 11, or as a complication of cyclophosphamide therapy.

ACUTE NEPHRITIC SYNDROME

Post-streptococcal glomerulonephritis

Acute glomerulonephritis occurs predominantly in schoolchildren. Although it characteristically occurs 7 to 14 days after a group A β-haemolytic streptococcal throat infection, an increasing percentage appear to have another, possibly viral explanation. In areas of the world with poor hygiene, glomerulonephritis following streptococcal skin infection with pyoderma is relatively common. Only certain serotypes of streptococcus are responsible and the detection of streptococcal antigen in the glomerular mesangium supports the concept of acute soluble complex injury. Reduced serum complement levels also indicate an immunological pathogenesis.

Many affected children are asymptomatic. Typical complaints include malaise, headache, and vague loin discomfort but it may be the smoky urine which at first causes alarm. Oedema tends to collect around the orbits and on the backs of the hands and feet. Urine microscopy shows gross haematuria with granular and red cell casts. Proteinuria is also present. In the majority of cases oliguria is only mild but severe fluid retention can occasionally produce acute hypertension, with encephalopathy and seizures, or heart failure.

Management. The confirmation of post-streptococcal glomerulonephritis establishes an excellent prognosis in most instances, and therefore all cases should have an antistreptolysin titre determination as well as a throat swab. The remainder of the family should also have throat swabs.

Treatment includes eradication of streptococcal infection with a 10 day course of phenoxymethyl penicillin. Hospital admission is required if there is any suggestion of oliguria, fluid overload or hypertension. The reduced GFR should be assessed by a plasma creatinine estimation and serial progress monitored by daily weight and fluid balance. Oliguria requires salt restriction and water intake balanced against insensible loss, 400 ml per m² surface area per day, plus the previous day's urine output. More aggressive management with diuretics and hypotensive drugs may be needed to control hypertension. Acute peritoneal dialysis is necessary to treat severe fluid overload, hyperkalaemia and a deteriorating clinical state.

The normal course is for the GFR to return to normal in 10 to 14 days. If oliguria persists or progresses, a renal biopsy is justified to define the nature of the glomerular lesion. Rapidly progressive glomerulonephritis with scarring and deteriorating renal function is fortunately rare in the young.

The long-term prognosis of post-streptococcal glomerulonephritis is assumed to be excellent, 92 to 98 per cent achieving resolution. There is still some caution about the eventual status of the non-streptococcal group.

Clinical features of HSP

Skin	haemorrhagic rash
Joints	pain and swelling
Bowel	pain and melaena
Kidney	haematuria

Henoch Schönlein purpura. Although approximately 70 per cent of children with Henoch Schönlein purpura have haematuria and or proteinuria, the glomerulonephritis is usually asymptomatic and nonprogressive with an eventual mortality of less than 1 to 3 per cent. This serious complication is, however, responsible for 5 per cent of children entering renal dialysis programmes. Children presenting with an acute nephritic syndrome or rapidly progressing to a nephrotic syndrome have an ominous future. Normal renal function 2 years after the initial insult is unlikely to deteriorate but there are exceptions. Renal histology is some guide to prognosis, the glomerular lesions varying from minimal change to focal or diffuse mesangial proliferation with crescents, and in the most advanced stages, sclerosis. There is no specific therapy for this nephritis and management is symptomatic. Children with urinary abnormalities after Henoch Schönlein purpura should continue to have urine examinations and blood pressure measurements at periodic intervals in order to detect the late development of hypertension and renal impairment.

NEPHROTIC SYNDROME

Oedema

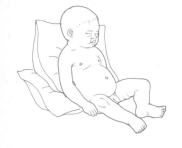

The nephrotic syndrome occurs when there is gross urinary protein loss resulting in hypoalbuminaemia and oedema. It is uncommon, with an incidence of 2 per 100 000 children (9–16 per 100 000 in Asian population) and a peak incidence between 1 and 5 years. Males are more commonly affected than females, 2.5:1. The cause is unknown. Approximately 85 per cent of caucasian children with nephrotic syndrome have the so-called 'minimal change' type.

Peri-orbital or dependent oedema and abdominal ascites are usually noticed first. There may also be abdominal pain, vomiting and diarrhoea. Hypovolaemia and circulatory collapse is a danger in the early phase of the illness since fluid shifts from the intravascular to the extracellular space, and it may be exacerbated by vomiting and diarrhoea. A careful review of pulse, blood pressure and haematocrit must be maintained until the situation stabilises. Intravenous plasma replacement may be necessary. These children are also susceptible to infection, particularly pneumococcal peritonitis and urinary tract infection. Fever in the presence of ascites justifies a diagnostic ascitic fluid tap for microscopy and culture.

Pathology. The term minimal change nephrotic syndrome is derived from light microscopy appearance. Electron microscopy shows fusion of the epithelial cell foot processes, a non-specific consequence of proteinuria. Although the pathogenesis of the renal insult leading to

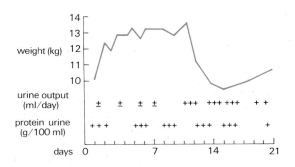

A typical clinical course with a dramatic weight loss following the diuresis

proteinuria is uncertain, it is thought to be a reduction in the fixed negative charge on the glomerular capillary wall. Renal biopsy is not required if the clinical picture matches minimal change nephrotic syndrome and there is a definite response to corticosteroids. Other pathological conditions such as focal segmental glomerulosclerosis and membrano-proliferative glomerulonephritis carry a more guarded prognosis.

Management. Diuretics should be used with care as they promote hyponatraemia and may further reduce the intravascular volume. Salt poor albumin infusion temporarily restores the circulating volume but is required in only a minority of children. Rest is normally guided by the patient's behaviour, and moderate fluid restriction is necessary only while the child is oedematous. Prophylactic penicillin should be given during the oedematous phase. The recovery is monitored by daily weights and proteinuria. Ninety per cent of children with minimal change disease will respond to corticosteroids within 8 weeks.

Frequent relapses may be controlled by alternate-day prednisolone, but if corticosteroid toxicity occurs there may be a case for a brief course of cyclophosphamide. Concern about the long-term gonadal effects of cytotoxic therapy restricts its usage.

Congenital nephrotic syndrome. Congenital nephrotic syndrome is very rare and either presents at birth with placental oedema or develops in the first year. It may be familial with autosomal recessive inheritance, and is more common in Scandinavia. Dialysis and transplantation can now be offered to children with this previously fatal condition.

Systemic causes of nephrotic syndrome. These include infections (e.g. malaria), poisons (e.g. mercurials), allergies (e.g. bee sting), and collagen vascular disorders (e.g. SLE).

A scheme for the management of the childhood nephrotic syndrome

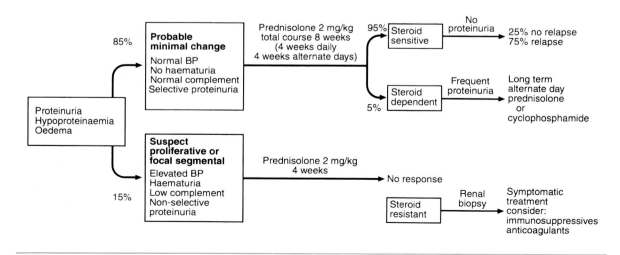

RENAL TUBULAR DISORDERS

It is essential to consider these disorders when urine analysis reveals glycosuria, aminoaciduria or impaired ability to concentrate or acidify urine.

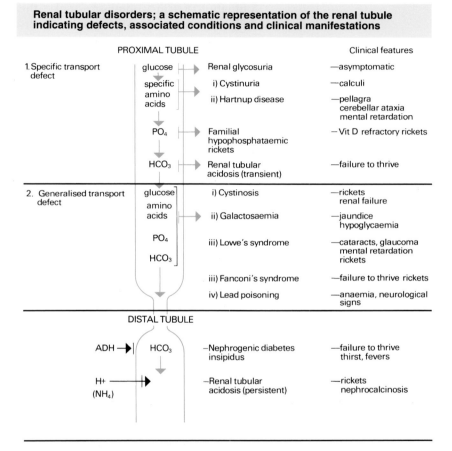

Renal tubular disorders; a schematic representation of the renal tubule indicating defects, associated conditions and clinical manifestations

PROXIMAL TUBULE | | Clinical features

Defect	Site	Condition	Clinical features
1. Specific transport defect	glucose	Renal glycosuria	—asymptomatic
	specific amino acids	i) Cystinuria	—calculi
		ii) Hartnup disease	—pellagra cerebellar ataxia mental retardation
	PO_4	Familial hypophosphataemic rickets	—Vit D refractory rickets
	HCO_3	Renal tubular acidosis (transient)	—failure to thrive
2. Generalised transport defect	glucose amino acids	i) Cystinosis	—rickets renal failure
		ii) Galactosaemia	—jaundice hypoglycaemia
	PO_4	iii) Lowe's syndrome	—cataracts, glaucoma mental retardation rickets
	HCO_3	iii) Fanconi's syndrome	—failure to thrive rickets
		iv) Lead poisoning	—anaemia, neurological signs

DISTAL TUBULE

Defect	Condition	Clinical features
ADH →	HCO_3 — Nephrogenic diabetes insipidus	—failure to thrive thirst, fevers
H+ (NH₄)	—Renal tubular acidosis (persistent)	—rickets nephrocalcinosis

ACUTE RENAL FAILURE

Acute renal failure is an uncommon but important problem in which the kidneys are no longer able to maintain biochemical homeostasis. Oliguria, less than 200 to 250 ml per m^2 surface area per day, is usually present. The possible causes fall into three main groups; pre-renal, renal, and post-renal.

Management. In practical terms the priorities are to distinguish pre-renal from established renal failure, and to exclude obstruction and pre-existing renal disease (acute on chronic renal failure). The presenting illness, gastroenteritis or septicaemic shock, may be very suggestive of circulatory failure and a pre-renal cause, but if oliguria has developed there is a risk that tubular nephropathy has already occurred. The examination of urine and plasma makes the distinction, as normal kidneys will concentrate urinary urea and reabsorb sodium. Proteinuria, cells and casts also suggest a renal lesion.

Pre-renal failure demands urgent vascular volume expansion and careful monitoring of fluid and electrolyte replacement. Renal failure may respond to intravenous, high-dosage frusemide but preparations should be made for peritoneal or haemodialysis, especially if the picture is complicated by hypertension, pulmonary oedema or worsening biochemistry. Gentamicin and other drugs with a primarily renal excretion should be used with caution.

Potentially reversible obstruction must not be overlooked and ultrasound, MCUG and radioisotopic procedures play a role.

Acute renal failure of childhood has in general a good outlook if dealt with expertly. However the survival is less good for acute renal failure complicating other life-threatening conditions such as severe infection or following surgery for complex disease.

Manifestations and management of acute renal failure

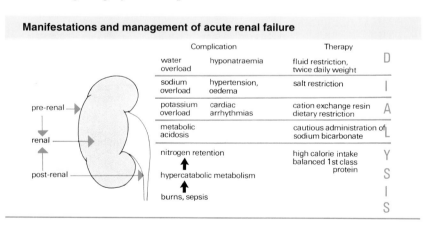

	Complication	Therapy	
	water overload	hyponatraemia	fluid restriction, twice daily weight
	sodium overload	hypertension, oedema	salt restriction
pre-renal →	potassium overload	cardiac arrhythmias	cation exchange resin dietary restriction
renal	metabolic acidosis		cautious administration of sodium bicarbonate
post-renal	nitrogen retention		high calorie intake balanced 1st class protein
	hypercatabolic metabolism		
	burns, sepsis		

Haemolytic uraemic syndrome (HUS)

This triad of acute renal failure, haemolytic anaemia with fragmented erythrocytes, and thrombocytopenia is the commonest cause of acute renal failure in infants and children. Small outbreaks occasionally occur in the UK. There are endemic foci in other parts of the world such as South America. Typically an episode of vomiting and diarrhoea is followed by pallor, haematuria and oliguria as acute renal failure supervenes. Seizures may reflect hypertension or direct central nervous system involvement. Other organs such as the gut, liver and heart can also be affected.

The epidemic form of HUS has been associated with a variety of bacterial and viral agents with current interest focused on intestinal infection with verotoxin producing *Escherichia coli*. While the pathophysiological mechanisms in HUS are still unclear it is suggested that an initial toxic insult to vascular endothelial cells may disturb the balance between prostacyclin production in endothelial cells and thromboxane synthesis by platelets.

The epidemic form of HUS generally has a good prognosis with supportive treatment alone, but sporadic cases in older children with no clear prodromal illness often result in residual renal impairment.

CHRONIC RENAL FAILURE

The incidence of chronic renal failure in children is much less than in the adult population but the effects on growth and development can be profound. Symptoms do not usually develop until 60 to 80 per cent of renal function is lost. There may be an insidious onset with growth failure, anorexia and nocturia, or an acute on chronic crisis may be precipitated by superimposed infection. Urinary tract infection or salt wasting can cause a rapid deterioration in renal function, while extrarenal infection with increased catabolic demands and vomiting may cause an acute decline in GFR.

Manifestations and management of chronic renal failure

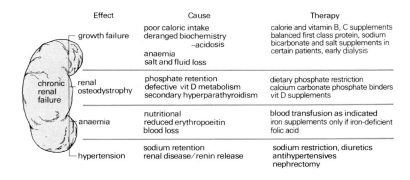

	Effect	Cause	Therapy
chronic renal failure	growth failure	poor caloric intake deranged biochemistry –acidosis anaemia salt and fluid loss	calorie and vitamin B, C supplements balanced first class protein, sodium bicarbonate and salt supplements in certain patients, early dialysis
	renal osteodystrophy	phosphate retention defective vit D metabolism secondary hyperparathyroidism	dietary phosphate restriction calcium carbonate phosphate binders vit D supplements
	anaemia	nutritional reduced erythropoeitin blood loss	blood transfusion as indicated iron supplements only if iron-deficient folic acid
	hypertension	sodium retention renal disease/renin release	sodium restriction, diuretics antihypertensives nephrectomy

These children should be supervised by a paediatric nephrology unit which can provide the optimal care consisting of specialist dietary advice, surgical liaison and psychosocial preparation if dialysis and transplantation become imminent. Growth impairment in chronic renal failure is a multi-factorial problem but aggressive feeding regimens with supplements in older children, and nasogastric or gastrostomy feeding in the first 2 years of life may help to prevent the short stature which has been a feature of such children.

Children develop end stage renal disease requiring dialysis and transplantation at the rate of approximately 4–6 million of the child population. Dialysis is seen only as an interim measure before transplantation which offers the best overall form of rehabilitation with growth potential. Recent experience with erythropoietin and growth hormone suggests that both the chronic anaemia and growth failure associated with chronic renal failure can be ameliorated by the use of these synthetic hormones.

Haemodialysis can be technically difficult in any child because of problems with vascular access. For most children the favoured method for chronic dialysis is continuous ambulatory peritoneal dialysis (CAPD) or chronic cycling peritoneal dialysis (CCPD). These provide opportunities for children of all sizes to be treated at home with generally freer diets and improved well being. Dialysis and transplantation are now feasible at any age, but such patients place considerable demands on family and treatment resources which can only be met by a fully integrated team approach that can decide the best treatment options for each individual.

THE TESTES

The testes develop as intra-abdominal structures, entering the inguinal canal during the seventh month of fetal life. At birth the testes are usually in the scrotum but in about 10 per cent of children they are undescended at birth and it is not uncommon for descent to be completed during the first two weeks of life. Descent is unlikely to take place after 1 year of age. The endocrine control of testicular descent is complex, involving gonadotrophins, androgens and Müllerian inhibitory factor.

Retractile testes

Normal testes in young boys are readily elevated to the upper scrotum by the cremasteric muscle. This commonly causes confusion and anxiety at routine medical checks. Careful records, and preferably parent held records, should confirm that the testes were both descended at the time of the newborn check. Retractile testes will descend if the boy is examined in a warm and relaxed atmosphere, and if he is asked to adopt a squatting position.

Undescended testes

Testes which fail to reach the scrotum may be classified into the following categories:

Incompletely descended testes (20 per cent). Incompletely descended testes lie along the path of descent but fail to reach the scrotum. They may be intra-abdominal or within the canal and hence impalpable. An emergent or high scrotal testis is easily palpable. These testes often appear grossly abnormal at operation, being small, soft and with a disassociated epididymis. Most are accompanied by a large hernial sac.

Maldescent and undescent of the testes

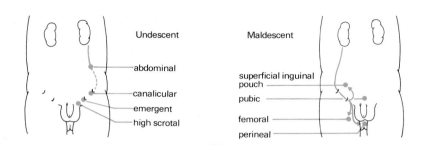

Spermatogenesis is poor and is probably not significantly altered by operation. Orchidopexy may be difficult as the vessels are usually short. Sometimes no testicular tissue can be found and is either the result of intrauterine torsion or true agenesis. In the latter case abdominal ultrasound should be performed to determine whether there is associated renal agenesis.

Ectopic or maldescended testes (80 per cent). Ectopic or maldescended testes pass through the inguinal canal and emerge from the superficial inguinal ring, thereafter following an abnormal course. Ectopic sites include the superficial inguinal pouch, perineal, femoral and pubic positions. Most ectopic testes are easily palpable. The testis is usually normal in appearance and a hernial sac is only occasionally present. Orchidopexy is easy because of adequate cord length. Spermatogenesis is almost normal with or without operation. The main indication for orchidopexy is to achieve optimal gonadal function. This is temperature dependent, the temperature of the scrotum being 1°C less than the intra-abdominal temperature. Previously orchidopexy was performed late in childhood but now most paediatric surgeons operate at the age of 2 to 3 years. The other indications for orchidopexy are cosmetic, psychological, and to

Features which distinguish maldescent from undescent of the testes

	Maldescent	Undescent
Frequency of occurrence	80% of cases	20% of cases
Presence of hernia	Some cases	100% of cases
Prognosis for fertility	Good	Poor
Technique of orchidopexy	Inguinal approach	Abdominal approach
Likelihood of getting testis into scrotum	Easy in all cases	Unpredictable
Normality of testis: naked eye and histology	Normal	Abnormal
Risk of torsion	Increased	Slightly increased
Risk of malignancy (*both* sides in unilateral presentation)	Slightly increased	Increased

reduce the risks of torsion, trauma and unrecognised malignancy. Testicular malignancy in the fourth decade of life is known to occur more frequently in individuals born with their testes outside the scrotum. Orchidopexy does not diminish the incidence of malignancy but does bring a previous impalpable testis into a palpable position.

Torsion of the testis

Approximately 20 per cent occur in the perinatal period and present as a discoloured scrotum. Unfortunately the diagnosis is often delayed and orchidectomy inevitable. However the opposite testis must be fixed in a stable position. The majority of torsions occur around puberty and present acutely as abdominal pain radiating to the testis or as intermittent testicular pain. There may be associated anomalies; a clapper bell testis due to high attachment of the tunica vaginalis or a long meso-orchium. The twist usually occurs in the spermatic cord. The undescended testis is also at risk of torsion. Urgent surgery is indicated when torsion is suspected.

Torsion of the hydatid of Morgagni. This is very common and can usually be distinguished from torsion of the testis because the pain is less severe, and as a consequence the history is usually longer than 6 hours. Sometimes it is possible to feel the torted hydatid and to demonstrate it by transillumination.

Varicoceles

Varicoceles occur infrequently in children. They do not usually need treatment during childhood.

Inguinal hernias and hydroceles

During its descent into the scrotum the testis is accompanied by a pouch of peritoneum, the processus vaginalis. The processus begins to close at birth and is normally obliterated during the first year of life. Both inguinal hernias and hydroceles are due to persistent patency of the processus. Where the processus remains very narrow, it allows peritoneal fluid to enter its cavity creating a hydrocele. If the hydrocele is present at birth and does not vary in size, it is called a non-communicating hydrocele and will usually resolve within 4 to 6 months of birth. Beyond this age it

Inguinal hernia and hydrocele

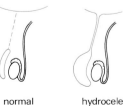

normal   hydrocele   communicating or scrotal hernia   non-communicating or inguinal hernia   hydrocele of cord

A hypochromic microcytic blood film is usually sufficient evidence to justify a trial of oral iron therapy. The history may provide clues to alternative diagnoses, for example recurrent vomiting indicating reflux oesophagitis or pica suggesting lead poisoning.

If oral iron is given for 1 month and the haemoglobin rises by 1.0 g/dl or more then iron deficiency was present. Children who fail to respond to an adequate course of iron warrant more detailed investigation including serum ferritin and haemoglobin electrophoresis, radiological studies of the gastrointestinal tract, and renal and thyroid function tests. Intestinal malabsorption may present with iron deficient anaemia, and there may be associated folate deficiency. There is some evidence that severe iron deficiency may itself impair the integrity and function of the intestinal mucosa.

Iron treatment should be continued for 3 months to replenish iron stores as well as to correct haemoglobin concentrations.

Iron balance in infancy

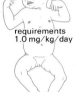

birth
total iron = 75 mg/kg.
75% circulating in blood

requirements
1.0 mg/kg/day

cow's milk	0.5 mg/l
breast milk	1.5 mg/l
mixed diet	4–9 mg/l
fortified milk preparations	5–12 mg/l

Iron preparations

Ferrous gluconate (Ferlucon) elixir	250 mg/5 ml dose contains 30 mg of elemental iron
Ferrous fumerate (Fersamal) syrup	140 mg/5 ml dose contains 45 mg of elemental iron
Ferrous sulphate (BPC) mixture	60 mg/5 ml dose contains 12 mg of elemental iron
Ferrous gluconate tablets	300 mg contains 36 mg of elemental iron
Ferrous sulphate tablets	200 mg contains 60 mg of elemental iron

APLASTIC ANAEMIA

A pancytopenia necessitates marrow examination which may show either reduced cellularity without infiltration, aplasia of the marrow, or invasion by malignant cells. Aplastic anaemia may be inherited or acquired.

Inherited aplastic anaemia. An autosomal recessive condition, Fanconi anaemia, is the most common of the inherited types, and presents in boys at 4–7 years of age and in girls between 6 and 10 years of age. Bruising and purpura are the usual presenting complaints with anaemia appearing more insidiously. Associated features include abnormal pigmentation, short stature, skeletal and renal malformations and there may be chromosomal breakages and a high Hb F. The condition is progressive but the deterioration may be delayed with androgens and corticosteroids. Most children with Fanconi anaemia die within a few years of diagnosis due to complications of pancytopenia and some develop acute leukaemia. Bone marrow transplantation from a compatible sibling or donor offers the main hope of therapy.

Acquired aplastic anaemias. These may occur at any age. Some cases follow the ingestion of certain drugs such as chloramphenicol; others follow hepatitis A, B or C and several other virus infections though there is frequently no obvious precipitating cause. If the bone marrow is moderately cellular at diagnosis there is a greater chance that spontaneous remission may occur. The majority with severe pancytopenia, respond poorly to corticosteroids and androgens, and are at risk of dying of infection. Compatible bone marrow transplantation is now the treatment of choice. Transplantation is more successful in those patients who have had the fewest blood transfusions and it is important therefore to explore the availability of suitable donors early in the course of the illness. Recently antilymphocyte globulin or antithymocyte globulin have brought about a prolonged remission in up to 40 per cent of children with aplastic anaemia; both deplete the T cell population. With the developments in bone marrow transplantation and ALG and ATG the prognosis has improved greatly during the last few years.

HAEMOLYTIC ANAEMIAS

Haemolytic anaemias may be congenital or acquired. Some of the acquired group produce problems in the first days of life and are due to maternal antibodies haemolysing the infant's cells. The diagnostic feature of haemolytic anaemias is a normal or low haemoglobin and a raised reticulocyte count.

The pathogenesis of haemolytic anaemias

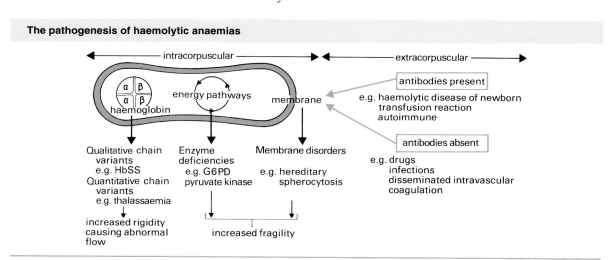

Hereditary haemolytic anaemias

The majority of haemolytic anaemias encountered in infancy and childhood are due to disorders of the red cells. They are characterised by anaemia, an increased reticulocyte count, an unconjugated hyperbilirubinaemia and if severe, skeletal changes secondary to compensatory marrow hyperplasia.

Hereditary spherocytosis

This is an autosomal dominant condition with a high new mutation rate in which the red cell membrane is abnormally permeable to sodium; the resulting spherocytes are destroyed in the spleen. The disorder may present as neonatal jaundice and has been confused with ABO incompatibility as spherocytes may be seen in this condition also. In later childhood hereditary spherocytosis may cause anaemia, chronic malaise and splenomegaly. The continuous high rate of bilirubin excretion leads to pigment gall stones. The haemoglobin concentration generally runs in the range of 9 to 11 g/100 ml, but may drop during an infection because of an increased rate of haemolysis and relative bone marrow hypoplasia. Jaundice may also become conspicuous in these episodes. The diagnosis is confirmed by demonstrating the increased osmotic fragility. Splenectomy is indicated if symptoms are severe. It is usually delayed for as long as possible because of the risk of overwhelming septicaemia in young splenectomised children. Continuous prophylactic penicillin and pneumococcal vaccine are recommended to prevent this hazard. Following splenectomy the red cell survival is returned to normal although spherocytosis persists.

Metabolic pathways of the red blood cell

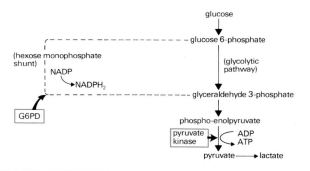

Hereditary red cell enzyme deficiencies

Two important pathways are essential for the normal function of the mature red cell. The hexose-monophosphate pathway provides a supply of reduced nicotinamide adenine-dinucleotide phosphate ($NADPH_2$) which is essential for protection against oxidative damage. The glycolytic or Embden-Meyerhof pathway provides the majority of energy for the cell. Deficiency of many of the enzymes in these two pathways has been described but the most important deficiencies are those of glucose-6-phosphate dehydrogenase (G6PD) and pyruvate kinase.

Glucose-6-phosphate dehydrogenase deficiency. There are many variants of this enzyme, each having a different geographical distribution. The form seen in black Americans results in haemolysis when the person is exposed to antimalarial and other drugs. The Mediterranean and Oriental variants often present in the newborn period with jaundice due to excess haemolysis and they may require an exchange transfusion. These conditions are also 'drug sensitive'. Ingestion of Fava

Typical timing of a drug induced episode

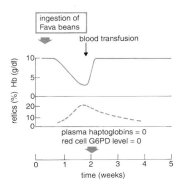

beans is a well recognised hazard in affected children. Patients with glucose-6-phosphate dehydrogenase deficiency should be given a list of drugs to avoid. The condition is X-linked, but females may have minimal symptoms, demonstrating the Lyon hypothesis, when the influence of the normal X chromosome overpowers the abnormal one.

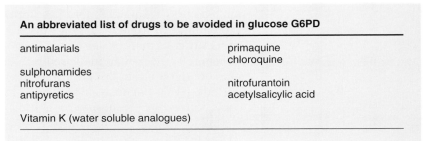

An abbreviated list of drugs to be avoided in glucose G6PD

antimalarials	primaquine
	chloroquine
sulphonamides	
nitrofurans	nitrofurantoin
antipyretics	acetylsalicylic acid
Vitamin K (water soluble analogues)	

Pyruvate kinase deficiency. This is considerably less common and affects mainly north European populations. It causes neonatal jaundice, anaemia and splenomegaly. Splenectomy is occasionally of benefit.

Disorders of haemoglobin synthesis

These fall into two main categories: those in which there is an amino-acid substitution in the globin portion of the molecule, the haemo-globinopathies; and those in which there is relative failure of globin chain synthesis, the thalassaemia syndromes. It is unusual for these conditions to present in the newborn period when fetal haemoglobin is the predominant haemoglobin type.

Changes in haemoglobins during development

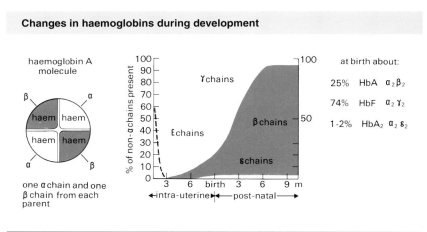

Sickle cell anaemia. Sickle cell anaemia is by far the most common of the haemoglobinopathies; 15 per cent of all black people carry the gene that causes valine to replace glutamine in the sixth position of the beta chain. The homozygous condition is referred to as sickle cell anaemia or disease, and the heterozygote as sickle cell trait. The disease is a serious condition with a number of important complications in addition to the chronic anaemia. Painful swelling of the hands and feet is a common early presentation. The splenomegaly of the younger child becomes less prominent as repeated infarctions produce an 'autosplenectomy'. There is reduced ability to concentrate urine within the first year of life, making dehydration a serious problem.

Crises are usually precipitated by infection and may be caused by dehydration, poor tissue perfusion, hypoxia and acidosis. The anaemia is sometimes exacerbated by temporary marrow failure secondary to parvovirus infection. Treatment is largely symptomatic with anti-biotics, warmth and adequate fluids. In developed countries the prognosis for a normal life is moderately good. The heterozygote is asymptomatic except under conditions of low oxygen tension as might occur at high altitude or under general anaesthesia.

Features of sickle cell disease

Crises

painful
haemolytic
aplastic
hepatic
megaloblastic

Acute infarction
abdominal
pulmonary
neurological
hands and feet syndrome
aseptic necrosis—femoral
and humeral heads

Clinical features

pallor; icterus

haemic murmur; hepatomegaly
splenomegaly (after 8 yrs of age only 10%)

chronic leg ulcers

renal involvement
haematuria
defective urine concentration

infections
pneumococcal septicaemia
salmonella osteomyelitis

In many parts of the world some children with homozygous sickle cell anaemia die in the first few years of life because of infections. A neonatal screening programme identifies the babies with Hb SS and prophylactic measures can dramatically reduce the mortality and the morbidity. These measures include penicillin daily, Pneumovax and folic acid. Haemophilus vaccine is recommended.

Thalassaemia syndromes are most common among Asian and Mediterranean races, and are subdivided into alpha and beta thalassaemia depending on the chain affected by the synthetic failure. Beta thalassaemia is the more common, the homozygous state resulting in a severe haemolytic anaemia with hypochromic microcytic cells. The compensatory bone marrow hyperplasia produces a characteristic overgrowth of the facial and skull bones. Although life may be sustained by repeated transfusion, this resource is unavailable to the majority of the world's affected children. Repeated transfusion introduces the hazard of chronic iron overload and tissue damage, leading to cardiomyopathy, diabetes and skin pigmentation. Continuous nocturnal desferrioxamine subcutaneous infusion is moderately effective in reducing the positive iron balance. Bone marrow transplantation is being explored as a definitive therapy and if there is an HLA compatible sibling would be the treatment of choice although the risks are considerable.

Normal and abnormal haemoglobins in later childhood

normal

different polypeptide chains in various haemoglobins

			% after age 3 yrs
HbA	α_2	β_2	(98-99%)
HbF	α_2	γ_2	(0-2%)
HbA$_2$	α_2	δ_2	(1-3%)

abnormal

HbS	α_2	β_2^s	sickle cell disease
HbAS	α_2	$\beta \beta^s$	sickle cell trait
Hb Barts	γ_4		thalassaemia
HbH	β_4		

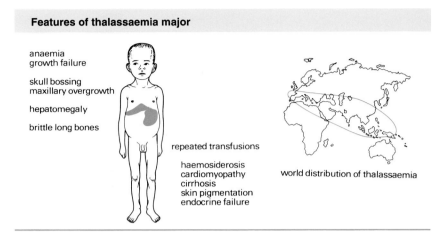

Features of thalassaemia major

anaemia
growth failure

skull bossing
maxillary overgrowth

hepatomegaly

brittle long bones

repeated transfusions

haemosiderosis
cardiomyopathy
cirrhosis
skin pigmentation
endocrine failure

world distribution of thalassaemia

In the first trimester fetal diagnosis for haemoglobinopathies is now available based on the techniques of trophoblast biopsy and restriction endonuclease analysis of fetal DNA.

Heterozygous beta thalassaemia produces a mild anaemia which may be confused with iron deficiency on the blood film. Haemoglobin electrophoresis both identifies abnormal haemoglobins and quantifies normal ones. Beta thalassaemias have an inability to make b chains, therefore there is little or no HbA ($\alpha_2\beta_2$) but slightly increased HbA2 ($\alpha_2\delta_2$).

BLEEDING DISORDERS

A variety of disorders may lead to excessive bleeding in childhood. The history may be important in distinguishing congenital from acquired problems. Previous surgery, including dental extractions, without

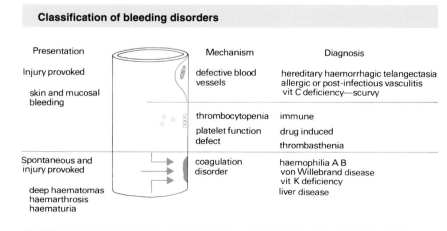

Classification of bleeding disorders

Presentation		Mechanism	Diagnosis
Injury provoked		defective blood vessels	hereditary haemorrhagic telangectasia allergic or post-infectious vasculitis vit C deficiency—scurvy
skin and mucosal bleeding		thrombocytopenia	immune
		platelet function defect	drug induced
			thrombasthenia
Spontaneous and injury provoked		coagulation disorder	haemophilia A B von Willebrand disease vit K deficiency
deep haematomas haemarthrosis haematuria			liver disease

undue bleeding provides good evidence against an inherited disorder. Tonsillectomy is notorious for putting a considerable strain on coagulation systems and may uncover mild haemophilia. A family history is often helpful in diagnosing sex-linked recessive disorders such as haemophilia or Christmas disease, but may be absent in up to a third of new cases. Von Willebrand disease and hereditary telangiectasia have a dominant pattern of inheritance. The character of the bleeding problem together with four basic tests of coagulation should make it possible to decide from which group of disorders a patient is suffering. These tests also serve as screening procedures in cases of suspected child abuse or before liver or jejunal biopsy.

Normal results in these four tests exclude all deficiencies other than factor XIII (fibrin stabilising factor) deficiency, and some rare platelet functional abnormalities.

Inherited deficiencies of each of the coagulation factors have been described; they are all rare with the exceptions of haemophilia A and B, and von Willebrand disease.

Haemophilia A and B (Christmas disease)

Classic haemophilia (A) occurs in approximately 1 in 14 000 males and is six times more common than haemophilia B, otherwise known as Christmas disease. In haemophilia A there is a functional defect in the factor VIII molecule, resulting in a reduced plasma factor VIII coagulant activity. It is transmitted as a sex-linked recessive, and carrier females are asymptomatic but may be detected because of an excess of immuno-reactive factor VIII over that which is biologically active. The severity of haemophilia is linked to the degree of deficiency of factor VIII; concentrations of factor VIII less than 1 per cent of normal causes severe problems, 1 to 5 per cent causes moderate problems, and 5 to 20 per cent only mild symptoms. Spontaneous bleeding into joints and muscles with resulting orthopaedic problems is the main hazard, and these tend to happen only in the more severe types.

It is essential to treat all bleeding incidents promptly by replacing the missing factor. Until relatively recently, this necessitated the use of fresh frozen plasma, but currently the availability of cryoprecipitate

Coagulation pathways

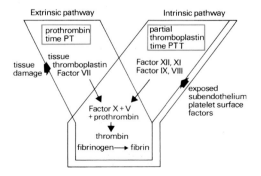

concentrates and purified dried human factor VIII have enabled the use of small volumes and therefore simplified treatment. Many families have now been trained to treat bleeding episodes at home. In general, the aim of replacement is to increase the factor VIII level to a biologically effective concentration of 10 to 20 per cent. Activity up to 50 per cent of normal may be necessary to combat severe trauma or surgery. Physiotherapy is needed to preserve the strength of muscles which might otherwise become weakened during periods of immobilisation and therefore increase the likelihood of the joint bleeding again as muscles are important in providing joint stability.

It is recognised that repeated factor VIII administration carries risks of transfusion hepatitis and chronic liver disease. AIDS is an additional threat but heat treatment is capable of excluding this agent from pooled factor VIII.

von Willebrand disease

von Willebrand disease is an autosomal dominant disorder. There is a reduction in factor VIII activity (VIIIR:Ag), and in platelet adhesiveness which causes a prolonged bleeding time which is normal in haemophilia A.

As in haemophilia milder forms of the disease with minor bleeding may respond to local measures (pressure, cold compresses) or tranexamic acid. Factor VIII concentrates are still the standard treatment, but recently it has become clear that desmopressin increases the relevant clotting factors two or threefold, and this can be used in both haemophilia A and in von Willebrand disease whenever a transient threefold increase in factor VIII is sufficient treatment.

Thrombocytopenia

Immune thrombocytopenic purpura. This is the most common of the thrombocytopenias and is thought to have an immunological basis as it often follows 1–2 weeks after a viral infection. There is a clear relationship with rubella. Platelet associated IgG antibodies are detectable in a significant proportion of cases. Problems usually develop when the platelet counts fall below $40 \times 10^9/1$, and in severe cases the count may be below $5 \times 10^9/1$. The common presenting features are petechiae and superficial bruising but mucosal bleeding may also occur. Rarely haemorrhage occurs into the brain or viscera. As the differential diagnosis includes acute leukaemia and aplastic anaemia, it is justifiable to perform a marrow examination immediately to demonstrate the normal or increased number of megakaryocytes which are characteristic of idiopathic thrombocytopenia.

In children, 85 per cent have an acute self-limiting course and the majority have recovered spontaneously by 6 months. In those who have only mild symptoms no treatment is necessary, but where there is a risk of severe generalised bleeding or bleeding into a solid organ, a short course of corticosteroids may help by producing a temporary elevation of the platelet count.

Most children need no treatment, unlike most adults with the similar disease. If it is felt that treatment is needed then 5 days of intravenous immunoglobulin will bring about an improvement in about half, splenectomy will be effective in about half as well.

Characteristic laboratory results

Test	ITP	von W.	Haemo-philia	Vit K def.
platelets	↓	N	N	N
bleeding time	↑	↑	N	N
PT	N	N	N	↑
PTT	N	N	↑	↑/N

Drug-induced thrombocytopenia is unusual in childhood but it is becoming increasingly recognised following the use of cotrimoxazole. Thrombocytopenia may occur in the neonatal period in a similar way to rhesus disease, that is to say that mother is platelet antibody negative, PLA -ve, while the baby is PLA +ve. This is called neonatal isoimmune thrombocytopenia. Intrauterine infection, maternal drug ingestion and idiopathic thrombocytopenia in the mother may also cause thrombocytopenia in the neonatal period. There is also a group of rare hereditary thrombocytopenias.

Wiscott-Aldrich syndrome

This is a sex-linked familial disorder in which boys present with early thrombocytopenia, eczema and susceptibility to infection, probably due to immunoglobulin abnormalities. Regular gammaglobulin administration reduces infection. It is often fatal in early childhood but is now amenable to bone marrow transplantation from an HLA compatible sibling.

Disseminated intra-vascular coagulation (DIC)

Severe disturbances such as septicaemia, shock and acidosis may promote simultaneous activation of both the coagulant and the fibrinolytic pathways, with a resulting consumption of platelets, fibrinogen, factors V and VIII but without the formation of insoluble fibrin. Soluble complexes of fibrin monomers circulate as fibrin degradation products and their detection is a further indication of consumptive coagulopathy. DIC should be suspected in a gravely ill child with both shock and generalised bleeding. Every attempt should be made to determine and treat the underlying cause. In the neonatal period this may be asphyxia, profound hypothermia, infection or severe rhesus disease. In infancy it may complicate meningococcal or haemophilus infections, and hypertonic dehydration and may lead to renal vein thrombosis, manifest by oliguria, haematuria and bilateral renal masses. The mainstay of treatment is fluid replacement, treatment of shock and antibiotics. Intravenous heparin to stop further clotting may be indicated.

BIBLIOGRAPHY

Nathan D G, Oski F A 1987 Hematology of infancy and childhood, 3rd edn. W B Saunders, Philadelphia
Stevens R F 1989 Handbook of haematological investigations in children. Wright, London

13 Malignancy

Causes of death 1–14 yrs

Organ growth curves

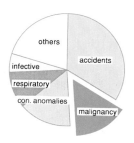

In childhood the incidence of malignant disorders is about 1 in 600, and leads to 14 per cent of all deaths in children aged 1 to 15 years. Cancers in children differ from those found in adults. The tumour types broadly reflecting the phases of tissue proliferation during normal growth and development. Acute lymphatic leukaemia is the commonest (33 per cent) whilst epithelium tumours (carcinomas) are rare (2 per cent). The majority of the solid tumours are embryonic in appearance, presumably because they are due to the malignant transformation of primitive tissues.

Knudson's hypothesis proposed that childhood malignancy arises as a result of at least two mutational hits, one of which is genetic. One example is bilateral familial retinoblastoma which is associated with a single gene defect on the long arm of chromosome 13. The malignant development is thought to be due to the loss of a regulator gene for tissue growth. The rarity of epithelial tumours in childhood is presumably due to the short exposure to environmental carcinogens as well as the importance of ageing processes in their development. Investigation of the possible mechanisms suggested by these associations are being pursued in a search for the oncogenesis to all forms of cancer.

Examples of conditions associated with malignancy in childhood	
General	Beckwith Weidemann syndrome
	Hemihypertrophy
	Multiple exostosis
	Neurofibromatosis
DNA repair defects	Ataxia telangectasia
	Fanconi anaemia
	Xeroderma pigmentosa
Immune deficiency syndromes	Common variable immune deficiency
	Severe combined immune deficiency
	Wiskott Aldrich syndrome
Chromosome abnormalities	11p13 deletion
	13q14 deletion
	Trisomy 21
Family cancer syndromes	Familial adenomatous polyposis
	Familial Hodgkin disease
	and there are many others

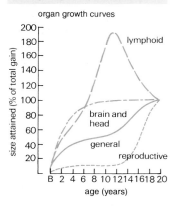

THE MANAGEMENT OF CHILDREN WITH CANCER

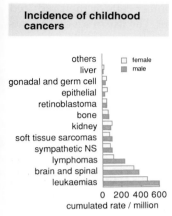

Incidence of childhood cancers

others
liver
gonadal and germ cell
epithelial
retinoblastoma
bone
kidney
soft tissue sarcomas
sympathetic NS
lymphomas
brain and spinal
leukaemias

☐ female
■ male

0 200 400 600
cumulated rate / million

Children with cancer need complex and disciplined management programmes to achieve the best chance of a cure and to minimise the pain and distress of the disease and its treatments. A comprehensive service includes ready access to specialist diagnostic facilities and experts in the planning, delivery and coordination of chemotherapy, surgery and radiotherapy. The management programme involves many health professionals whose clinical skills must be complemented by an awareness of the psychosocial aspects of the care of each individual child. Because cancer in children is relatively rare, multi-centre, national and international trials are required to evaluate new treatment techniques. In the UK the Medical Research Council (MRC) coordinates childhood leukaemia (UK Acute Lymphatic Leukaemia trials — UKALL) and bone tumour trials. The UK Childhood Cancer Study Group (UKCCSG) with the European paediatric oncology group (SIOP) coordinates the majority of trials for other solid tumours.

Support for child and family

If cancer is suspected the management must be prompt and thorough. The child and family initially need support to help them come to terms with the diagnosis. As soon as it is possible they must be told about the nature of the cancer, its prognosis and its treatment. Anxieties should be anticipated at all stages of treatment and beyond. When the intensive treatment comes to an end, concern moves to a fear of relapse. The child and family often need help socially, emotionally and financially. Relationships within the family are bound to be disturbed, the other children in the family may be forgotten. Good management includes the care and support of the whole family as well as the unfortunate child. In the UK, the Malcolm Sargeant fund and a number of local parent driven charities provide invaluable support by funding dedicated social workers and counsellors as well as offering financial assistance.

Symptom management

Cancer and its investigation and treatment can produce distress, discomfort and occasionally severe pain both at the time of diagnosis, at the time of relapse and during terminal care. The team should have expertise in the management of such disabling symptoms. The effective use of analgesics, local anaesthetics and chemotherapy/radiotherapy should ensure good control of almost all distressing symptoms in most children. The dying child should, wherever possible receive care at home with the support of the community paediatric nursing service. As a back-up, there should be ready and easy access to a familiar ward.

There are three established treatment modalities that can be directed against cancer: chemotherapy, surgery and radiotherapy.

Chemotherapy

The majority of chemotherapy agents kill cancer cells by interfering with the replication and division of DNA during cell division. They are most commonly given intravenously, although some individual agents are given orally, topically, intrathecally and even directly into pleural or abdominal cavities. Their effectiveness depends on their being more cytotoxic to the cancer cells than to normal dividing cells. This may relate to the higher rate of cell division by cancer cells or their reduced ability to recover between courses of treatment. The use of several agents simultaneously reduces the likelihood of chemoresistance developing.

Toxicity. Some drug doses are limited by the toxicity of the drug on normal tissues. The common toxicities are hair loss, and bone marrow and immunosuppression. During the severe and prolonged neutropenias any fever is treated with broad spectrum antibiotics until an infecting agent has been identified or excluded. Mucosal and systemic fungal infections are common. Immunosuppression exposes the child to the risk of suffering severe forms of common infectious illnesses like measles and chicken-pox. The increasing immunisation rates have gone some of the way to reduce these risks. Active immunistaion and anti-viral drugs also help. The gut, brain, liver, kidney and heart are also affected by specific agents in either a dose-related or idiosyncratic fashion. Management is simplified by the use of permanent indwelling central venous catheters for the delivery of blood products, intravenous drugs and parenteral nutrition.

Bone marrow transplantation. Higher doses of chemotherapy can be used if bone marrow is available to be given after the drugs have been cleared from the circulation, thus 'rescuing' the patient from prolonged myelosuppression. The bone marrow may have been previously 'har-vested' from the patient (autologous bone marrow rescue) or 'harvested' from a histocompatible donor (heterologous bone marrow transplant). Both methods of bone marrow 'rescue' are hazardous because of pro-found immunosuppression and the severity of associated organ toxicities. Heterologous transplantation has the added risk of graft versus host disease (GvHD) where the new marrow does not recognise its host as self and reacts against it, producing skin rashes and a variety of other organ toxicities requiring further immunosuppression for their control.

Bone marrow growth factors. Recent research has identified bone marrow growth factors (colony stimulating factors) which stimulate blood cell production. These growth factors can reduce the duration of chemotherapy-induced neutropenia. It is hoped that this might limit the duration of chemotherapy-induced bone marrow suppression for patients with curable disease and permit a safe increase in dose intensity for patients with more resistant disease.

Surgery

In earlier years, surgery was the first line treatment for most solid tumours. With the success of modern chemotherapy however, pri-mary surgical resection is becoming a rare event. Instead tumour biopsy with open or closed approaches is followed by tumour shrinkage with chemotherapy and subsequent tumour resection. This approach has reduced the extent of local surgical damage and increased the chance of complete resection. However surgery is required to insert

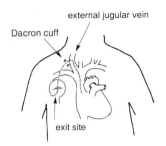

Central venous line

external jugular vein

Dacron cuff

exit site

permanent indwelling central venous catheters to facilitate the delivery of intensive chemotherapy, intravenous fluids and blood sampling. The use of these catheters is not without risk as they can become infected both within the lumen and in the soft tissues around them. They are also prone to blockage and displacement. These risks can be reduced by adopting meticulous techniques.

Radiotherapy

Radiotherapy is effective against most malignancies. External beam radiotherapy can be delivered precisely and safely to any area of the body. Delivery of radiotherapy does require an immobilised patient, which in younger children *can* be achieved by careful preparation with the help of videos and specially directed play therapy. Failure means sedation or anaesthesia. Radiotherapy is only effective in the region where it is applied and so it is mainly used to treat areas of known disease, although total body irradiation can be used in conjunction with bone marrow rescue techniques. It damages the growing tissue and local effects can be disfiguring.

Distortion of growth in the pelvis following irradiation

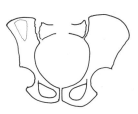 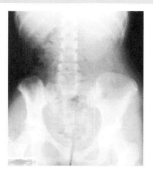

Cranial irradiation has been used extensively to treat sanctuary sites of leukaemia in the brain. The side effects of such treatment include short term memory defects, difficulties with mental arithmetic and poor attention span. These symptoms are more severe in those children who were irradiated at a younger age. Repeated irradiation for CNS relapse of leukaemia or high dose radiotherapy for intracranial malignancies may damage the hypothalamic–pituitary axis leading to a variety of endocrine disturbances such as growth hormone deficiency, hypothyroidism and precocious puberty. Attempts are being made to target radiotherapy more specifically by injecting radioisotopes attached to antibodies or chemicals taken up by the tumour.

Long term follow up

Long term follow up is essential to monitor patients for signs of early relapse and the secondary effects of their treatment. Secondary effects include specific organ toxicities such as cardiomyopathy after anthracyclines, sterility after the use of alkylating agents and renal toxicity after the use of platinum compounds. Second tumours do occur with an increased frequency compared to the rest of the population. This is probably due to a combination of circumstances including the underlying genetic predisposition and the carcinogenic effects of radiotherapy and certain chemotherapeutic agents.

Prognosis

The overall long term survival rates have now reached 65 per cent; many children can be cured and look forward to adult life. It has been estimated that with current success rates, those cured of cancer will constitute 1 in 1000 people aged 20 years by the turn of the century. The quality of life for these survivors and the consequences for the adult medical services must be a high priority in future health planning.

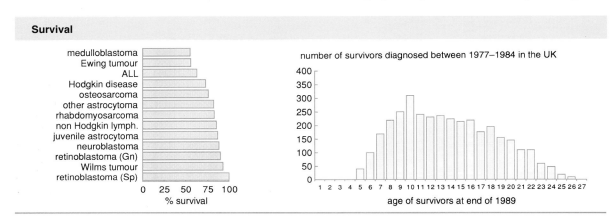

ACUTE LEUKAEMIA

This is characterised by a malignant clonal proliferation of white cell precursors (blast cells) which occupy and inhibit the function of the bone marrow. They may circulate in the blood and form leukaemic deposits in many tissue. There are two main categories of acute leukaemia, lymphatic and myeloid. In acute lymphatic leukaemia (ALL), the blast cells resemble primitive precursors of lymphoid origin whilst in acute myeloid leukaemia (AML) they resemble myeloid precursors.

Acute lymphatic leukaemia

ALL accounts for 85 per cent of childhood leukaemias. It can occur throughout childhood where it is equally common in both sexes, and the peak incidence is around 5 years of age.

Aetiology. A variety of causes for the development of ALL have been proposed. ALL is more common in Down syndrome and in syndromes involving chromosomal instability like Fanconi anaemia. Exposure to excessive radiation has also been associated with the development of ALL as seen in survivors of radiation from nuclear devices. A viral aetiology has also been proposed although no specific virus has been identified.

Clinical features of acute leukaemia

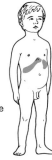

Symptoms

anorexia/lethargy
fever/infection
bleeding
gum hypertrophy
bone/joint pain
symptoms of raised intercranial pressure
hypothalamic symptoms

Physical signs

pallor
ecchymoses/petechial haemorrhages
hepatosplenomegaly
lymphadenopathy
papilloedema
cranial nerve palsies
testicular enlargement
superior vena cava obstruction

Clinical presentation. The onset is usually insidious although acute presentations, over a few days, occur in about 15 per cent. Examination of the blood or bone marrow will show an excess of lymphoblasts in conjunction with the depressed production of red cells, other white cells and platelets. Occasionally lymphoblasts are only seen in the bone marrow and not the blood (aleukaemic leukaemia). A full range of diagnostic tests should be performed to evaluate each case with respect to prognosis. The majority of cases are typed as 'common ALL' or 'pre B ALL', according to cellular surface markers. The cerebrospinal fluid should be sampled to look for evidence of CNS disease.

Prognostic features. Multifactorial analysis of large numbers of children with leukaemia has identified a variety of clinical and cellular characteristics which predict prognosis. Those justifying adjustments to standard treatment approaches are indicated below.

Prognostic features in acute lymphoblastic leukaemia

Patient features	Therapeutic action
Age < 1 year	Intensify systemic treatment, ?HBMT, delay/omit radiotherapy
Sex	Girls do better than boys: no change to treatment approach
White cell count > 50 × 10^9/l	Intensify systemic and CNS treatment, ?HBMT
CSF involvement	Intensify CNS directed therapy
Cellular features	
Cell morphology (L3)/cytochemistry B cell	Intensify treatment systemic treatment, ?HBMT
T cell type:	Risk linked to blast count
B cell type: – mature B cell	Intensify chemotherapy, ?HBMT
– common ALL antigen	Standard risk
– pre B cell	Standard risk
Null cell (commonly infant leukaemia)	Intensify chemotherapy, ?HBMT
Cytogenetics	
t(8:14)(q24: q32) commonly mature B cell	Intensify treatment, ?HBMT
t(4: 11)(q21: q23)(congenital leukaemia)	Intensify treatment, ?HBMT
t(9: 22) Philadelphia chromosome	Intensify treatment, ?HBMT

HBMT = heterologous bone marrow transplant

Treatment sequence

1. Remission induction
2. Consolidation/
   intensification
3. CNS directed therapy
4. Consolidation/
   intensification
5. Continuing treatment

The first four steps take 6 months, the whole programme 2 years

Treatment. Multi-agent chemotherapy and high dose steroids are the mainstay of treatment which is initially directed at inducing a bone marrow remission. The early stages of such treatment may be associated with life-threatening disturbances of fluid and electrolytes due to rapid lysis of tumour cells leading to renal impairment (tumour lysis syndrome). Subsequent therapy is directed at eradicating residual leukaemic cells which may be present in the bone marrow or the CNS and involves the use of blocks of intensive systemic treatment (consolidation therapy); CNS directed treatment with methotrexate (IV and IT) and CNS irradiation; and protracted low dose continuous treatment for a total treatment time from diagnosis of up to 2 years.

Prognosis. These complex treatment schedules have evolved over a number of years and have resulted in dramatic, successive improvements in survival rates, such that overall there is now a greater than 60 per cent chance of long term survival. Further improvements are expected with recent developments in treatment. Intensification of chemotherapy with heterologous bone marrow transplantation from a matched related donor may be performed in children with the adverse features in first remission or after relapse in other groups. However, only a minority of children have suitable donors, so this form of therapy is not widely applicable. The risks for unrelated donor transplants are considerably greater and are justifiable only when the prognosis is extremely grave.

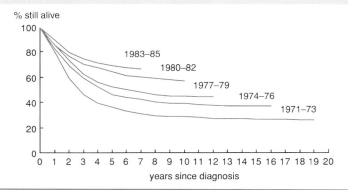

Actuarial survival curves for UK children with acute lymphatic leukaemia

% still alive

1983–85
1980–82
1977–79
1974–76
1971–73

years since diagnosis

Acute myeloid leukaemia

AML accounts for 15 per cent of childhood leukaemias, it occurs equally in both sexes and is evenly distributed throughout childhood. Its aetiology in childhood is largely unknown, although previous exposure to radiation or chemotherapy agents is known to be a precipitating factor. Its clinical presentation closely mirrors that of ALL. There are no clinical or biological variables which predict for survival. Intensive, high dose, chemotherapy of often shorter duration is used and has recently produced encouraging improvements in survival. CNS disease is a rare event and CNS directed treatment does not need to be as intensive.

The prognosis has improved in recent years and up to 50 per cent of children are now thought to be curable. Where possible, matched, related, heterologous bone transplantation is performed, often in first remission.

Chronic leukaemias (myeloproliferative disorders)

The most common myeloproliferative disorder is chronic myeloid leukaemia (CML), and there is an adult (ACML) and a juvenile type (JCML). Both are characterised by an excessive production of mature white cells.

ACML presents with symptoms of anaemia, massive splenomegaly, and the very high white cell count consists of predominantly mature granulocytes. Cytogenetic studies of bone marrow commonly identify the Philadelphia chromosome t(9:22). There is a high incidence of malignant transformation to acute leukaemia at a median of 4–5 years from diagnosis. JCML, on the other hand is characterised by skin rashes, lymphadenopathy, fevers, bleeding and an elevated HbF. The white count is mildly elevated with a marked monocytic component. Children die from infection or disease progression; acute blast transformation is not a recognised feature of the disease.

ACML can be controlled with oral chemotherapy, titrated against the blood count for a limited time period. JCML is not amenable to such an approach. Where related, matched donors exist, heterologous bone marrow transplantation is recommended for both of these disorders. The poor long term prognosis justifies the consideration of transplantation from matched, unrelated donors.

Myelodysplastic disorders

These disorders represent a poorly defined collection of bone marrow diseases where there is disordered blood cell production, often with malformed, disordered or suppressed cell production. They are associated with a variety of characteristic chromosomal abnormalities and a variable predisposition to malignant transformation into acute leukaemia.

LYMPHOMAS

Malignant lymphomas are a group of lymph system tumours which can be broadly classified into the Hodgkin and non-Hodgkin types.

Hodgkin disease

Is characterised by areas of lymph tissue hyperplasia, containing giant multinucleate Reed-Sternberg cells, reactive inflammatory infiltrate and granulomata. The patients have clinical and laboratory evidence of a predominantly cellular immune deficiency which may be instrumental in the development of the disease. They present mainly in later childhood, adolescence and young adulthood with enlarged lymph nodes and systemic upset.

Diagnosis is dependent upon lymph node biopsy and thorough

Clinical features of Hodgkin disease

Signs and symptoms

weight loss (>10% body weight) (B)
night sweats (B)
persistent fever (B)
pruritis
lymph node enlargement:
    cervical 70%, axillary 20%, inguinal 10%
hepatosplenomegaly

B = presence of B symptoms

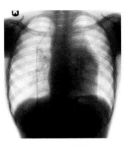

mediastinal mass

staging investigations to look for evidence of disease in the rest of the lymph system, adjacent non-lymphoid structures and the bone marrow. Treatment with local radiotherapy for stage 1 disease and multi-agent chemotherapy for more extensive disease results in a very favourable prognosis for most cases (90 per cent chance of long term cure). However there remains the chance of relapse many years after diagnosis.

Non-Hodgkin lymphoma

This group of disorders is characterised by a malignant clonal proliferation of lymph tissue which can be sub-classified both histologically and immunologically. The majority of NHL in children are highly malignant tumours which are either undifferentiated and mainly T-cell type (40–50 per cent), or lymphoblastic and B cell type (30–35 per cent). T cell lymphomas more commonly arise in the mediastinum whilst B cell lymphomas may arise within the cervical region or abdomen.

Clinical features of non-Hodgkin lymphoma

Investigations

tumour biopsy
bone marrow
CSF sample
pleural/ascitic fluid cytology
blood uric acid
renal function tests

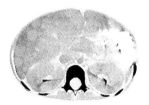

abdominal B cell lymphoma with
extensive liver involvement

Clinical presentation is commonly with fever, malaise and symptoms of lymph node enlargement in any part of the body. The disease may present with dramatic enlargement of lymph nodes causing pressure symptoms like superior vena cava obstruction, or it may be insidious in onset. It is not uncommon for the disease to be multifocal including the CNS, yet with no apparent primary tumour. Treatment is dependant upon multi-agent chemotherapy, the lymphoblastic lymphomas responding well to ALL treatment with the same dangers of the tumour lysis syndrome and they have a similar prognosis. The undifferentiated tumours require more intensive chemotherapy and the consideration of bone marrow transplantation, if the disease is extensive. The outlook is improving and there is now up to a 50 per cent chance of long term survival even in patients with extensive disease

NEUROBLASTOMA

Neuroblastoma is a malignant tumour of sympathetic neuroblasts which may arise in any part of the sympathetic nervous system. It is a puzzling tumour in that prognosis is better in the youngest infants and there may be natural remission. Urinary vanillyl-mandelic acid (VMA) provides a reliable marker for diagnosis and monitoring during treatment. VMA has also been used as the basis for population screening in infancy. Half the children present in the first 2 years of life and it is rare after the age of 5.

Clinical presentation is dependant upon the site of the primary tumour and the extent of tumour metastasis. Seventy-five per cent of the tumours have metastasised at the time of presentation. The children are frequently miserable, failing to thrive and may have extensive bruising, mimicking the appearance of a physically abused child. Diagnosis is dependant upon the presence of a typical mass, elevation

Clinical features of neuroblastoma

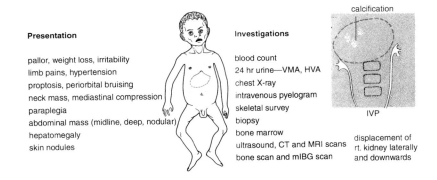

Presentation

pallor, weight loss, irritability
limb pains, hypertension
proptosis, periorbital bruising
neck mass, mediastinal compression
paraplegia
abdominal mass (midline, deep, nodular)
hepatomegaly
skin nodules

Investigations

blood count
24 hr urine—VMA, HVA
chest X-ray
intravenous pyelogram
skeletal survey
biopsy
bone marrow
ultrasound, CT and MRI scans
bone scan and mIBG scan

calcification

IVP

displacement of rt. kidney laterally and downwards

CT scan showing calcified mass anterior to left kidney

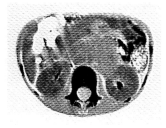

of VMA and identification of tumour cells in the marrow or biopsy of a tumour mass. Presentation in the newborn period is remarkable for its rapid progression and potential for spontaneous resolution.

Treatment is dictated by stage at presentation; localised tumours are resected and adjuvant chemotherapy given to eradicate residual disease. Infants with stage 4 disease are treated expectantly, chemotherapy being given if tumour progression is relentless or potentially life-threatening. More disseminated disease requires high dose multi-agent chemotherapy. Despite this, the over 1 year age group is associated with a poor prognosis (20–30 per cent survival). Novel treatment approaches are being explored, including targeted radiotherapy using mono–iodobenzylguanidine (mIBG), a breakdown product of noradrenaline, specifically taken up by neuroblasts.

Neuroepithelial tumours

Peripheral neuroepitheliomas or malignant peripheral neuro-ectodermal tumours (MPNET) are a collection of malignant tumours which are thought to arise from the embryonic neural crest and may be located within soft tissues or bone. They are small round cell neoplasms, clinically distinct from neuroblastoma, most commonly presenting in the thoraco-pulmonary region. Treatment, in the majority of cases, is with primary chemotherapy followed by surgical resection and subsequent irradiation of residual disease. Outcome is dictated by the presence or absence of metastatic disease at the beginning of treatment and the amenability of the primary lesion to complete surgical resection or high dose irradiation.

BRAIN AND SPINAL TUMOURS

Brain and spinal tumours are the second commonest group of malignant disorders. Their aetiology is largely unknown, although they may be associated with family cancer syndromes, pre-existing brain malformations and previous treatment for other malignancies.

Brain tumours

These may occur throughout infancy and childhood and present with signs and symptoms related to raised intracranial pressure, focal neurological defects and endocrine disturbances. Classically their presentation is late, early symptoms being attributed to a variety of non-specific clinical and psychological disorders. Computerised tomography (CT) and magnetic resonance imaging (MRI) have revolutionised the investigation of suspected brain and spinal tumours. CT/MRI guided stereotactic biopsy holds great promise for accurate diagnosis of conventionally inaccessible lesions.

Two-thirds of the tumours present infratentorially with cerebellar or brain stem dysfunction. Astrocytic, embryonal and ependymal

Classification

Astrocytic tumour
  astrocytoma
  glioblastoma
Ependymal tumour
(Ependymoma)
Embryonal tumour
  medulloblastoma
  medulloepithelioma
  primitive neuroectodermal
   tumour (PNET)
  retinoblastoma
Choroid plexus tumour
Pinealoma/pineocytoma
Cerebral lymphoma
Intracranial germ cell tumour
Pituitary adenoma
Craniopharyngioma

Distribution of brain tumours

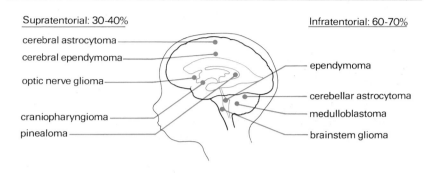

Supratentorial: 30-40%

cerebral astrocytoma
cerebral ependymoma
optic nerve glioma
craniopharyngioma
pinealoma

Infratentorial: 60-70%

ependymoma
cerebellar astrocytoma
medulloblastoma
brainstem glioma

tumours predominate. There is an increased chance of posterior fossa tumours metastasising down the spinal column, the embryonal group being most malignant in this regard. Metastasis outside the CNS does rarely occur. Supratentorial tumours may either be located within the hypothalamic–pituitary axis, producing endocrine or visual disturbances, or distant from this axis, producing symptoms of epilepsy or spasticity. Supratentorial tumours are most commonly astrocytic or ependymal with varying degrees of malignant potential.

Clinical features of brain tumours

Raised intracranial pressure

headache (early morning)
vomiting
mood changes
papilloedema
VI cranial nerve palsy
head tilt

Endocrine

short stature
hypogonadism
precocious puberty
diabetes insipidis

Focal neurological signs

cerebral
  seizures
  spasticity
  focal fits
cerebellar
  ataxia
  nystagmus
  diplopia
brain stem
  facial weakness
  dysphagia
  ocular palsies
  spasticity

Spinal tumours

These are rare, but require prompt recognition if irreversible cord damage is to be avoided. They most commonly present with disturbances of gait or sphincter or back pain. The latter symptom almost always has a sinister significance in childhood and adolescence. Spinal tumours may arise from neural tissue within the spinal cord, the most common are astrocytic or ependymal in origin. Alternatively, extrinsic, non-neural tumours may cause cord compression; neuroblastoma, lymphoma and Ewing tumour being the most common.

Treatment. Successful treatment of CNS tumours relies heavily upon the successful control of raised intracranial pressure, primary tumour resection and subsequent chemo/radiotherapy. Chemotherapy is currently being explored more widely in the younger age group, where CNS radiotherapy is particularly damaging and difficult to deliver.

The prognosis for these tumours is dictated both by the location of the tumour and its potential for local growth and metastatic spread. Overall, there is a 50 per cent chance for long term survival although this figure does not disclose the degree of neurological handicap that may exist in the survivors.

SOFT TISSUE SARCOMAS

The most common of these is the rhabdomyosarcoma, a highly malignant tumour thought to arise from the primitive mesenchyme and showing characteristics of striated muscle. Such tumours can arise anywhere in the body but they are most common in three regions: 1) the head and neck, 2) the retroperitoneum and genitourinary tract and 3) the upper and lower extremities. Their presenting features are dictated by the location of the tumour; they may metastasise widely. Treatment is with primary chemotherapy, followed by consideration of surgical resection and radiotherapy depending upon the consequences of such treatment in the anatomical location.

Other soft tissue sarcomas may have features of smooth muscle (leiomyosarcoma), adipose tissue (liposarcoma), fibrous tissue (fibrosarcoma), synovium (synovial cell sarcoma) and blood vessels (angio-/lymphangiosarcoma).

RENAL TUMOURS

The commonest renal tumour is the nephroblastoma (Wilms tumour). It is a tumour of embryonic kidney tissue which may arise within embryonic rests (nephroblastomatosis). It presents most commonly from birth to 5 years of age, 10 per cent of cases are bilateral. It is most notable for its association with a number of congenital anomalies as well as cytogenetic abnormalities on chromosome 11p. Its genetic pattern is most commonly sporadic although a number of hereditary cases have been reported.

The history of the evolution of treatment approaches in this tumour acts as a model for the development of novel approaches in other tumours of childhood. Use of the staging system has permitted tailoring of treatment to the requirements of individual patients, thereby minimising the duration and consequences of therapy.

Clinical features of Wilms tumour

Presentation
fever, poor appetite, vomiting
abdominal mass 90% (lateral, superficial)
haematuria 30%
abdominal pain 20%

Investigations
urine analysis, blood count
chest X-ray, PA and lateral
renal ultrasound and/or CT scan
chromosomes

Staging
1. encapsulated tumours completely removed
2. microscopic invasion of capsule
3. involvement of regional lymph nodes
   or tumour rupture
4. metastatic tumour
5. bilateral renal tumour

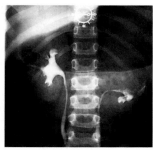

large mass arising from L kidney

A number of other renal tumour types are recognised in childhood, including mesoblastic nephroma, an almost universally benign tumour of infancy, rhabdoid tumour, clear cell sarcoma and renal cell carcinoma.

GERM CELL TUMOURS

Germ cell tumours

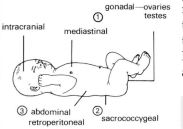

gonadal—ovaries
① testes
intracranial mediastinal
③ abdominal ② sacrococcygeal
retroperitoneal

Germ cell tumours may be malignant or benign. They arise from precursors of sperm and ova but retain the potential to produce tissues resembling any somatic or supporting structure. They arise either within the gonads or extra-gonadally, where they are found predominantly in the midline, including CNS tumours arising from the pineal gland and hypothalamus. There are two age incidence peaks, at less than 3 years and around puberty.

Use of AFP measurements to monitor for early relapse in a presumed stage 1 testicular germ cell tumour

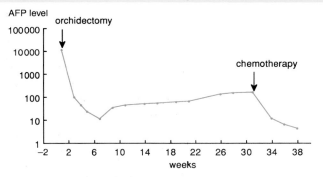

Note the satisfactory response after chemotherapy

The commonest presentation is with a congenital sacrococcygeal teratoma. The tumours often secrete alpha fetoprotein (AFP) or beta human chorionic gonadotrophin (HCG) which can be used as tumour markers to monitor response to treatment and detection of early relapse. Disseminated tumours and those incompletely resected are treated with chemotherapy to which they are very sensitive. With such treatment a greater than 90 per cent chance of cure is possible in most cases.

BONE TUMOURS

Osteosarcoma and Ewing tumour are the two most common malignant bone tumours. Clinical presentation is with local swelling, pain and occasional pathological fractures. Osteosarcomas arise more commonly in the femur around the knee or in the proximal humerus of adolescents and young adults. Ewing tumours present commonly in flat bones of the axial skeleton and the mid shaft of long bones and usually in children under 10 years of age. Osteosarcoma exhibits strong evidence of a genetic predisposition. There are frequent reports of familial cases as well as an association with a previous history of retinoblastoma. Ewing sarcoma cells are characterised by t(11:22) corresponding to the cytogenetic abnormality in neuroepithelioma.

Osteogenic sarcoma (left) and prosthesis in place after surgery (right)

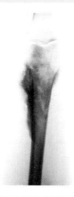 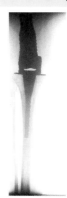

Treatment is dictated by the bone involved and tumour responsiveness to chemotherapy. Axial tumours are often difficult to resect. Tumours of long bones are more amenable to surgery and recent techniques have increased the likelihood of salvaging the limb. Initial chemotherapy is used to reduce the tumour extent and allow for resection followed by prosthetic bone replacement. With such approaches there is an overall 50 per cent chance of cure in these tumours.

OTHER TUMOURS

Hepatic tumours

Hepatoblastoma is an embryonic tumour affecting children less than 3 years of age and is associated with hemihypertrophy and family cancer syndromes. Hepatocellular carcinoma occurs later in childhood and is associated with pre-existing cirrhosis brought about by infection (hepatitis B), long standing biliary obstruction, α_1–antitrypsin deficiency or some inborn errors of metabolism, e.g. hereditary tyrosinaemia. A combination of primary chemotherapy and surgical resection has resulted in improved success rates and liver transplantation should be considered in tumours unsuitable for resection.

Retinoblastoma

This retinal tumour is the best known hereditary tumour. Sixty per cent of tumours arise as a result of sporadic mutations and are almost always unilateral. The remaining 40 per cent are bilateral tumours which are thought to be hereditary and associated with deletions of the retinoblastoma gene at 13q14. Only 10 per cent of these cases have a positive family history. Those with the hereditary form are at increased risk of subsequently developing osteosarcoma in their thirties, particularly within irradiation fields. Presentation is most commonly before 2 years of age with a white pupil, strabismus, a painful red eye or poor vision. Prognosis for survival is determined by the extent of local spread and for vision, by the location of tumours and treatment necessary for their control. Risk of continued tumour formation persists until around 4–5 years of age.

Carcinomas and others

There are many other rarer tumours of childhood including adrenal, thyroid and nasopharyngeal carcinoma. Adrenal carcinoma is important for its association with family cancer syndromes and hemihypertrophy. Differentiated thyroid cancer is notable for its increased incidence in patients after therapeutic irradiation and the medullary cell tumours of the thyroid for their association with the multiple endocrine neoplasia syndrome type II. Finally, in nasopharyngeal carcinoma, the most common of these three, the Epstein Barr virus is implicated in its aetiology.

HISTIOCYTIC DISORDERS

This group of disorders includes a variety of conditions which may be life threatening but are not thought to be true malignancies. The commonest condition is Langerhans cell histiocytosis which may present in many ways depending upon the system within which the disease process is active. Symptoms at presentation result from proliferation of components of the histiocyte–macrophage system which may occur anywhere in the body. Such proliferations may take a variety of forms including skin rashes, bony lesions, lymphadenopathy, diabetes insipidus, a variety of organ dysfunctions due to histiocytic infiltrates and associated systemic upset with fever. The classical clinical syndromes which describe the presentations include, in order of increasing severity, eosinophilic granuloma of bone, Hand-Schuller-Christian disease and Letterer-Siwe disease. It is thought to be a disorder of immune regulation. The natural history is for the disease to burn itself out during childhood and adolescence so treatment approaches must be tailored to cause minimal long term damage.

Familial erythrophagocytic lymphohistiocytosis presents with pancytopenia and splenomegaly in the first year of life, there being family history of children dying with similar conditions. Other syndromes are thought to be precipitated by previous viral infections. Malignant histiocytosis is the only truly malignant histiocytic condition which presents as a lymphomatous condition. These conditions are usually managed by paediatric oncologists because of their multisystem nature and the potential value of cytotoxic treatments in their management.

BIBLIOGRAPHY

Nathan D G, Oski F A 1987 Hematology of infancy and childhood, 3rd edn. W B Saunders, Philadelphia
Plowman P N, Pinkerton C R 1992 Paediatric oncology. Chapman & Hall, London
The National Registry of Childhood Tumours at the Childhood Cancer Research Group. John Radcliffe Infirmary, Oxford

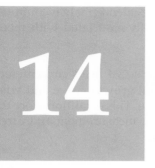

14 Growth

Accurate measurements of height, weight and head circumference plotted on record charts provide an invaluable illustration of growth and development. Growth reflects not only general health but also the nutritional and emotional environment of a child, and disordered growth may be the only obvious manifestation of disease or deprivation.

HEAD GROWTH

At birth the head circumference, 32 to 37 cm, is three-quarters of its adult value, 52 to 57 cm, and the majority of postnatal growth occurs in infancy. The anterior fontanelle, which normally measures approximately 2.5 by 2.5 cm at birth, may no longer be palpable by 6 months but often remains patent until 18 months.

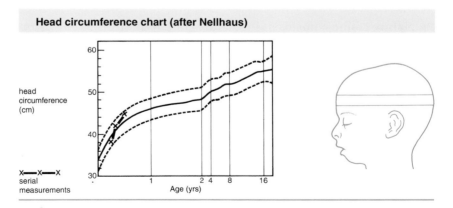

Head circumference chart (after Nellhaus)

Microcephaly

Microcephaly is commonly associated with brain hypoplasia or previous brain damage.

Macrocephaly

Macrocephaly refers to a large head from whatever cause. With hydrocephalus the increased volume is due to accumulation of CSF within the ventricular system. In megalencephaly the brain itself is larger than usual and this is responsible for the large head. Megalencephaly is commonly benign and often familial but is occasionally associated with mental handicap.

Hydrocephalus

Hydrocephalus must be considered when serial head circumference measurements deviate away from a normal growth curve and where there are signs of raised intracranial pressure. This condition more than any other emphasises the need for accurate measurement and careful plotting on an appropriate chart.

Asymmetrical skulls

Asymmetrical skulls are caused by inequality of growth rates at the coronal, sagittal and lambdoid sutures. The inequality may be due to an innocent cause like the postural effect which leads to mild plagiocephaly or rarely it may be due to premature fusion of the sutures, craniosynostosis.

Asymmetrical skulls and craniosynostosis

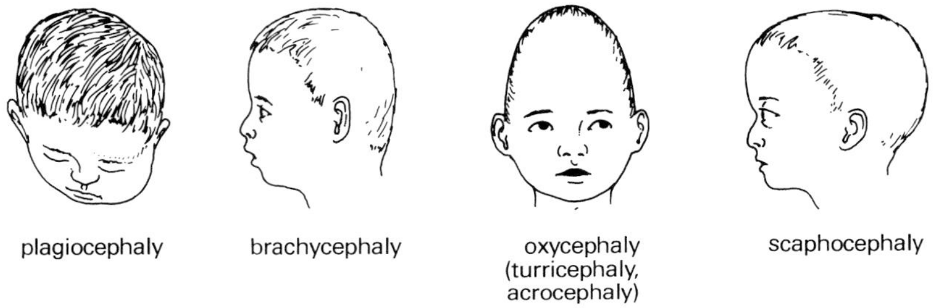

plagiocephaly   brachycephaly   oxycephaly (turricephaly, acrocephaly)   scaphocephaly

Premature craniosynostosis   Premature craniosynostosis occurs as an isolated congenital deformity, as a component of certain inherited syndromes, and secondary to metabolic disorders such as hypophosphatasia and idiopathic hypercalcaemia. It has also been reported after excessive thyroxine replacement therapy. Localised forms of craniosynostosis produce characteristic skull shapes and in some there are potentially damaging pressure effects upon the brain, eyes, and cranial nerves. Infants suspected of having this condition require prompt referral to a neurosurgical centre experienced in assessing and treating these problems. Craniectomy or reconstruction of the sutures is usually performed in the first few months of life, and may have to be followed by cosmetic procedures.

HEIGHT AND WEIGHT

Height and weight are interpreted by plotting accurate measurements against population standards for age. A child's position on the chart is described in terms of centile. This is a useful illustration of the child's size compared to normal but it is an approximation. There are secular

Measurement of length: infants

A baby (0-2 yrs) needs two people

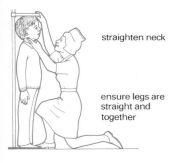

adjust   flatten legs   hold head

Measurement of height: children

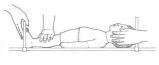

straighten neck

ensure legs are straight and together

trends which reduce the relevance of standards derived decades earlier, and standards cannot readily accommodate a multiracial society. It is important therefore to follow the rate of a child's growth to determine whether he or she remains parallel to or deviates away from population centiles. A low height velocity is more indicative of pathology than a low height centile.

Height velocity for age charts show three main components; infancy, childhood and puberty. Height velocity in infancy, up to age 12 to 18 months, starts high and decelerates rapidly. This phase is a continuation of fetal growth in which nutrition is the dominant influence. Childhood is a period of slow decline in height velocity although it should not fall below 5 cm per year.

There are many factors involved in childhood growth but growth hormone is a key regulator. Cell receptors for growth hormone increase after 12 months, a finding which matches the clinical observation that isolated growth hormone deficiency slows childhood but not infancy growth.

Puberty and increased sex hormone release results in height acceleration, peaking at approximately 10 cm per year. This change in the tempo of growth has a very variable timing with respect to chronological age but is linked to sexual maturation and bone age. Interestingly puberty alters the rate at which an individual reaches adult height but does not alter final height. An otherwise normal hypogonadal boy or girl will go on growing at an ever diminishing rate until they eventually reach the height for which they were genetically programmed.

SHORT STATURE

Short stature, defined as a height below the third centile, occurs in many healthy children but each case should be carefully evaluated and particular attention must be paid to those who are severely short with a height less than minus three standard deviations, those whose parental heights suggest that they should be above the third centile, and those in whom serial measurements show progressive deviation from the normal. The investigation of these children must take into account the multiple genetic and environmental factors which influence growth.

Genetic and environmental causes of short stature

Familial short stature. Adult height is subject to polygenic inheritance and has therefore a normal distribution. In assessing a problem of short stature it is useful to plot the parents' height centiles on the child's growth chart. In calculating the mid-parental height for a boy add 12 cm to his mother's height; for a girl subtract 12 cm from her father's height. It must be remembered that parental short stature may have resulted from inherited disease, for example skeletal dysplasia, or from still relevant environmental influences.

Growth charts (after Tanner and Whitehouse)

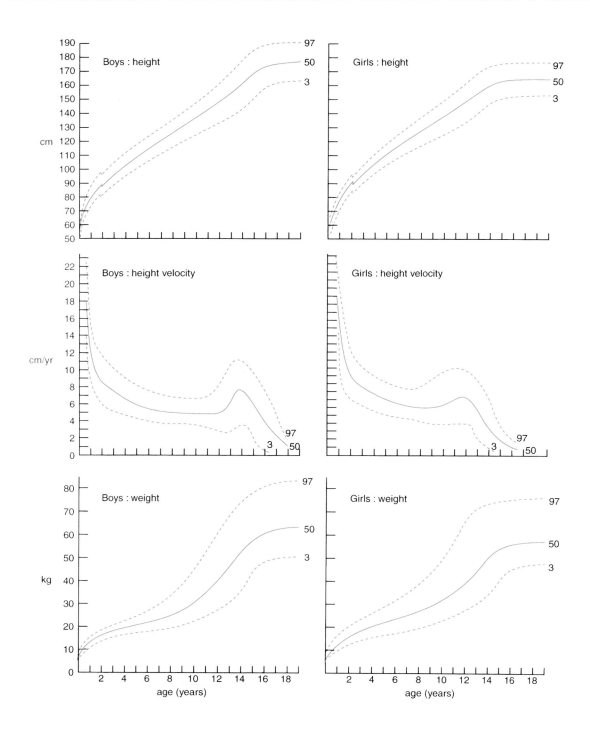

Longitudinal growth assessment

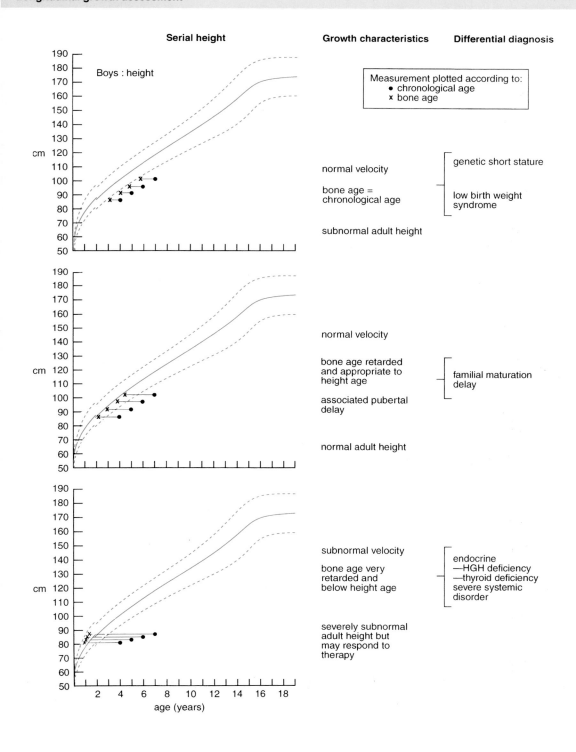

Serial height

Growth characteristics

Differential diagnosis

Boys : height

> Measurement plotted according to:
> • chronological age
> x bone age

normal velocity

bone age =
chronological age

subnormal adult height

genetic short stature

low birth weight
syndrome

normal velocity

bone age retarded
and appropriate to
height age

associated pubertal
delay

normal adult height

familial maturation
delay

subnormal velocity

bone age very
retarded and
below height age

severely subnormal
adult height but
may respond to
therapy

endocrine
—HGH deficiency
—thyroid deficiency
severe systemic
disorder

age (years)

Causes of short stature (after Lacey and Parkin)

6 chromosomal abnormalities
1 cystic fibrosis
1 chronic renal failure
1 Fallot tetralogy
1 juvenile rheumatoid
1 Hurler syndrome
4 mental handicap

1 growth hormone deficiency

98 ten-year-old children below 3rd centile

Constitutional delay of growth and puberty (CDGP). Delayed maturation and a delay in the pubertal phase of growth is a common cause of short stature which emerges as a problem in secondary school age children, especially boys. These youngsters remain prepubertal and in the decelerating phase of childhood growth, while their contemporaries are developing sexually and accelerating in height. The problem is magnified if it is superimposed on familial short stature. CDGP is often genetically determined and hence the importance of enquiring about patterns of puberty in close relatives. In the absence of a positive family history it is important to exclude environmental or health factors which have either restrained growth in the past or may still be active. Bone age estimation typically shows approximately 2 years delay and when height is adjusted for this delay it falls into a range which matches the target height predicted from parental stature.

For most affected youngsters explanation, and reassurance about their acceptable final height, is all that is necessary. Boys tend to be more vulnerable to psychological problems associated with CDGP. Height is a more conspicuous asset in the male. Girls have height acceleration as an early component of puberty whereas boys have to wait until the second half of puberty, equating to testicular volumes of above 8 ml. When behavioural problems and social isolation blight a teenage boy's passage through what is already a turbulent period, then there is justification for artificially altering the tempo of puberty and height acceleration with a short course of either testosterone depot injections or oxandrolone.

Low birth weight conditions. The majority of preterm and small-for-gestational age infants achieve normal adult size. A minority have permanently restricted growth. They are a heterogenous group consisting of infants exposed to external influences such as congenital infection or maternal drugs, or having intrinsic disorders, for example chromosomal anomalies. A number of syndromes include low birth weight and subsequent growth restriction. Russell-Silver syndrome combines these features with a triangular facies, small mandible and body asymmetry.

Social deprivation. Short stature is most prevalent in the lower social classes and reflects the superimposition of a disordered environment on genetic potential. It is not easy to define the latter as successive generations have usually been exposed to the same adverse factors. Growth hormone release is depressed in emotionally deprived children but rapidly reverts to normal when they are provided with love and reasonable care. These disturbed children may also show bizarre, compulsive eating behaviour, to the extent that they develop distended abdomens and bouts of vomiting.

Nutritional starvation produces a different response with exaggerated growth hormone secretion but a block at tissue level where there is diminished synthesis of the growth factors which mediate in the peripheral anabolic effects of growth hormone.

Russell-Silver syndrome

Russell-Silver syndrome
small face
short stature
low birth weight
asymmetry (50%)
short 5th finger (75%)
mental retardation (20%)

Systemic causes

Those sufficient to restrict growth are usually severe and can be diagnosed by careful history and examination. Exceptions are chronic renal disease and malabsorption. Coeliac disease is a particular problem in that it may mimic hypopituitarism producing subnormal height velocity, delayed bone age and suppressed growth hormone responses. A jejunal biopsy may therefore be necessary in doubtful cases.

Endocrine causes of short stature

Growth hormone deficiency. The mechanisms responsible for the release and action of growth hormone (GH), are complex and are only gradually being unravelled. At the hypothalamic level a cascade of neurotransmitters modulates the balance between growth hormone releasing factor, GRF, and growth hormone releasing inhibitory factor or somatostatin. This sequence controls the pulsatile pattern of normal GH release. GH does not act directly to promote linear growth but does so via insulin-like growth factor-1, IGF-1. The action of IGF-1 on cartilage growth plates is in turn dependent on binding proteins and the status of cell receptors.

Growth hormone deficiency may be congenital or acquired, and it may be isolated or part of a generalised pituitary failure. Familial disorders account for less than 10 per cent. Congenital abnormalities may result from pituitary malformation or damage of the pituitary stalk; high definition MRI imaging is throwing new light on these anatomical associations. Congenital isolated GH deficiency may represent the extreme end of a normal distribution of GH secretory capacity, and therefore there is no clearcut distinction between children with so-called GH deficiency and those with normal short stature. Congenital panhypopituitarism may be associated with midline facial fusion defects or with hypoplasia of the optic nerves, septo-optic dysplasia. Acquired hypopituitarism occurs as a result of pituitary area tumours or infiltration, following basal meningitis and after severe head injuries. It is being increasingly recognised in children who recover from brain tumours or acute leukaemia treated with cranial radiotherapy.

The diagnosis of GH deficiency depends on demonstrating that a child has a subnormal growth rate and a delayed bone age, and that the clinical picture is compatible with subnormal GH production rather than other indentifiable restraints. In a minority of patients, associated pituitary hormone deficiencies or imaging evidence of an anatomical abnormality in the pituitary region will confirm the diagnosis. Traditionally provocation tests such as insulin-induced hypoglycaemia and clonidine or arginine have been used to measure GH release. A clearly subnormal GH response is diagnostically useful, but many short children produce borderline levels which do not assist in the decision whether or not to treat with biosynthetic GH. Height acceleration after starting GH treatment is a further useful step in consolidating the diagnosis. Children with severe GH deficiency and subnormal height velocities have a striking response to modest dosage GH and, if diagnosed sufficiently early, can be restored to a trajectory which takes them to an acceptable adult height. Short children with intermediate GH secretory capacity and near normal height velocities require higher dosage GH therapy to gain significant height acceleration, and it is still uncertain whether they can achieve final height advantage which justifies long-term, costly therapy.

Craniopharyngioma. This is a rare but important condition to exclude whenever there is a possibility of secondary hypopituitarism. The tumour is composed of expanding cystic remnants of Rathke's pouch, a dorsal protrusion of the embryonic stomatodoeum, and its strategic location results in life threatening pressure effects. Headache and defective vision are more common initial complaints than short stature, but visual field assessment and a lateral skull X-ray are essential in the assessment of short children.

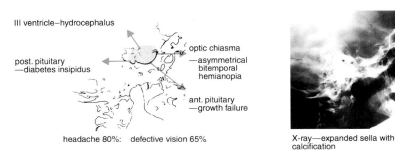

Pressure effects and clinical features of craniopharyngioma

III ventricle–hydrocephalus

optic chiasma
—asymmetrical bitemporal hemianopia

post. pituitary
—diabetes insipidus

ant. pituitary
—growth failure

headache 80%:   defective vision 65%

X-ray—expanded sella with calcification

Juvenile hypothyroidism results in progressive growth failure and is characterised by severe retardation of skeletal development. It is readily confirmed by performing thyroid function tests and responds well to thyroxine replacement.

Adrenal insufficiency, hypoparathyroidism and pubertal disorders account for a small number of children with short stature. Corticosteroid therapy at a dosage in excess of prednisone 5 mg per day or its equivalent interferes with linear growth. Alternate day single dose corticosteroid regimens permit more normal growth.

Investigation of short stature

In the majority of children the history will reveal a genetic or social basis for their problem and detailed investigation is therefore inappropriate. Those lacking such an explanation, having definitely abnormal growth, or having additional signs or symptoms, require serial accurate measurements. In addition to an accurate measurement of height, which provides the basis for longitudinal growth assessment, there must be some comparison of trunk versus leg length to allow recognition of disproportionate short stature. Pubertal staging, optic fundi and visual field assessment are essential parts of the physical examination. Laboratory investigations are guided by the clinical findings but in general are limited to total blood count, plasma electrolytes, creatinine, calcium, phosphate, alkaline phosphatase and thyroid function. Turner syndrome is not rare and hence there is a case for chromosomal analysis in short girls. Radiographs of the left wrist and hand for bone age determination and a skull X-ray for pituitary fossa examination complete the initial assessment.

It is unnecessary to subject children to more formal assessment of growth hormone secretion, such as insulin-induced hypoglycaemia, until they have had at least 6 months of longitudinal growth assessment. Exact height measurement at 3 monthly intervals enables the height velocity to be determined. A subnormal velocity confirms the case for further detailed investigation. The combination of serial height measurements and bone age determinations is not only a useful tool in the diagnosis of short stature, but provides a parameter by which therapy may be judged.

Disproportionate short stature

Calculation of the ratio of upper and lower body segment lengths will reveal cases of disproportionate short stature. Skeletal disorders account for the majority of this group and may be classified into those where abnormality originates in the skeleton, or has a systemic metabolic basis, for example mucopolysaccharidoses. They may also be divided into those with short limbs or short trunks, the latter usually having kyphoscoliosis. Exact diagnosis, confirmed by radiological and metabolic studies, is essential for genetic counselling.

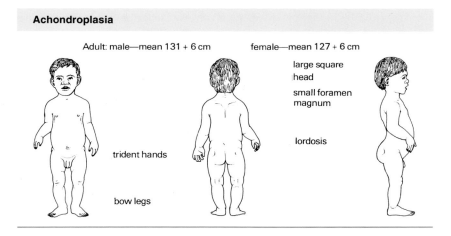

Achondroplasia

Adult: male—mean 131 + 6 cm   female—mean 127 + 6 cm

large square head

small foramen magnum

lordosis

trident hands

bow legs

EXCESSIVE HEIGHT

The great majority of tall children come from tall families and accept their stature as normal. An unusually tall child may have an underlying disorder but these are usually readily excluded. Occasionally, girls apparently destined to have an adult height above 5 feet 10 inches (178 cm) are brought for advice and possible medical intervention. Prediction of final height is not easy as it is influenced by the time of menarche and the rate of skeletal maturation as well as by the linear growth rate in childhood. Tables are available for predicting adult height but they are liable to errors of approximately 5 cm either way. Exogenous oestrogen therapy has been used to promote accelerated skeletal maturation and a premature cessation of linear growth in girls but the benefits are often marginal, and there is concern about the risks of interfering with the humoral mechanism of puberty and of increasing the incidence of reproductive tract neoplasia. The orthopaedic approach to this problem, epiphyseal stapling, retains its place in a very small group of children with asymmetrical growth. Irradiation of the growing epiphyses has rightly been abandoned because of the high risk of inducing osteosarcomata.

Pathological causes of excessive height

Endocrine disorders	Other disorders
Pituitary — eosinophilic adenoma	Cerebral gigantism (Soto syndrome)
Thyrotoxicosis	Marfan syndrome
Precocious puberty (early stages)	Homocystinuria

BIBLIOGRAPHY

Beighton P 1988 Inherited disorders of the skeleton, 2nd edn. Churchill Livingstone, Edinburgh
Brook C GD 1989 Clinical paediatric endocrinology, 2nd edn. Blackwell Scientific Publications, Oxford

Endocrine

Although the fetus is totally dependent on a maternally regulated environment, fetal endocrine systems differentiate and commence autonomous activity in the first trimester. The placenta is relatively impermeable to peptide hormones so that most fetal hypothalamic–pituitary–endocrine gland circuits evolve independently of any direct interference from maternal hormone levels. The adrenal cortex is an exception in that the placenta actively participates in steroid metabolism and this is reflected in the major transition from fetal to adult cortex activity with birth.

Trophic hormones are first detectable in the anterior pituitary between 5 and 8 weeks' gestation, and serum levels of thyroid stimulating hormone (TSH) and the gonadotrophins (LH and FSH) reach adult levels by 16 to 20 weeks. This early surge of trophic hormone activity may relate to endocrine gland development prior to the establishment of sensitive feedback mechanisms.

Although the conventional endocrine system is the key to understanding control of growth and development in postnatal life, it is less directly involved with fetal organisation. Fetal life is dominated by cellular division and differentiation, events which are controlled by local or paracrine systems in which populations of cells release and respond to local growth factors. The paracrine system is a complex interplay of multiple peptide growth factors, binding or transport proteins, and cell receptor sites. Growth factors may have a broad specificity, acting on a wide variety of cells in many tissues, for example insulin-like growth factors (IGF-I, IGF-II), or may be tissue specific, for example nerve growth factor (NGF). Molecular biology has provided the tools to explore this vital area. Not only is the research unravelling the regulation of fetal growth, it is casting new light on the disturbances of cellular control that lead to tumour formation. Oncogenes are nucleotide sequences which code for peptides capable of transforming normal cells into neoplastic cells. The term oncogene was originally applied to retrovirus genomes incorporated into host cells but we now know that the genes are homologous to normal genetic constituents. These normal regulator genes have been termed proto-oncogenes and their peptide products are growth factors. Bioengineered growth factors offer considerable promise as therapeutic tools.

The conductor!

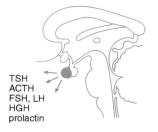

TSH
ACTH
FSH, LH
HGH
prolactin

PUBERTY

Puberty is the series of physical and physiological changes which convert a child into an adult capable of reproduction. Although it is conventionally regarded as phase dominated by increasing gonadal activity and the appearance of secondary sexual characteristics, it is better to regard it as part of the continuum of growth and maturation. Disorders of puberty have to be judged against the whole tempo of a child's development. There is considerable variation in the tempo of growth and development. As a rule girls have earlier puberty, and growth acceleration is one of the first components. Ninety-five per cent start puberty between the ages 9 and 13 years, and have onset of periods, menarche, between 11 and 13 years. Height growth is largely completed at menarche. Boys tend to have later puberty but this is partly because the initial stage, testicular growth, is less obvious. Normal male puberty commences as early as age 9 years or may be delayed to 14 years. Height acceleration occurs in the second half of the male puberty. The 12.5 cm sex difference in mean adult heights arises from the more prolonged male prepubertal growth period and also from greater pubertal height gain. For boys with late puberty the penalty is that their height gain may be substantially delayed.

Normal breast stages, girls (after Marshall and Tanner)

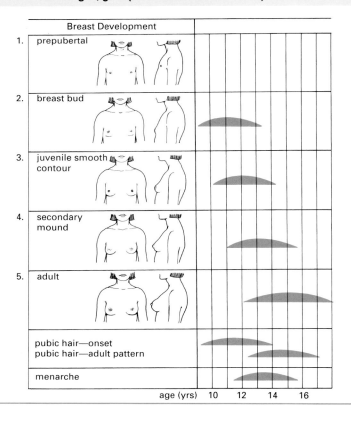

A standardised system for staging secondary sexual characteristics has been provided by Marshall and Tanner. Testicular volume can be calibrated using a Prader Orchidometer, the prepubertal testis being no more than 3 ml rising to between 12 and 20 ml in the adult. Another essential tool in the assessment of pubertal problems is the left hand and wrist bone age.

Physiology of puberty

The newborn infant is capable of releasing high levels of gonadotrophins, testosterone and oestradiol but this transient hormonal activity is subsequently inhibited by a very sensitive gonadohypothalamic feed-back mechanism. Puberty follows the elevation of the threshold for this feedback inhibition but the mechanisms responsible for this re-adjustment are not known. The pineal gland may be partly responsible for hypothalamic suppression of gonadotrophin release as tumours which destroy this gland or its connections sometimes result in precocious puberty. Longitudinal studies show that from the age of 6 years nocturnal pulses of LH release gradually increase in frequency and amplitude. Ovarian ultrasound examination also reveals increasing follicular activity from mid-childhood. The onset of puberty is not an abrupt event but is preceded by several years of endocrine adjustment. Adrenarche describes the increase in adrenal androgen release which commences

Normal genital stages, boys (after Marshall and Tanner)

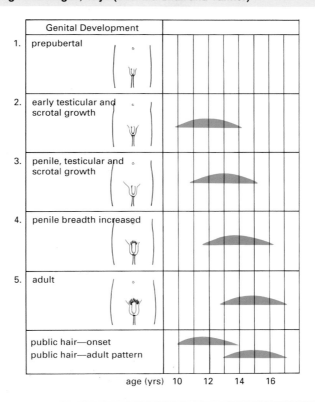

between 6 and 8 years of age. Gonadarche and adrenarche are closely parallel events but the exact link between the two remains a mystery. Adrenal androgens, particularly in girls, are responsible for sexual hair growth and skeletal maturation.

Precocious puberty

Precocious puberty is termed 'true' or intracranial when it is controlled by the hypothalamic-pituitary axis, and 'false' when an extracranial or exogenous source of hormone is responsible.

Early puberty in girls is relatively common and there may be a family history. Detailed assessment is unnecessary unless puberty commences before the age of 6 years or menses before 8 years, or if puberty pursues an abnormal sequence of events with virilisation or is accompanied by other problems such as neurological symptoms, hypertension or abnormal growth. Of girls commencing puberty early, 90 per cent have no demonstrable abnormality. Detailed ultrasound imaging of the ovaries and uterus is an invaluable tool in confirming diagnosis and monitoring progress.

Precocious puberty in boys, onset before age 9 years, is almost always pathological and requires detailed investigation. Testicular palpation is a useful guide; infantile testes in a rapidly growing pubertal boy point to an adrenal pathology. Symmetrically enlarged testes favour an intracranial problem, and a single large testis suggests a gonadal tumour.

Treatment is determined by the underlying cause, and by the potential disruption to the child's life from an unwanted puberty. In the majority of patients, who have lost normal neurohypothalamic restraint on puberty, control may be regained by using a superagonist of LHRH which causes suppression of pituitary gonadotrophin release. Although this can be successful in halting and reversing sexual maturation, it fails to restore the growth potential lost because of advanced bone age, a constant feature of precocious puberty.

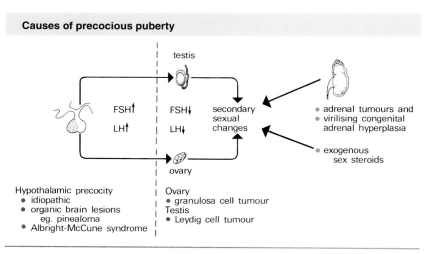

Causes of precocious puberty

testis

FSH↑   FSH↓   secondary sexual changes   • adrenal tumours and virilising congenital adrenal hyperplasia

LH↑   LH↓   • exogenous sex steroids

ovary

Hypothalamic precocity
- idiopathic
- organic brain lesions
  eg. pinealoma
- Albright-McCune syndrome

Ovary
- granulosa cell tumour

Testis
- Leydig cell tumour

Premature thelarche. Infant and young girls may have transient, cyclical and often asymmetrical breast development unaccompanied by growth acceleration or other pubertal features. Ovarian ultrasound examinations show parallel follicular development confirming that there is temporary activation of the FSH-oestradiol axis. The uterus remains small. Isolated thelarche is usually self-limiting and innocent so that reassurance is appropriate. Occasionally there may be further episodes and progression into early puberty.

Premature adrenarche or pubarche. There is a normal increase in adrenal androgen release in mid-childhood reflecting the maturation of the zona reticularis. This hormonal activity is thought to account for the modest growth spurt which normally occurs around age 6 to 8 years. The adrenal androgens may reach a level sufficient to produce early appearance of pubic hair as well as more pronounced growth acceleration and bone age advance. This is more commonly recognised in girls and is seldom indicative of progression into early puberty. Adrenarche and maturation of the gonads, gonadarche, have separate regulation. If pubic hair or growth acceleration becomes increasingly conspicuous, or occurs in a child of less than age 6 years, then steps should be taken to exclude congenital adrenal hyperplasia or an adrenal tumour.

Disordered puberty after cranial radiotherapy. A growing population of children are survivors of tumour therapy regimens incorporating cranial radiotherapy. A delayed side-effect is loss of the neural integration of growth and puberty. Girls in particular subsequently present with inappropriately early puberty often combined with relative growth hormone deficiency. They may be faced with short stature unless treated with LHRH analogues and growth hormone.

McCune–Albright syndrome. This curious entity links irregular skin pigmentation, fibrous dysplasia of bones and autonomy of endocrine glands, notably the ovaries. The ovaries may become very enlarged with large solitary cysts. The resulting early puberty follows an atypical pattern with vaginal bleeding occurring earlier than predicted from breast changes. Children may present with pathological bone fractures.

Delayed puberty

A convenient definition of delayed puberty is absence of early signs by age 14 years. However attention should also be payed to youngsters who fail to progress through puberty within an acceptable timescale. Assessment of delay must take into account the whole tempo of growth and maturation. Pubertal delay may be the conspicuous problem which brings a child to the doctor, but there is often an established pattern of low height velocity and bone age delay. Most frequently this is an inherited characteristic, constitutional delay of growth and puberty, and there is a family history of late puberty. In an important minority the delay has been imposed by either environmental or health restraints. If the delay cannot be explained by family history or identifiable restraint, then investigations need to be directed at establishing whether there is a fault either in the hypothalamo-pituitary regulation of gonadotrophin release or in the gonadal response.

Hypogonadotrophic hypogonadism. This may be inherited either in isolation or together with deficient smell sensation, Kallman syndrome. Clues at birth include micropenis and cryptorchidism, but there is a wide spectrum of severity and the condition may not be recognised until adult life. Acquired causes include tumours in the hypothalamo-pituitary region.

Hypergonadotrophic hypogonadism. High LH and FSH levels indicate that the gonadal response and feedback is impaired. Ovarian ultrasound and testicular palpation assist in defining the gonadal pathology. In girls an important cause is Turner syndrome, but ovarian dysgenesis can also occur in isolation. Boys may have congenital faults of testicular differentiation, or can lose the testes as a result of intrauterine torsion and infarction.

Complete testicular feminisation. This is the consequence of complete androgen insensitivity in the receptors of internal and external genitalia so that genetically XY individuals with testes present as female. Affected children may present in early life with an inguinal hernia containing a testis, but they not uncommonly first come to attention because of amenorrhoea in the presence of an otherwise entirely acceptable female puberty. Examination reveals a blind-ending vagina and an absent uterus. Management is based on supporting an unambiguously female person, but the testes need to be removed and oestrogen replacement provided.

Haematocolpos. Increasing abdominal distension and monthly discomfort without bleeding calls for examination of the vulva, as an imperforate hymen may produce retention of menstrual products.

DISORDERS OF SEXUAL DIFFERENTIATION

The primordial gonad is undifferentiated and biopotential. The gonad differentiating gene carried on the short arm of the Y chromosome is responsible for testicular differentiation which becomes apparent from 6 weeks. From 8 weeks the testes impose their control on the internal genitalia. The Leydig cells by secreting testosterone promote the development of Wolffian ducts to give rise to epididymis, vas deferens, seminal vesicles and ejaculatory ducts. The Sertoli cells produce Müllerian inhibitory factor which diffuses more locally to suppress the paramesonephric ducts. In a later phase, a product of testosterone, dihydrotestosterone, causes the male differentiation of the external genitalia. In the absence of an intact Y chromosome, the basic organisational drive is towards the female pattern; ovaries, disappearance of Wolffian structures and persistence of Müllerian or paramesonephric derivatives as Fallopian tubes, uterus and upper vagina. Functioning ovaries are not necessary for the differentiation of female internal and external genitalia. Turner syndrome girls have streak gonads and yet they complete otherwise normal internal and external sexual differentiation.

The relative complexity of male differentiation makes it more vulnerable to error, and leads to a long list of causes as well as a wide spectrum of severity of male pseudohermaphroditism. Problems may range from an obviously male infant with hypospadias and cryptorchidism to an apparent female. Female differentiation is more robust but can be modified by the presence of excessive androgens during fetal life producing virilisation, female pseudohermaphroditism. Congenital adrenal hyperplasia is the commonest cause of virilised females.

Ambiguity is a major management challenge not least because of family pressures. Specialist advice is needed to select appropriate investigations. In general these include chromosome analysis, adrenal and gonadal steroid measurements, and imaging to define the internal genitalia. The priorities are to define the basic fault at sex chromosome, gonadal, adrenal or end-organ level; to ensure that there are no life-threatening implications such as adrenal failure; and to select the gender most likely to provide an acceptable life. Reconstructive surgery is very successful in correcting a virilised girl, but it can do little to convert a genetic male with a minute phallus into an acceptable boy. The latter child is far better reared as a girl.

Classification of ambigious genitalia

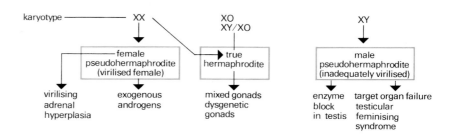

ADRENAL GLANDS

During intrauterine development the adrenal cortex is considerably enlarged due to a thick inner fetal zone. This zone, which accounts for 80 per cent of the cortex at full term, involutes rapidly after birth leaving the outer adult zone to synthesise essential mineralocorticoids and glucocorticoids. The fetal cortex acts in a mutually dependent relationship with the placenta to synthesise oestriol and dehydro-epiandrosterone. The measurement of these steroids in the maternal serum or urine provides an index of feto-placental health. The increasing development of the adult zone at term may be a factor in initiating the onset of labour.

Congenital adrenal hyperplasia. This group of inherited, autosomal recessive disorders is caused by the absence of essential enzymes in the pathway of cortisol and aldosterone synthesis. The resulting interruption of the adrenohypothalamic feedback stimulates excessive cortico-trophin (ACTH) release and overactivity of the biosynthetic steps prior to the block, with an accumulation of androgenic steroids. The commonest variety is 21-hydroxylase deficiency, approximately 1 in 5000 live births. Affected female infants are virilised at birth with clitoral hypertrophy and variable fusion of the labia minora. The most masculinised girls may be confused for males with hypospadias and cryptorchidism. Prompt recognition of this problem is less easy in males and they may not be diagnosed prior to an adrenal crisis in the second week of life. The crisis, often preceded by vomiting and poor weight gain, is biochemically characterised by low serum sodium and high potassium. Grossly elevated serum ACTH and 17-hydroxyprogesterone levels suggest the 21-hydroxylase deficiency. This may be confirmed by elevated concentrations of urinary pregnanetriol and 17-oxosteroids. A salt-losing crisis demands urgent therapy with intravenous saline, glucose and hydrocortisone. Long-term management must aim to suppress the hyperplastic adrenal glands and provide replacement hydrocortisone and a salt-retaining steroid, fludrocortisone. The correct replacement is that which permits normal linear growth and maintains serum 17-hydroxyprogesterone and adrenal androgens within acceptable limits. Surgical correction of the masculinised female perineum is commenced in the first year.

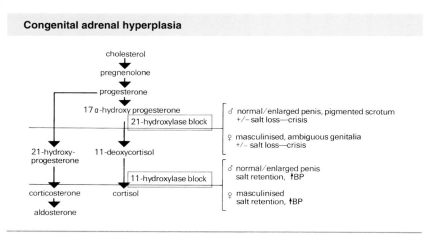

Congenital adrenal hyperplasia

Adult men and women are capable of normal fertility but should remain on hydrocortisone and fludrocortisone. Among the rarer forms of congenital adrenal hyperplasia, 11-beta-hydroxylase deficiency results in virilisation and salt retention with hypertension. Affected children may present with excessive growth, but the advanced bone age considerably limits their final adult stature.

Cushing syndrome. This disorder is due to sustained high circulating cortisol levels of either exogenous or endogenous origin. Iatrogenic disease is now less common with the introduction of effective alternatives to systemic corticosteroid therapy in for example asthma. Endogenous Cushing syndrome is fortunately rare in childhood but is likely to be due to a potentially malignant adrenocortical tumour. It should be considered when acne and masculinisation accompany the usual signs of cortisol excess. Distinction must be made between these potentially malignant unilateral tumours and the rarer problem of bilateral adrenal hyperplasia due to pituitary microadenomata. In the majority of cases the nature of the adrenal pathology will be demonstrated by CT scans. Adrenal tumours require unilateral adrenalectomy and additional radiotherapy if there is histological evidence of capsule invasion. In acquired bilateral adrenal hyperplasia, management is directed against the pituitary adenomata using high voltage radiation or trans-sphenoidal microsurgery.

Not infrequently obese girls with striae are suspected of having an underlying 'hormonal problem' such as an adrenal tumour. The vast majority are healthy and owe their obesity to their nutrition. A useful guide is to appreciate that nutritional obesity is generally accompanied by above average stature. Cushingoid features linked to growth failure are suspicious.

Adrenal cortical failure (Addison disease). This uncommon disorder has an autoimmune basis and may occur in association with diabetes mellitus, thyroiditis and hypoparathyroidism. Children either present with an insidious onset of weakness, weight loss and increased pigmentation or become acutely ill following a brief episode of diarrhoea and vomiting. An adrenal crisis demands urgent therapy with intravenous glucose and saline together with hydrocortisone. Long-term replacement consists of hydrocortisone (15–20 mg/m^2 surface area/day) and fludrocortisone (0.1 to 0.2 mg daily). With all patients on corticosteroid replacement therapy, the child must be provided with a steroid warning card and the parents advised of the necessity of increasing the dosage during times of illness.

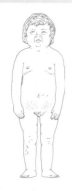

Cushing syndrome: clinical features

face and trunk obesity
heightened facial colour
hirsutism
hypertension
mood changes
muscle wasting
osteoporosis
striae
bruising
androgen effects suggest an adrenal tumour eg. acne and clitoral hypertrophy

THYROID

The thyroid originates from a ventral extension of the endoderm foregut which migrates caudad to lie at the level of the upper trachea. Developmental failures may be classified as hypoplasia or maldescent.

Hypoplasia varies from absence of detectable thyroid and early severe hypothyroidism, to lesser degrees which remain asymptomatic until later childhood. An ectopic gland may account for a lingual mass or produce a thyroglossal cyst. A sinus may occur along the line of descent.

Physiology

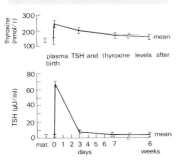

Neonatal thyroid function

plasma TSH and thyroxine levels after birth

The fetal thyroid contains colloid and iodoproteins by 10 weeks gestation; plasma TSH is detectable at this stage and there is evidence for early activity of the pituitary-thyroid axis. The fetal thyroid preferentially releases 'reverse T3', a molecule which differs from tri-iodothyronine by the location of a single iodine atom. Reverse T3 is thought to be inactive and its place in physiology has not been established. There is minimal transplacental passage of maternal thyroxine to the fetus.

Following birth there is a surge of TSH release later paralleled by increased thyroxine (T4) and tri-iodothyronine (T3). TSH levels return to the normal adult range by 1 week but T4 and especially T3 show a slower decline to adult values. The definition of normal neonatal thyroid function is essential for the development of screening programmes to detect congenital hypothyroidism.

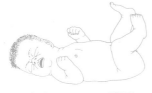

Congenital hypothyroidism

coarse facies
dry skin
hoarse cry
hypotonia
umbilical hernia
constipation
prolonged jaundice

TSH ↑↑
thyroxine ↓

Congenital hypothyroidism. Congenital hypothyroidism is relatively common, 1 in 3000 live births. It is usually a sporadic condition and it is uncommon for there to be recurrence in siblings. Central nervous system development is critically dependent on T4 and T3, especially in late pregnancy and early infancy, and hypothyroidism is an important cause of preventable mental handicap. It has recently been discovered that the hypothyroid fetus partially compensates for deficiency by diverting the minimal transplacental supply of T4 to the brain where it is converted to T3 by a specific cerebral deiodinase. Delivery interrupts this tenuous source of T4. The signs of hypothyroidism, notably prolonged jaundice, are usually present by age 2 weeks but are often overlooked. Fortunately screening for elevated TSH levels at age 1 week has proved to be both sensitive and specific. Thyroxine therapy introduced by age 3 weeks and titrated to parallel growth enables the majority of children to achieve development closely resembling normal.

Endemic goitre and hypothyroidism. Iodine deficiency remains the commonest cause of thyroid disease worldwide. It results in a spectrum of severity including profound neurological cretinism, deaf–mutism, myxoedema with dwarfism, and goitres. Genetic variation and diet, notably cassava consumption, influence susceptibility to iodine deficiency. Iodization programmes and iodine depot injection in early pregnancy can dramatically reduce the prevalence of these disorders.

Goitrous hypothyroidism. This is rare outside of endemic regions. A group of inborn errors of thyroid metabolism may present in the newborn period or more commonly come to light in later childhood with the emergence of a goitre. Antithyroid drugs given to control maternal hyperthyroidism in pregnancy can result in a fetal goitre. Iodine containing drugs can also induce fetal hypothyroidism, and topical iodine

Ectopic sites of the thyroid gland

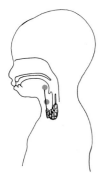

should be avoided in preterm infants particularly as they are already at risk of borderline hypothyroidism.

Juvenile hypothyroidism. Current neonatal hypothyroid screening programmes detect the majority of congenitally hypoplastic and ectopic glands that previously resulted in presentation after infancy. Autoimmune thyroiditis is now the more frequent cause of children, usually girls, who present with primary hypothyroidism. Features include goitre, progressive growth failure with marked bone age delay, lethargy and constipation. The secondary epiphyseal dysgenesis can produce orthopaedic problems, notably slipped upper femoral epiphyses. Intellectual development does not usually suffer because the thyroid deficiency occurs after the critical phase of brain development; paradoxically parents may complain of their children's behaviour after thyroxine treatment has transformed them from hypothyroid induced docility into normal teenagers! Thyroxine is the standard therapy for hypothyroidism. Infants require a relatively higher dose, 5 µg per kg per day, diminishing to 2 to 3 µg per kg in later childhood. The dose is monitored by checking height and bone age increments as well as biochemical parameters. Therapy must be life long.

Neonatal hyperthyroidism. This is an uncommon disorder but must be anticipated in all infants of mothers with a history of thyrotoxicosis. Maternal thyroid stimulating immunoglobulins may traverse the placenta to overstimulate the fetal thyroid producing irritability, fever, diarrhoea and poor weight gain. Although transient the condition is potentially fatal and may require antithyroid therapy or propranolol.

Juvenile hyperthyroidism. This is uncommon but the features are similar to those seen in adults with the addition of excessive growth and occasional abnormal choreiform movements. The diagnosis is confirmed by elevated plasma thyroxine levels. Medical management using carbimazole is the treatment of choice. An initial two year course may result in spontaneous remission in 25 to 75 per cent of cases, and a further course should be completed before considering surgical management. Radioactive iodine is to be avoided in childhood.

Isolated thyroid nodules. These must be carefully investigated by isotope scans and biopsy to exclude carcinoma.

PARATHYROID GLANDS

Hypoparathyroidism

Transient hypoparathyroidism is a common neonatal event and the resulting hypocalcaemia may cause convulsions or apnoeic episodes. Permanent hypoparathyroidism is rare and has to be distinguished from conditions in which there is organ unresponsiveness to circulating parathyroid hormone, the pseudohypoparathyroidism syndromes.

Features of hypoparathyroidism

Acute hypocalcaemia	Chronic hypocalcaemia
convulsions	convulsions
neuromuscular excitability	calcification of basal ganglia
Chvostek sign	headache, vomiting (raised intracranial pressure)
Trousseau sign	photophobia
carpopedal spasm	cataracts
	poor dentition
	chronic diarrhoea
	Investigation: serum calcium $\downarrow$
	serum phosphorus $\uparrow$
	alk. phos.—normal

True hypoparathyroidism. True hypoparathyroidism is confirmed by demonstrating undetectable plasma PTH levels, and increased urinary phosphate or cyclic AMP excretion during an infusion of parathyroid hormone.

Pseudohypoparathyroidism syndromes. These syndromes are refractory to parathyroid administration and the children may show the other features; short stature, round facies, short metacarpals, ectopic calcification and mental retardation.

Pseudopseudohypoparathyroidism. This is part of the group of X-linked disorders in which the typical physical abnormalities are not accompanied by biochemical derangement.

Classification of hypoparathyroidism

Transient neonatal	Prematurity, cerebral injury
	Maternal diabetes
	Maternal hyperparathyroidism
Permanent life-long	Isolated hypoplasia
	Di George syndrome. Thymus aplasia, defective immunity, candidiasis, cardiac lesions
	Autoimmune — associated diabetes mellitus, Addison disease, chronic hepatitis, etc.
	Post-thyroidectomy
Pseudohypoparathyroidism syndromes	

Treatment of hypoparathyroidism. Acute symptomatic hypocalcaemia requires urgent correction with intravenous calcium, 0.1 mmol elemental calcium per kg bodyweight per hour. Ten per cent calcium gluconate should be diluted to 2 per cent for use and the infusion must be carefully monitored.

Permanent hypoparathyroidism and pseudohypoparathyroidism are treated with supraphysiological doses of vitamin D or related compounds which act by promoting intestinal calcium absorption and by mobilising bone calcium. The dose of vitamin D is adjusted to maintain the plasma calcium level in the low normal range (2.15 to 2.40 mmol/l). Chronic overdosage carries the risk of nephrocalcinosis and renal failure.

DIABETES

Diabetes mellitus is the disorder which results from insulin deficiency. In most juvenile diabetics, this is due to irreversible islet beta cell damage. Diabetes is rare in infancy but the incidence rises so that by age 16 years, 2 per 1000 are affected. Children account for only 4 to 6 per cent of the total diabetic population but the life-long implications of the disease emphasise their importance.

Aetiology

Duration of symptoms before diagnosis

0–2 wks	20%
2–6 wks	52%
6 wks plus	28%

The failure of islet beta cells appears to reflect both genetic and environmental factors. HLA-DR3 and DR4 are linked to increased incidence and are present in 95 per cent of type 1 or insulin dependent diabetics. The HLA system is carried on chromosome 6 and is linked with determinants of immune function. There is growing evidence of auto-immune beta cell damage, paralleled by circulating islet cell antibodies for months or even years before clinical diabetes becomes manifest. It is however unclear how environmental influence converts inherited susceptibility into overt disease. Viral involvement is favoured by seasonal peaks of presentation, case clustering and the occasional isolation of coxsackie B virus from newly recognised but fatal diabetes. We are no nearer defining a specific group of viral pathogens against which immunisation might be developed. Other still speculative evidence favours early dietary exposure as an environmental trigger.

Clinical features

Clinical features of childhood diabetes

Early	Late
polyuria	vomiting
(secondary	abdominal pain
nocturnal	hyperventilation
enuresis)	(metabolic
thirst	acidosis)
lethargy	shock
weight loss	coma
anorexia	
(increased	
appetite unusual)	
constipation	

The symptoms are characteristic and the diagnosis is seldom in doubt if hyperglycaemia, glycosuria and ketonuria are detected. Young diabetics always require prompt diagnosis and therapy, but the correct diagnosis may be confused by a coincidental febrile illness and the hyperventilation mistakenly interpreted as being due to pneumonia. Diabetes may be confirmed by a single blood glucose estimation and glucose tolerance tests are rarely necessary. Early diagnosis saves lives and allows an organised introduction to the principles of diabetic management; often as an out-patient. Ketoacidosis obviously necessitates urgent admission.

Diabetic ketoacidosis. The basic principles of treatment consist of insulin therapy, fluid and electrolyte replacement and the correction of provoking factors. Low dose insulin regimens are favoured as these provide for more predictable control of blood sugar and largely avoid hypoglycaemia and hypokalaemia. Although metabolic acidosis may be prominent it is unnecessary to administer sodium bicarbonate unless there is severe circulatory failure.

Long-term management   It is not possible to return diabetics to a physiologically normal state with current methods of insulin administration. Management must be a compromise aimed at the following objectives: a happy child leading a full life and equipped for a normal adult role; normal growth; education and motivation to maintain the best possible diabetic control. Current clinical and experimental studies support the belief that optimal control reduces the long-term risk of microvascular disease. In practice good control means freedom from symptoms and satisfactory blood glucose profiles confirmed by regular glycosylated haemoglobin levels. This can only be achieved at the expense of occasional hypoglycaemic episodes. The essentials of management are diet, appropriate insulin and education in the techniques and understanding of diabetes.

A scheme for the management of diabetic ketoacidosis

1. **Initial management**
   Assess circulatory status
   Weigh
   Insert i.v. line and send samples to laboratory
   Stop oral intake and insert nasogastric tube
   Attach ECG monitor

2. **Identify provoking factors,** e.g. infection

3. **Treat shock**
   i.v. N saline or plasma

4. **Fluid and electrolyte management**   **Insulin management**
   Calculate total fluid requirement
   (deficit + maintenance + losses)
   Replace   1/3 0–4 hr
                    1/3 4–12 hr
                    1/3 12–24 hr

   • Extracellular replacement:
     i.v. N saline + KCl until blood glucose < 14 mmol/l
                                                            i.v. short-acting insulin
                                                            initial dose 0.25 U/kg
                                                            continue 0.10 U/kg/hr
                                                            using infusion pump until blood glucose < 14 mmol/l

   • Intracellular replacement: reduce insulin to 0.05 U/kg/hr
     i.v. 0.2 N saline in 5% glucose + KCl   (adjust according to blood glucose)

   • Graded re-introduction of oral fluids 2-hourly milk/   start 8-hourly short-acting insulin 0.5-2.0 U/kg/day
     sugar drinks

   • Regular diet   establish on medium-acting insulin

Diet. The modern diabetes diet emphasises good nutrition based on a normal proportion of appropriate carbohydrates, particularly those high in fibre. This approach has replaced the restricted carbohydrate intake which placed too great a reliance on fat-based calories. Dieticians assist the family in adjusting their previous diet and provide a meal and snack structure based on readily recognised 10 g portions.

Insulin. Most young children are managed on a regimen of twice daily combined short and medium duration human insulins. There is the choice of mixing the two insulins in the syringe, which allows for titration according to blood glucose profiles, or of using premixed preparations which have the advantage of reducing errors inherent in drawing up the insulins separately. A range of user friendly pen injection devices has also been introduced. These reduce the tedium of injection preparation, and allow for older children and adolescents to be recruited to regimens based on three or four injections daily. These more intensive schemes provide insulin in a way which resembles normal physiology more closely and, if used with regular blood glucose monitoring, have the potential for providing excellent control.

Injections are the focal points of a diabetic child's day, and considerable attention must be given to teaching and reinforcing good technique. School age children should be capable of performing their own injections. Common faults include too shallow needle insertion which is more painful, and targetting injections on a favourite site which promotes unsightly fat hypertrophy. Fat hypertrophy interferes with insulin absorption and adds to the unpredictability of insulin effect.

Monitoring. Regular capillary blood glucose measurement is now part of the modern diabetic way of life. The problem is to devise a compromise between the child's variable lifestyle and worthwhile data collection. There are often short and medium term problems in achieving desirable control but hopefully the child and family will grasp the longer term objectives of understanding and achieving good diabetes control.

A selection of insulins

Type		Approximate time of action (hours)		
		Onset	Peak	Duration
Short-acting (neutral insulin)	Actrapid Velosulin Humulin S	½	1–3	6–8
Medium-acting (isophone insulin)	Protaphane Insulatard Humulin I	1–1½	2–12	18–24
Medium-acting (insulin zinc suspension)	Monotard Humulin Zn	2–3	6–14	22–24

Problems in diabetic control

Poor control and so-called brittle diabetes with recurrent ketoacidosis and hypoglycaemia may arise from several causes.

Hypoglycaemia. Parents have a great fear of insulin reactions and this naturally leads to caution in attaining near normoglycaemia especially in the evening tests. All diabetic children must have immediate access to glucose tablets or drinks. Families should be provided with glucagon injection for emergency management of hypoglycaemia.

The dawn phenomenon. This refers to the common finding of refractory hyperglycaemia in the early part of the day. It results from waning insulin action after the previous evening's injection exacerbated by circadian rhythms of growth hormone and cortisol release.

Factors which influence diabetic control

Behaviour. Parents require advice on how to cope with injection trauma, dietary delinquency, fake tests and pseudo-hypoglycaemia. Clinic visits must not be regarded as times of judgement. Adolescents may become introspective and depressed about the future so that poor control and carelessness may be a symptom of their distress.

Diabetes and growth. Children with diabetes can look forward to a normal adult stature, although comparison between identical twins discordant for diabetes shows some loss of final height. Modest pubertal delay is more frequent; marked delay especially in girls is an indication for excluding coexistent auto-immune hypothyroidism.

Long-term complications

Epidemiological studies of previous generations of childhood onset diabetics provide sobering statistics; a mortality rate 2 to 6 times in excess of non-diabetic controls, and a sad catalogue of blindness, limb amputations, renal failure, heart attacks and suicide. These problems arise from a combination of microvascular and accelerated macrovascular disease. Diabetic kidney disease stands out as a particular threat for an approximate 25 to 40 per cent of diabetics who are genetically susceptible to this complication. Markers for this group include a positive family history of cardiac and cerebrovascular disease, and higher blood pressure. Fortunately there is already evidence that more recent cohorts of patients are less likely to manifest kidney disease and related problems; whether this is an effect of improved management or a reflection of changing population behaviour is unclear. It is clear that greater attention to blood pressure control in young adults who demonstrate microproteinuria can reduce the rate of renal deterioration. Hopefully the combination of good metabolic control with intensive insulin regimens, avoidance of smoking and kidney protecting drugs such as ACE inhibitors will further benefit diabetics.

Diabetic retinopathy is the single most common cause of blindness in developed countries. Capillary occlusion is the first stage in a sequence of events which develop after 10 years of diabetes in the majority of patients. Few develop retinopathy before age 15 years, suggesting that the pubertal years are important in the genesis of microvascular disease. Vision threatening retinopathy is now largely preventable by regular eye checks and photocoagulation. Subcapsular snowstorm cataracts are a rare complication in childhood diabetes.

HYPOGLYCAEMIA

Causes of hypoglycaemia in infancy and childhood

Substrate deficiency (ketones usually present)

- ketotic hypoglycaemia
- hepatic enzyme deficiencies
    glycogen storage diseases
    galactosaemia
    hereditary fructose intolerance
- exogenous hepatotoxins and poisons
    Reye syndrome
    alcohol, aspirin
    unripe Akee fruit
- endogenous hepatotoxins
    tyrosinosis
    maple syrup urine disease
- endocrine deficiencies
    pituitary, adrenal

Hyperinsulinism (ketones absent)

- pancreatic
    nesidioblastosis
    insulinoma
    mesenchymal tumours
- prediabetes mellitus
- insulin administration

Hypoglycaemia is rare after the newborn period but must be considered in the assessment of non-febrile seizures, particularly those occurring early in the morning and after prolonged fasts. A blood glucose of less than 2.2 mmol/l is diagnostic and the urine should also be tested for ketones, a helpful step in distinguishing the two main categories of disorders which cause recurrent hypoglycaemia: substrate deficiency and hyperinsulinism. In children in whom there is no obvious explanation, a carefully monitored period of starvation with serial determinations of plasma glucose, insulin, cortisol, growth hormone, beta-hydroxybutyrate and lactic acid is the most useful investigation.

Ketotic hypoglycaemia. This is the commonest cause of hypoglycaemia after the first year. Affected children are usually small, slim and more susceptible to attacks during coincidental illness. Nocturnal fits associated with vomiting and unconsciousness develop and ketonuria is prominent. Monitored starvation results in a more pronounced hypoglycaemia and ketonaemia than normal, but insulin levels are very low. Limited gluconeogenic reserves probably account for this disorder. Hypoglycaemia can be avoided by regular bedtime snacks and additional glucose drinks during illness. The problem resolves spontaneously in later childhood.

Nesidioblastosis is a rare problem of young infants in which developmental disorganisation of the islet cells and inappropriate insulin release results in refractory hypoglycaemia. The latter may be partially controlled using continuous infusions of glucose, and diazoxide. The most successful long-term therapy is a 75 to 80 per cent resection of the pancreas.

Insulinomas account for most cases of hyperinsulinism in older infants and children, and again extensive resection of the pancreas is indicated.

BIBLIOGRAPHY

Brook C G D 1989 Clinical paediatric endocrinology, 2nd edn. Blackwell Scientific Publications, Oxford
Tattersall R B, Gale E A N 1990 Diabetes: Clinical management. Churchill Livingstone, Edinburgh

16 Skin

Man consists mainly of water and it is his skin which stops him from drying out. In addition, the skin protects the body from physical, chemical and biological insult. The superficial layer of the epidermis, stratum corneum, with its compact horny cells provides an effective barrier to the passage of substances in either direction. The dermis, with its high collagen content, gives skin its ability to stretch and mould. Its numerous blood vessels and sweat glands are important in the control of body temperature.

The epidermis develops in the third week of fetal life, and is initially composed of two layers, an outer periderm and an inner basal layer. The periderm is equipped with absorptive microvilli and actively transfers substances between amniotic fluid and fetal tissues. It is normally shed long before term, but occasionally it persists as a horny cocoon, creating the so-called 'collodion baby'. The basal or germinative layer gives rise to the definitive multi-layered epidermis, and this differentiation is largely complete when keratinisation establishes the stratum corneum in the sixth month of fetal life. An extremely premature infant has thin, poorly keratinised epidermis, and is therefore vulnerable to excessive skin water losses after birth.

The sebaceous glands are active from mid gestation, and their secretion, together with the residue of the periderm, accounts for the vernix caseosa. The vernix provides a greasy coating to the newborn skin and

The arm of a 'collodion baby'

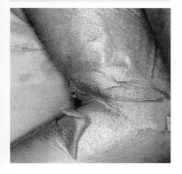

Lesions

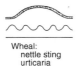

Scales:
psoriasis
ringworm

Macule: (flat disc)
freckles
measles

Papule:
wart

Lump:
cavernous
haemangioma

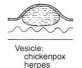

Wheal:
nettle sting
urticaria

Vesicle:
chickenpox
herpes

Bulla:
2nd degree
burns

Ulcer:
ruptured vesicle
injury

may have bactericidal properties. Term infants are able to sweat within 2 to 5 days after birth, but there may be a delay of 2 to 3 weeks in the premature. Sebum and sweat retention are common in the newborn.

RASHES OF EARLY INFANCY

Erythema toxicum on cheek

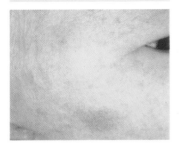

Seborrhoeic dermatitis

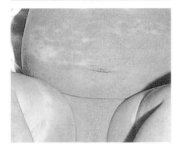

Erythema toxicum. This is possibly the most frequent skin eruption in the first weeks of life, and reflects sweat gland immaturity and the tendency for babies to overheat. It arises as crops of papules or papulo-vesicles over the face, trunk and napkin area. It generally resolves rapidly with appropriate clothing and ventilation, but may occasionally become secondarily infected.

Seborrhoeic dermatitis is a distinctive erythematous and scaly, non-eczematous eruption of unknown cause. It usually starts during the second or third month of life as cradle cap or napkin dermatitis which spreads rapidly, sometimes giving psoriasis-like lesions over much of the body. The child is never ill and is not distressed by it. In its mildest form, just one or two lesions may be present in the flexures giving rise to an erroneous diagnosis of atopic eczema. Very mild corticosteroid and antiseptic combinations such as 1 per cent hydrocortisone and 3 per cent clioquinol will usually clear it.

Rashes in the napkin area are very common and not always indicative of poor mothering. The main causes are napkin dermatitis, candidiasis and seborrhoeic dermatitis.

Napkin dermatitis. Napkin dermatitis is caused by prolonged contact with wet napkins. Bacterial conversion of the urine to ammonia creates

Ammoniacal napkin rash: sparing flexures

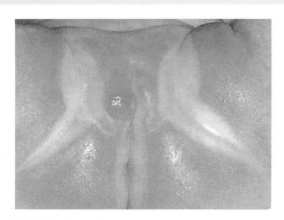

Monilial infection: involving flexures

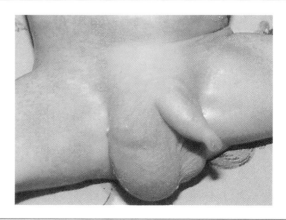

an alkaline irritant. Simple measures are usually effective; frequent napkin changes, careful washing at each change and the application of a protective cream such as zinc and castor oil ointment. The napkin should be rinsed thoroughly after washing and used with disposable napkin liners.

Candidiasis. Candidiasis is commonly superimposed on a napkin rash and warrants treatment with nystatin ointment.

ATOPIC ECZEMA

Atopic eczema affects 3 per cent of children and usually has its onset between 2 and 18 months of age. There is often a family history of other atopic disorders, hay fever or asthma. Itching is very prominent and scratching frequently results in secondary infection. It has a fluctuating course with approximately 50 per cent resolving by 18 months and few continue to have a problem beyond childhood. Although skin prick tests for specific allergens are often positive, they provide little guide to clinical management as multiple factors are usually involved. There is some preliminary evidence that breastfeeding and total avoidance of cow's milk protein in the first few months of life may reduce the incidence of atopic problems in genetically susceptible infants.

Atopic eczema

Infant

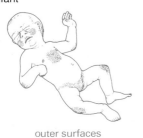

outer surfaces

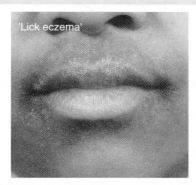

'Lick eczema'

Childhood

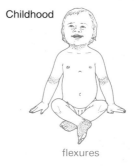

flexures

Management Atopic eczema is a very taxing illness for child and family. Disturbed nights, irritability and the often alarming appearance add to the burden. The parents have an active role in management and need careful sympathetic instruction. The skin is often dry because of an associated ichthyosis; the avoidance of all soap and the use of emulsifying ointment in its place helps to correct this. Corticosteroid ointments applied once or twice daily benefit the affected areas but should be used sparingly and the potency kept to the minimum necessary to control the disease. One per cent hydrocortisone cream or ointment, or betamethasone cream diluted to 1 in 10 with cetomacrogol cream, are usually adequate for all but the most stubborn patches. Secondary infection may be treated with a topical antibiotic, for example chlortetracycline or neomycin combined with a corticosteroid. If the child is pyrexial, or deeper spread of infection occurs, a systemic antibiotic should be given. The control of scratching and the provision of undisturbed nights are valuable assets. Antihistamines, for example trimeprazine tartrate or promethazine, used as night sedation are well tolerated and valuable if given as a short course during exacerbation. Other useful measures include using cotton underclothes rather than wool, avoiding heat, and light bandaging of the limbs at night. The hands must never be tied to prevent scratching. There is no contraindication to immunisation against diphtheria, whooping cough, tetanus and poliomyelitis, but these should be given when the eczema is in a less acute phase. Primary infection with herpes simplex virus may give a very severe reaction known as Kaposi varicelliform eruption.

INFECTIONS AND INFESTATIONS

Bacterial

Impetigo. This is a highly contagious superficial skin infection which passes rapidly through a vesicular phase and usually presents with typical golden brown crusts. Topical therapy with the application of 3 per cent chlortetracycline cream is adequate for limited infections. More extensive lesions require a systemic antibiotic, for example erythromycin. Refractory or atypical cases raise the possibility of an underlying cause such as scabies, scalp pediculosis or an immune deficiency.

Bullous impetigo of the newborn. This may have serious complications, for example osteomyelitis and pneumonia, and the mortality is high. Systemic antibiotics are required, for example flucloxacillin.

Impetigo: face

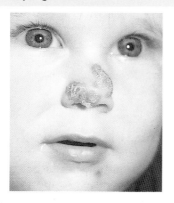

Bullous impetigo: abdomen

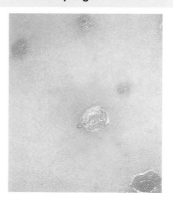

Erysipelas: leg

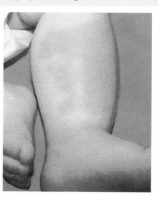

Toxic epidermal necrolysis (Lyell disease, Ritter disease or staphylococcal scalded skin syndrome). Toxic epidermal necrolysis results from epidermal cleavage due to toxins of staphylococcus phage type 71. Typically, young infants and children develop acute inflammation and soreness which evolves into a generalised exfoliation, the scalded skin syndrome. Even ordinary handling can result in skin loss and extreme care is necessary in the nursing of these children.

Viral

Primary herpes simplex. Primary herpes simplex infection is usually asymptomatic but it can produce a gingivostomatitis in young children. It presents with fever, irritability, and difficulty in swallowing. The latter is caused by extensive shallow ulcers of the buccal, gingival and pharyngeal mucosas. Occasionally there may be a vulvovaginitis or a keratoconjunctivitis. Herpetic encephalitis is a rare but grave complication. Gingivostomatitis requires careful nursing to ensure an adequate fluid intake. Idoxuridine paint may accelerate healing if it can be successfully applied to the ulcerated mucosa.

Herpes zoster. This is not uncommon in children and usually settles without leaving post herpetic neuralgia. Povidone-iodine paint will reduce infectivity and the likelihood of secondary infection.

Viral warts. Viral warts affect most children at some time during childhood. They are harmless and self limiting, and treatment is only indicated if there is discomfort. This is most likely on the pressure bearing areas of the soles. The application of a salicylic acid based wart paint is usually all that is required.

Molluscum contagiosum. This is more likely to affect covered areas of the body. The individual lesions can be cleared by pricking the centre with a sharpened stick dipped in liquid phenol.

Herpes	Filiform warts	Molluscum

Fungal skin infection

Fungal infections due to the usual human dermatophytes are uncommon in childhood; a diagnosis of athelete's foot is nearly always wrong. Susceptibility to animal ringworm, especially Microsporum canis

Tinea capatis	Ringworm (kerion)

Tinea capitis
(microsporum canis)

circulating scaling
patches with hair
loss

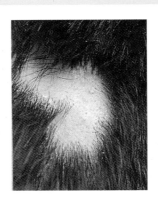

Kerion
(trichophyton verrucosum)

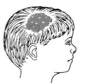

inflamed, pustular
boggy mass

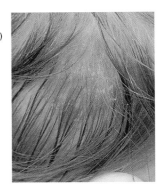

from cats and dogs, is quite high and scalp involvement is unique to children.

Infestations

Scabies is due to a mite which is spread by close family contact and invades the horny layer of the skin where it lays its eggs. The burrows are generally over hands, wrists, elbows, feet and genitalia but can occur on the face of babies. Infestation provokes an intense itch and a secondary erythematous papular rash. The mite may be identified using a low power lens and a needle. The whole family should be treated by a single application of benzyl benzoate emulsion to all the skin surfaces below the neck. A less irritating alternative is 1 per cent gamma benzene hexachloride.

Pediculosis capitis or head lice infestation is common in our schools. It may present as a persistent itch with secondary dermatitis or be found on routine hair examination. The oval nits are easily seen firmly adhering to the hair shaft. The mature lice are less often visible. The application of 0.5 per cent malathion solution is effective against the lice and nits.

Scabies	Head lice

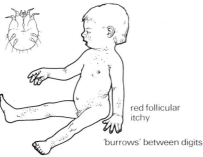

red follicular
itchy

'burrows' between digits

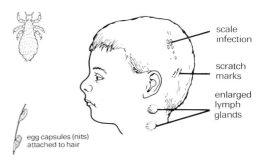

scale
infection

scratch
marks

enlarged
lymph
glands

egg capsules (nits)
attached to hair

CONGENITAL SKIN LESIONS

Birth marks

Strawberry naevus (superficial cavernous angioma). A third of these elevated lesions occur on the face and become conspicuous and grow rapidly in the first month of life. In spite of parental pressure, management must be conservative with the reassuring knowledge that spontaneous disappearance occurs by the age of 5 or 6 years.

Capillary naevus (port wine stain). This defect in dermal blood vessels can occur anywhere but is commonest on the upper half of the body. There is no tendency to fade or spread. Usually it is an isolated cosmetic problem, but occasionally there may be meningeal involvement as well, for example in the Sturge-Weber syndrome.

Pigmented naevi. These naevi are rarely evident at birth and start to appear at the age of 2 years. In childhood they are usually flat or only slightly elevated. Histologically they show junctional activity but malignancy is extremely rare. With maturation the majority lose their junctional elements and become intradermal and completely benign. Extensive macular pale brown 'café au lait' spots are a feature of neurofibromatosis.

Strawberry naevus	'Salmon patch'	Sturge-Weber syndrome

1 month

1 year

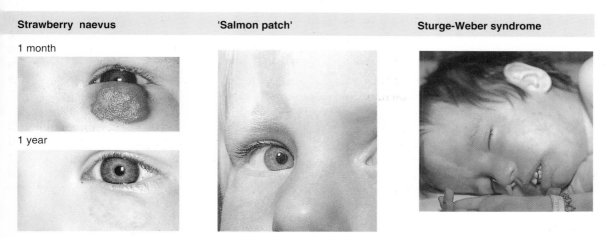

Ichthyosis. The most frequent form is an autosomal dominant condition characterised by dry finely scaling skin. It may coincide with and complicate atopic dermatitis. Restoration of skin moisture with an emollient cream is the basis of treatment.

Congenital anhidrotic ectodermal dysplasia. This is a rare, sex-linked, recessive condition producing loss of sweat glands, dental hypoplasia, and sparse hair, eyebrows and eyelashes. These children are intolerant of heat.

Epidermolysis bullosa. This condition is a pathological susceptibility to blistering and there are a number of genetic varieties. The severity ranges from blistering with unusual trauma to serious life threatening scarring and deformity, despite careful handling.

Incontinentia pigmenti. This rare condition is almost exclusively restricted to females and is usually obvious at birth. Groups of vesicles evolve through warty papules to bizarre patterns of pigmentation. There is associated eosinophilia, dental and eye abnormalities.

Xeroderma pigmentosum. This autosomal recessive condition is manifest by dry photosensitive skin liable to freckling, keratoses and malignant transformation.

Acrodermatitis enteropathica. This produces progressive mucocutaneous ulceration and is associated with bowel pathology. It responds to treatment with zinc.

'Café au lait' spots	Epidermolysis bullosa	Incontinentia pigmenti

 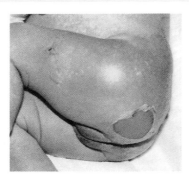 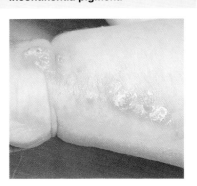

OTHER COMMON SKIN DISORDERS

Psoriasis

This commonly presents as an acute guttate rash following an upper respiratory tract infection. An eruption of small discrete red scaling lesions may develop rapidly and cover much of the body. Resolution usually occurs after 2 months or so, but the existence of the psoriatic tendency has been indicated and the more typical plaques on elbows, knees and scalp may develop at any time. Treatment should be kept to a minimum compatible with asymptomatic control. The application of coal tar and salicylic acid ointment after bathing is a useful measure.

Pityriasis rosea

This is an acute self limiting eruption giving rise to erythematous scaling macules with a central distribution. It may superficially resemble guttate psoriasis but is distinguished by a herald patch, which appears

Guttate psoriasis   **Pityriasis rosea (insert 'herald patch')**   **Granuloma annulare**

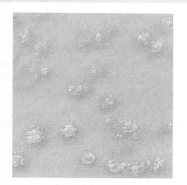  

3 or 4 days before the main eruption, and by the frequent presence of itching and fine scaling. A mild corticosteroid ointment may help resolution.

Granuloma annulare. These skin lesions consist of asymptomatic dermal nodules usually on the fingers or toes. It is a harmless condition but resolution may be slow, taking years rather than months.

Alopecia areata. These areas of localised hair loss on the scalp have a characteristic margin of exclamation mark hairs. The alopecia is usually self-limiting and possibly related to periods of school or other stress. Rare cases progress to alopecia totalis. It should be distinguished from habitual hair pulling, trichotillomania, and ring-worm of the scalp in which there is an obvious inflammatory element.

Acne. Acne occasionally occurs in a child less than 18 months old and reflects physiological adjustments in the responsiveness of sebaceous glands to postnatal hormone changes. Its occurrence later in childhood, but before the onset of puberty, requires further investigation in case of underlying adrenal pathology. It is, of course, very common in adolescence but the problem should not be discounted because it may dominate life and give rise to self-imposed isolation. It is linked to the onset of sebaceous gland activity and the production of free fatty acids in follicles which are blocked, with resulting comedones or black-heads, inflammation and pustules. Treatment is directed at removing the keratin plugs, for example with benzoyl peroxide, and suppression of lipolytic bacteria with long-term low dose antibiotics, usually tetracycline 250 mg twice daily.

Erythema nodosum. These tender erythematous nodules occur most frequently over the pretibial region. They appear in crops and may be associated with fever and arthralgia. An underlying problem may be streptococcal infection, tuberculosis, *Mycoplasma pneumoniae*, food or drug sensitivity. In the majority no underlying condition will be found.

Erythema multiforme is a local vascular reaction which may be triggered by viral infections like herpes simplex and mycoplasma or drugs. As the name suggests the rash takes many forms. The characteristic lesion is like a target or iris in shape, the rash is symmetrical and affects the limbs more than the trunk. When the reaction involves the mucous membranes, the Steven Johnson syndrome, the systemic reaction is more severe and there is a significant morbidity and mortality. In this situation steroids, acyclovir and immunoglobulin may all be justified.

Erythema nodosum	Erythema multiforme	Steven-Johnson syndrome

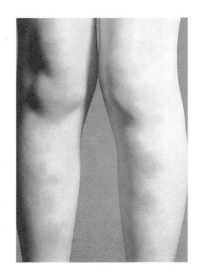
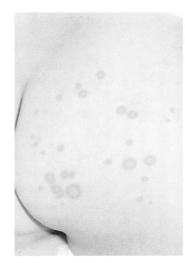
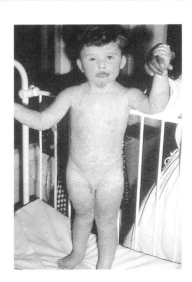

BIBLIOGRAPHY

Verbov J 1988 Essential paediatric dermatology. Clinical Press, Bristol
Weston W L 1979 Practical paediatric dermatology. Little, Brown & Co., Boston.

17   Bone and Joint

The immature joint

- diaphysis
- metaphysis
- epiphyseal cartilage
- epiphyseal ossification centre

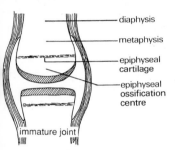

immature joint

Bone tissue can be detected in the 8-week fetus. It arises from precursor mesenchymal cells which either evolve into osteoblasts and osteocytes capable of primary ossification, or into chondroblasts and chondrocytes which give rise to an initial cartilagenous model. Tissue oxygen concentration, mechanical stress and hormonal agents are some of the factors known to dictate the type of bone development. In the limbs there are also complex interactions between skeletal formation and the ectodermal covering. Mineralisation which is essential to bone structure depends on the transplacental passage of calcium, phosphorus and vitamin D or its metabolites. This mineral transfer is maximal in later gestation and the calcium content of the fetus is doubled in the last month. The calcium deficit created by premature delivery increases the requirement for vitamin D in the postnatal period. Following delivery, the skeleton continues its growth, both in length and weight. It also undergoes considerable remodelling, particularly in the first two years when the rate is 10 times that which occurs in adult life. Maturation is accompanied by progressive endochondral ossification with the appearance of epiphyseal centres and the disappearance of the growth cartilages. This maturation is subject to genetic and environmental controls and may be quantified to provide the bone age, a valuable parameter in assessing growth and its disorders.

Polyarthritis in childhood	
Infection	Bacterial: pyogenic – tuberculosis Viral: rubella, mumps, parvovirus Arthropod borne: Lyme disease
Post-infectious	Post streptococcal arthritis and rheumatic fever
Allergic	Henoch Schönlein purpura
Collagen vascular disease	Juvenile chronic arthritis, systemic lupus erythematosis, dermatomyositis, Kawasaki disease
Haematological disease	Leukaemia, haemophilia, sickle cell disease
Gastrointestinal disease	Ulcerative colitis, Crohn disease
Trauma and synovitis	

ARTHRITIS

A swollen painful joint requires prompt evaluation as it may be the first sign of severe systemic illness. Young children present with fever, limp or reluctance to use their limbs rather than specific joint symptoms. When many joints are involved it is a polyarthritis. A monoarthritis is when a single joint is involved in which case a pyogenic infection must be excluded.

Pyogenic arthritis. In pyogenic arthritis the joint is usually hot, swollen and acutely tender and more than one joint may be involved. Movement of the affected joints is restricted and very painful. The joint must be aspirated and the fluid examined by microscopy and culture, and also blood samples taken for culture at the same time. Osteomyelitis adjacent to a joint may produce a sympathetic effusion but the tenderness will be on the bony metaphysis rather than over the joint. The commonest infecting organism is *Staphylococcus pyogenes*, and flucloxacillin given intravenously is the treatment of choice. Surgical drainage is frequently required if the diagnosis is delayed beyond 48 to 72 hours from the onset of symptoms. During the acute phase of the illness the joint is splinted, but later physiotherapy and mobilisation is essential to prevent joint flexion from developing into a permanent deformity.

Septic arthritis and osteomyelitis in infants develop and destroy rapidly

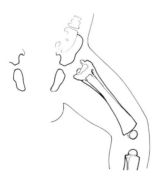 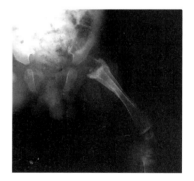

Rheumatic fever. See Chapter 9.

Tuberculous arthritis is now very rare in Europe but occasionally presents in the spine and the larger synovial joints.

Viral arthritis may be confused with juvenile chronic arthritis or rheumatic fever.

Henoch Schönlein purpura is a diffuse, self-limiting allergic vasculitis. It is common in young children but the precipitating factors have not been fully identified. The clinical picture is readily recognisable; the majority resolving quickly and requiring only analgesics. A minority have more severe gastrointestinal manifestation and may warrant a brief course of corticosteroid therapy. For renal lesion see Chapter 11.

Allergic polyarthritis. A transient allergic reaction consisting of an urticarial rash and synovitis is not uncommon. It may follow mild upper respiratory tract infections, drug or dietary allergen exposure.

Juvenile chronic arthritis

Chronic arthritis in children comprises a collection of disorders of unknown aetiology although there is growing evidence of genetic susceptibility with links to HLA tissue types. The diagnosis of JCA must be based on clinical features and other disorders manifesting arthritis have to be excluded. There are three main forms of presentation: the systemic variety is the rarest, then more frequent a polyarthritis and the commonest form a pauciarticular onset in which joint involvement is limited to less than five joints. All these diseases are rheumatoid factor test negative. Some teenage girls present with an aggressive disease — juvenile rheumatoid arthritis which is seropositive and has features similar to the adult disease.

Systemic juvenile chronic arthritis (Still disease) may not have any joint symptoms at onset. The diagnosis is made on clinical grounds with no single laboratory marker. It should be considered in an ill child with any of the following features — a remitting fever, variable rash, hepatosplenomegaly, anaemia, weight loss or abdominal pain. Acute leukaemia, metastatic neuroblastoma or septicaemia can produce similar features so a marrow examination and full septic screen may be necessary.

Clinical features of JCA

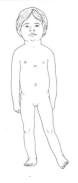

Lymphadenitis
transient pink maculopapular
   rash (prominent with fever)
pleurisy
pericarditis
hepatosplenomegaly
abdominal pain
variable symmetrical
   polyarthritis

Investigations:
   moderate normochromic
   normocytic anaemia
   ESR raised
   rheumatoid factor negative
   platelet count raised

Example of the fever and response to an antipyretic

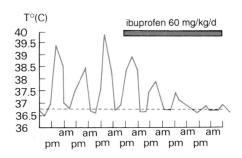

Polyarticular juvenile chronic arthritis presents with painful swelling and restricted movement in both large and small joints. It has a symmetrical distribution and characteristically involves the temporomandibular joints, the cervical spine, flexor tendons of the hands as well as limb joints. Systemic features are usually minimal weight loss and mild anaemia.

Pauciarticular onset juvenile chronic arthritis is a heterogeneous group of disorders with two main groups. In addition the arthropathy of psoriasis or inflammatory bowel inflammation (Crohn disease and ulcerative colitis) can present like this before becoming a polyarthritis.

Young girls frequently present with a swollen knee or ankle. They may have a positive anti-nuclear factor test and they are at high risk of developing chronic iridocyclitis. The latter should be screened for, as it can be asymptomatic until blindness occurs. This group generally has a good outcome but some progress to develop asymmetric polyarthritis.

Older boys may present with a swollen knee, tenosynovitis and a family history of HLA B27 related disease which may progress to a disease pattern of juvenile ankylosing spondylitis.

Management. The priorities in therapy are to reduce joint inflammation, maintain function and to prevent deformity. Non-steroidal anti-inflammatory drugs are used such as naproxen or ibuprofen. The latter in high dosage is useful for the control of fever in the systemic disease. Aspirin can be used but it has a narrow therapeutic range, drug absorption is variable and side effects can be troublesome. Intra-articular steroids can suppress activity in single joints. Topical corticosteroids are used for iridocyclitis and oral or intravenous steroids are used to control features such as pericarditis in severe systemic illness. Hydroxychloroquine, penicillamine or gold injections may be given for chronic joint destruction. Recently methotrexate and immune regulatory drugs are being used earlier in the disease.

Physical therapy is more important than the drug treatment. Daily exercises, hydrotherapy, day and night splints are all part of a personalised programme which is essential to maximize long term joint mobility. With this most children can enter adulthood with an independent life even if their disease remains active.

Prognosis differs in the various sub-groups but overall 75 to 80 per cent should have no or only minor disability after 15 years.

OSTEOMYELITIS

Common sites

- humerus
- femur
- tibia
- calcaneum

Osteomyelitis affects the metaphyses of long bones and is usually haematogenous in origin. The principal exception is that at the proximal femur, as the metaphysis is intracapsular, the infection may spread to the bone by direct inoculation from a primary pyoarthrosis of the hip joint. The growth plate normally acts as a barrier to extension of infection from a primary metaphysal focus to the associated epiphysis. *Staphylococcus pyogenes* accounts for 90 per cent, with *Haemophilus influenzae* and *Streptococcus pyogenes* as less common isolates. Children with sickle cell disease are susceptible to salmonella infections and the site is frequently atypical.

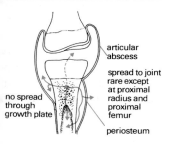

The anatomy of osteomyelitis

articular abscess

spread to joint rare except at proximal radius and proximal femur

periosteum

no spread through growth plate

Clinical features. The infected limb is painful and held immobile, pseudoparalysis. Swelling and occasionally redness may be seen if diagnosis is delayed. Examination of all inexplicably febrile children must include careful palpation of the limbs looking for areas of local swelling and tenderness. The adjacent joint may contain a sterile, sympathetic effusion. Repeated blood culture is the most satisfactory method of determining the responsible organism and therefore establishing its antibiotic sensitivity. X-rays are not of diagnostic help in the first 10 to 14 days. The first radiological signs are subperiosteal new bone formation and spotty rarefaction. Radionuclide bone scan will almost always demonstrate a zone of high emission at a much earlier stage and has proved to be a most useful tool to confirm diagnosis and localise the pathology.

Management. Prompt, effective parenteral antibiotic therapy is essential for a successful outcome. Neglected cases are liable to develop irreversible bone necrosis, draining sinuses and limb deformity. Appropriate antibiotic regimens include high-dosage, intravenous flucloxacillin or fusidic acid (to cover staphylococcal infection) with ampicillin (to cover Gram negative organisms) until there is an unequivocal clinical response and then effective oral therapy for up to 6 weeks until all the clinical, radiological and haematological parameters indicate healing of the disease. Lack of response in the first 48 hours of therapy is an indication for surgical exploration and drainage.

NORMAL POSTURAL VARIATIONS

These are common problems which arouse much parental anxiety. Reassurance is usually more appropriate than expensive shoe modifications or unnecessary physiotherapy.

In-toe gait. This may originate in the foot (metatarsus varus), in the

Causes of in-toe gait

femoral anteversion

tibial torsion

metatarsus varus

tibia (tibial torsion), or in the femora (persistent anteversion of the femoral neck). These conditions are symmetrical, pain free and are accompained by normal mobility. They generally resolve in 3 to 4 years.

Out-toe gait. Out-toe gait is also common in the first 2 years of life and may be unilateral. It always corrects spontaneously.

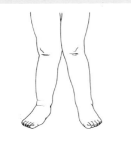

Genu valgum

Genu varum (bow legs). Outward curving of the tibia is usually associated with internal tibial torsion, is not uncommon and always corrects with growth. Severe examples should raise the suspicion of rickets (nutritional in susceptible groups, or the congenital hypophosphataemic form) or Blount disease, a rare developmental abnormality of the proximal tibial epiphysis.

Genu valgum (knock-knees). This is frequent in the 2 to $4\frac{1}{2}$ year age-group and is usually innocent if symmetrical and independent of any other abnormality. Severe and progressive cases raise the possibility of rickets which is most frequently seen among Asian immigrant children. Rickets may be confirmed by the X-ray appearance of the typical frayed metaphyseal changes and by an elevated serum alkaline phosphatase.

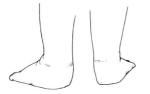

Pes planus

Flat feet. The medial arch of the foot develops within 2 to 3 years of walking. It is largely obliterated by a fat pad in younger children. Persistent flat feet may be familial or reflect joint laxity. It is insignificant if the foot is pain free, mobile and develops an arch when standing on tiptoe. Neurological problems and pathological joint laxity are occasional underlying causes. Severe convex flat foot is occasionally due to congenital vertical talus, in which condition early surgical treatment can avoid crippling deformity in later life.

SCOLIOSIS

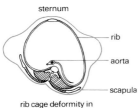

The anatomy of scoliosis

rib cage deformity in structural scoliosis

Scoliosis, a term coined by Galen, refers to a spinal curve in the coronal plane. Scoliosis may be postural or structural. Structural curves are fixed and associated with vertebral rotation which produces, in the thoracic region, rib asymmetry detectable most easily when the child bends forwards. A postural curve will correct with adjustment of posture and is not accompanied by rotation. Such a curve will not evolve to a structural scoliosis.

Structural scoliosis. This may be idiopathic, either infantile ('early onset') or adolescent ('late onset'), congenital (with hemivertebrae or unsegmented lateral bony tethers) or secondary to other disease, such as osteogenesis imperfecta, Marfan syndrome or neurofibromatosis. Neuromuscular imbalance, as in poliomyelitis, cerebral palsy, or muscular dystrophy, can also result in a severe scoliosis.

Structural scoliosis: clinical detection

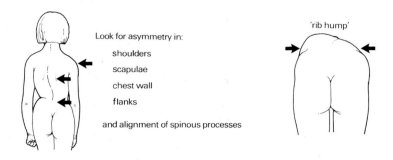

Look for asymmetry in:

shoulders

scapulae

chest wall

flanks

and alignment of spinous processes

'rib hump'

Idiopathic adolescent scoliosis. Eighty to 85 per cent of all structural scoliosis falls into this group, affecting mainly girls in the age range 10 to 14 years. Great efforts have been made in the last decade to detect such cases early by programmes of school screening and this has resulted in many early curves being treated successfully by bracing; it is not, however, established that this has reduced the need for surgery. Thus, the value of screening programmes is uncertain and as the late onset curve, even allowed to progress unchecked, is unlikely to produce life-threatening cardio-respiratory compromise from thoracic deformity, the problem is primarily a cosmetic one, albeit severe. The WHO has suggested that screening for cosmetic problems is not a justifiable resource allocation.

Physiotherapy has no place in the treatment of structural scoliosis. Curves of up to 40° or 50°, depending on age of onset, are usually treated by a thoraco-lumbo-sacral orthosis (TLSO) which controls progression in about 70 per cent of cases.

HIP DISORDERS

Congenital dislocation of the hip

Early detection of the lax hip at birth is important as it permits a relatively simple and safe treatment protocol with a high expectancy of a normal hip as the outcome. Delay in diagnosis leads to progressively severe dysplasia of both the femoral head and the acetabulum resulting in the need for more complex management, including the possibility of a long surgical programme.

The precise aetiology is unknown. There is a high incidence of both shallow acetabulum and of congenital joint laxity in the first order relatives of CDH patients. There is wide variation in the geographical incidence of the condition. Established, irreducible CDH, in the absence of a neonatal screening and treatment programme is found in about 1.5 per 1000 live births in most European groups. The Lapps and the North American Indians, who swaddle their infants with the hips extended and the legs together, have a much higher incidence; the Island Lake Manitoba Indian community, who still use the cradleboard have a 4 per cent incidence of CDH. It is a rare condition among ethnic groups who carry the infant with his legs astride the mother's pelvis, as in black Africans and the Chinese. It is against this background that it is believed that posturing the hips in subtotal abduction-in-flexion (the 'human' position as opposed to the 'frog' position) is believed to prevent the evolution of the lax neonatal hip into a fully established, irreducible dislocation. Screening for neonatal hip laxity and treatment by splintage is likely, with a well-controlled programme, to reduce the incidence of late-diagnosis CDH.

Neonatal screening. These techniques must be learnt by practical instruction from an experienced clinician. The infant should be well-fed, warm, relaxed and lain on a firm surface. The hips and knees are flexed to 90° with one examining hand to each leg. The thumb should be on the inner side of the baby's knee and the ring and little fingers behind the greater trochanter. Gentle but firm pressure is applied in the line of the femur, so that a lax hip would be dislocated posteriorly. The thighs are then abducted fully with a gentle motion, at the same time lifting the greater trochanter forwards; this motion is less like opening a book and more like opening a surgical 'peel pack'. It is the movement which has to be learned. If a hip is lax, the reduction which occurs as the legs are abducted will be felt as a clunk or jumping sensation. Many normal hips 'crack' or click (like pulled finger joints!) and only experience can teach the distinction between clunks and clicks.

Ortolani test for congenital dislocation of hip

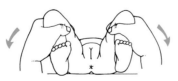

hips flexed 90°   knees flexed

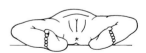

clunk+

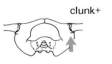

A variant of this test is to steady the pelvis with one hand with the thumb over the pubic symphysis and the fingers of the same hand behind the buttocks, and then with the other hand holding the examined leg as before, attempt to rock the head of the femur backwards and forwards in and out of the socket. This test must be applied in different degrees of abduction until the 'lax arc' is found. Any doubt about a hip should lead to referral to an orthopaedic surgeon with paediatric experience. Any child whose hip has been suspect should be X-rayed at 3 to 6 months of age. Infants statistically at risk are relatives of other lax hip children, first born females, babies born by breech delivery (or by LSCS after a breech intrauterine position) and those with foot deformities or sternomastoid 'tumour'. Babies at high risk of hip instability can have ultrasound examination to detect or monitor problems.

Congenital dislocation of hip: radiology and management

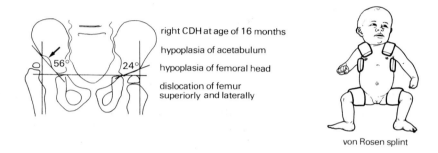

right CDH at age of 16 months

hypoplasia of acetabulum

hypoplasia of femoral head

dislocation of femur
superiorly and laterally

von Rosen splint

Congenital dislocation of the hips (bilateral)

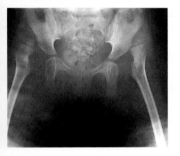

Management. The infant whose hips remain suspect by the second or third week of life should be splinted and referred for orthopaedic follow-up. The use of an appropriate splint (von Rosen or Craig type), properly applied and adjusted, for a period of about 3 months will in most cases be all that is required. X-rays must be used to confirm normal hip joint development until independent walking. X-rays are of little use under 3 months of age. The finding of limited abduction in flexion at the hip is a feature of the established dislocation and is, therefore, not a sign which develops until about 3 to 4 months of age. Conversely, the clunk will disappear at about 3 weeks of age when the hip first becomes irreducible.

It is unfortunately true that dislocated hips are still missed in spite of the widespread introduction of screening procedures. Suspicion is raised by a child with a shortened leg, or with a gait in which the affected foot is placed flat on the ground while the opposite knee is flexed. It does not generally delay the onset of walking but may well cause frequent falls. Bilateral cases have a symmetrical gait and tend to present even later if missed in the neonatal period. Attempted reduction of the hip involves initial traction followed by more prolonged splintage or in the event of failure, operative intervention. The latter may involve open reduction, femoral osteotomy and acetabular reconstruction.

Transient synovitis

This is the most common cause of limp, with hip and/or knee pain, in young children. It is a unilateral, self-limiting condition of ill-defined aetiology although many follow a mild upper respiratory tract infection. Boys in the age group 2 to 12 years (average 6 years) are most susceptible. It usually has a sudden onset with limp, and pain of variable severity. Abduction, full extension and internal rotation are restricted and there may be tenderness over the anterior aspect of the hip. There is usually no leucocytosis, and the ESR is normal or only mildly elevated. X-rays are normal. The diagnosis can only be made after exclusion of an infective process at or adjacent to the hip joint, Perthes disease, slipped upper femoral epiphysis or even a primary neoplasm, benign or malignant.

Transient synovitis seldom lasts for more than a few days or weeks and treatment consists of simple analgesics and bed rest often with simple skin traction. Approximately 6 per cent of cases considered to have transient synovitis subsequently develop features of Perthes disease.

Perthes disease

Necrosis of femoral head

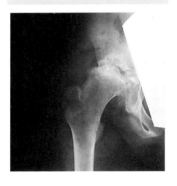

This results from episodes of segmental avascular necrosis of the femoral head. The necrotic bone is gradually replaced by new bone, but recovery can be complicated by residual deformity of the femoral head. It is most common in the 4 to 8-year age group and the ratio of boys to girls is 5:1. The underlying cause has not been established but it is suspected that the femoral head disorder is part of a more generalised growth disturbance in which skeletal development is retarded.

Limp, with or without pain, is the presenting complaint and hip mobility, especially abduction and internal rotation, is limited. The hip X-ray reflects the natural history of the bone necrosis; initial increase in density followed by fragmentation and reossification. The identification of the femoral head at risk of deformity is central to management; the head at risk is usually treated by 'containment' in the acetabulum either by femoral osteotomy or bracing. The healing phase during which the head requires protection lasts 2 to 4 years.

Slipped upper femoral epiphysis

A slipped epiphysis

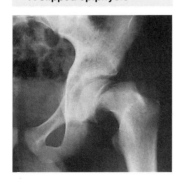

This condition, occurring during the adolescent growth spurt (10 to 14 years in girls; 12 to 16 in boys), is a posterior slipping of the epiphysis of the femoral head in relation to its metaphysis, a shearing failure of the growth plate resulting. The slip may be acute after minimal trauma (massive trauma is required to displace a normal proximal femoral epiphysis) or gradual. Atypically early presentation should lead to the search for an underlying endocrine disease, the commonest being hypothyroidism. The condition is bilateral, but not necessarily synchronous, in about 25 per cent of cases. Obese children with delayed secondary sexual development, or tall thin boys, appear to be especially susceptible. Pain in the hip, the thigh or the knee associated with limp in this age group demands urgent referral for investigation. Slipped upper femoral epiphysis is a true emergency, as massive further slipping may supervene without warning at any time.

Treatment is by pin fixation in situ for mild slips and by either open reduction and fixation or femoral osteotomy for major slips. Manipulation should never be attempted: it either fails to improve the position or, if it produces a reduction, avascular necrosis of the femoral head is then highly likely.

KNEE DISORDERS

The knee is a common source of complaint among adolescents. In assessing the cause of knee pain, the hip must also be examined as hip pain is often referred to the knee.

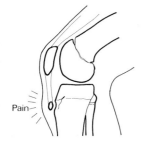

Tender tubercle!

Pain

Osgood Schlatter syndrome is a painful, tender swelling of the tibial tubercle due to repeated minor avulsion trauma at the site of insertion of the patellar tendon – a traction apophysitis. It is an example of an overuse syndrome and is caused by excess physical exertion before skeletal maturity. Most cases will resolve with a total embargo on sport, swimming, physical education, cycling, etc. for up to 6 months. Return to these activities should then be graduated and moderated if a recurrence is to be avoided. Resistant cases usually resolve after a period of rest for 6 to 8 weeks in a plaster cylinder cast.

Chondromalacia patellae indicates softening of the articular cartilage of the patellae usually as the result of indirect trauma, for example unaccustomed games activity. The retropatellar pain is worse on rising from prolonged sitting or on stairs, and is accompanied by crepitus. Avoidance of repetitive knee bending and physical recreation is usually adequate advice. Occasional cases have patellar misalignment worthy of surgery.

TALIPES (CLUBFOOT)

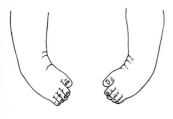

Equinovarus

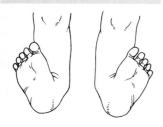

Calcaneovalgus

Talipes equinovarus. The fixed clubfoot is one of the most complex deformities facing orthopaedic surgeons as it represents disruption of complicated interrelationships between bone, ligament and muscle. The incidence is 1.2 per 1000 live births, rising by 20-fold where there is an affected first degree relative. Males are more at risk by a ratio of 3:1, and 50 per cent of cases are bilateral. All cases must be examined carefully to exclude an underlying neurological problem.

Treatment is largely determined by the rigidity of the deformity and by the secondary changes. In the earliest stages, gradual manipulative correction is combined with strapping. Over a period of 6 to 8 weeks this results in correction of approximately 60 per cent of cases. If the hind foot remains in an equinus position operation is required to release the responsible soft tissue shortening. Manipulation and strapping are continued until the foot will evert and dorsiflex beyond the neutral position. In the final stages, Denis Browne's bootee splints, in which open-ended boots are attached to a crossbar, are worn at night. The whole course of treatment may continue until at least 5 years of age. A true correction must be obtained by 3 months of age and if this goal has not been reached, then surgical soft tissue release is usually undertaken without delay. Failure to achieve early true correction may result in the need for corrective bone surgery later in childhood.

Talipes calcaneovalgus. In this deformity the foot is dorsiflexed and everted but the underlying structural abnormality is less profound and the foot is more amenable to simple manipulation.

GENETIC BONE AND JOINT DISORDERS

Marfan disease (autosomal dominant). This disease consists of arachnodactyly, hypermobile joints, ocular abnormalities, and a high arched palate. There are commonly associated deformities of the spine and chest. The prognosis is determined by associated cardiovascular problems such as dilated aortic root, dissecting aortic aneurysm and billowing mitral valve incompetence.

Cleido-cranial dysostosis (autosomal dominant). The features include absence of part or all of the clavicle, and delayed ossification of the skull with persistent open skull sutures. Affected children also tend to be short.

Diaphyseal aclasis, multiple cartilagenous exostoses (autosomal dominant). This disorder of the growth plate results in multiple cartilage capped osteomas arising at the ends of long bones. The multiple bony swellings make their appearance in infancy and increase in number and size during growth. They may cause pain, deformity and growth impairment. A proportion of patients, probably less than 5 per cent, are liable to malignant sarcoma transformation in adult life.

Osteogenesis imperfecta (autosomal dominant, occasionally recessive). In this condition there is an underlying failure in collagen metabolism resulting in multiple fractures of fragile bones, lax joints and thin skin. Blue sclerae, scoliosis, hypoplastic teeth and progressive deafness are also features. The congenital form may be so severe that the fetus dies *in utero* or shortly after birth. The later onset variety is compatible with a reasonable prognosis and may present in adolescence as 'osteoporosis'.

Osteopetrosis or marble bone disease (autosomal recessive or autosomal dominant). The recessive form is more severe causing bone marrow failure and early death. The dominant or less severe form presents in childhood as facial paralysis, bone fractures and osteomyelitis. Bone marrow transplantation has had limited success in reintroducing normal osteoblast and osteoclast function.

BONE TUMOURS AND ALLIED DISORDERS

Features suggestive of a bone tumour include pain, swelling or a limp. Fortunately the majority of underlying lesions are benign; atypical osteomyelitis, incomplete fracture of normal bone, a simple cyst or an osteoid osteoma. Ewing tumour and osteosarcoma are described in the chapter on malignancy.

Simple bone cysts (unicameral cysts) are most frequently seen in the metaphyseal regions of long bones and are discovered usually only when they fracture and cause pain. The X-ray features are characteristic. They fill in spontaneously and disappear shortly after skeletal maturity. The fractures heal readily but the cyst often remains. Treatment is usually by washout of the cyst using two wide-bore needles inserted under anaesthetic and X-ray control, followed by the instillation of triamcinolone acetate.

Osteoid osteoma may present with intermittent and often nocturnal pain. X-rays show extensive periosteal thickening with a focus of dense new bone surrounding a centrally placed radiolucent nidus. The majority are so painful that surgical removal of the nidus is required. These lesions concentrate bone-seeking radionuclides such as technetium-99 m compounds and this can be exploited to locate them at surgery by the use of sterilisible miniature gamma ray detectors. Recurrence is virtually unknown after successful removal of the nidus tissue.

BIBLIOGRAPHY

Bleck E E 1987 Orthopaedic management in cerebral palsy. Mac Keith Press, Oxford
Cassidy J T, Petty R E 1990 Textbook of paediatric rheumatology, 2nd edn. Churchill
    Livingstone Inc., New York
Weiner D S 1992 Pediatric Orthopaedics. Churchill Livingstone Inc., New York

18 Brain, Cord, Nerve, Muscle

Brain growth

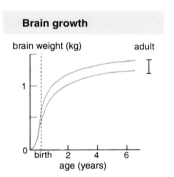

All who are concerned with the safe passage of children from conception to adulthood, have as a prime goal the preservation of normal brain development. Potential hazards have effects which are largely determined by the degree of differentiation of the nervous system. In the first trimester genetic and environmental influences may disrupt embryogenesis and produce malformations which either abort or reach term as gross anomalies, for example anencephaly and spina bifida. In later fetal life and during infancy insults are more likely to produce focal, irreversible pathology in differentiated tissue, lesions which may well be the basis of cerebral palsy.

In addition to interference with structural differentiation, the brain is also susceptible to problems during its various growth spurts. In the human fetus maximal neuronal proliferation occurs in the mid-trimester and is relatively protected from maternal malnutrition and placental dysfunction, but it is vulnerable to viral infection, radiation, drugs and excessive alcohol. Glial multiplication and myelination occurs over a more extended period from the third antenatal trimester through the first 2 years of life and is therefore exposed to the effects of intra- and extrauterine malnutrition, perinatal asphyxia and inborn errors of metabolism. We are only on the threshold of understanding how these hazards may influence the subtler components of growth, dendritic proliferation and synaptic connectivity.

INTRACRANIAL INFECTION

Acute infection of the meninges may be viral (aseptic meningitis), or bacterial (acute purulent meningitis) in origin. Meningitis may also be due to tuberculosis and rarer pathogens such as fungi and protozoa. Leukaemic cell infiltration can cause a sterile meningitis.

Acute purulent meningitis Purulent meningitis is relatively common in childhood especially in preschool years, 35 per cent of childhood cases occurring in the first and 80 per cent in the first 5 years of life. In the UK one in 500 children suffer from purulent meningitis between the age of 1 month and 10 years. It is essential to make an early diagnosis as delay increases the risk of death or neurological complications.

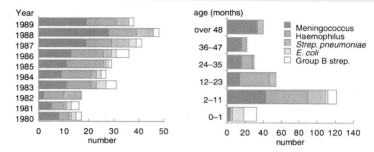

The causes of bacterial meningitis in the middle of England over the last 10 years and at different ages (data from Dr Heather Fortrum)

Tests for neck stiffness

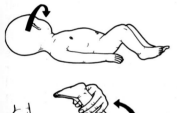

The characteristic features of meningeal irritation, neck stiffness and Kernig sign are often absent in children under 18 months of age. Such young infants are more likely to present with a fever, poor feeding, vomiting and drowsiness. Some in this age group have a convulsion as the first sign of illness. An infant who has a fever with convulsion almost invariably warrants a lumbar puncture because of the difficulty of excluding meningitis on clinical grounds in this age group. The development of complicating meningitis may be the reason why a child with an otitis media or other upper respiratory tract infection fails to respond to an antibiotic and becomes increasingly drowsy. On the other hand children with an upper respiratory tract infection, cervical lymphadenitis or pneumonia may show meningismus, that is they have the signs of meningeal irritation in the absence of intracranial disease. However lumbar puncture is not without risk in the child with meningitis, indeed in some instances it is considered to be too risky and treatment is started after blood cultures have been taken.

Lumbar puncture

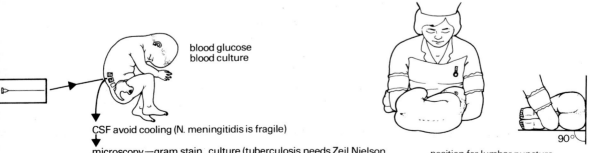

blood glucose
blood culture

CSF avoid cooling (N. meningitidis is fragile)

microscopy—gram stain, culture (tuberculosis needs Zeil Nielson or immunofluorescent stain)

chemistry—protein and glucose

position for lumbar puncture

90°

Treatment. For children older than 3 months intravenous treatment with a third generation cephalosporin such as cefotaxime 200 mg/kg/day is appropriate until the microorganism and its antibiotic sensitivities have been identified. *Haemophilus influenzae* is normally sensitive to cefotaxime but requires this dosage to be maintained for at least 10 days. *Neisseria meningitidis* and *Diplococcus pneumoniae* are usually very sensitive to parenteral benzylpenicillin, 300 mg/kg/day for 10 days.

Children with meningococcal infections often have a widespread purpuric rash and are liable to develop septicaemic shock. Purpura in a febrile child suggests meningococcal septicaemia and must always be regarded seriously, for treatment should be commenced as soon as possible. Prophylactic treatment with rifampicin to eradicate nasopharyngeal carriage and minimise the risk of contact cases is required for the index case and household contacts of all cases of meningococcal meningitis and in those cases of *H. influenzae* meningitis where there is a child under 3 years of age in the household.

Complications. Meningitis may be complicated by convulsions which require treatment with anticonvulsant drugs. Inappropriate antidiuretic hormone release often accompanies intracranial problems and can lead to hyponatraemia which may be prevented by careful restriction of intravenous and oral fluids. Subdural effusions are probably frequent but the majority are small and insignificant. Occasionally, an enlarging head circumference and bulging fontanelle suggest a larger accumulation. This may be visualised by transilluminating the skull, or ultrasound or CT scanning, and confirmed by performing a subdural tap when a fluid containing a high protein content can be aspirated. A rapidly increasing head circumference may also be a consequence of hydrocephalus due to inflammatory obstruction of the CSF pathways. About 10 per cent of all children surviving meningitis have long-term neurological abnormality; convulsions, deafness, spasticity, mental handicap or other learning difficulties.

Recurrent meningitis raises the possibility of a congenital mid-line sinus, or a post-traumatic dural defect providing communication with an air sinus. An immune deficiency should also be considered.

Neonatal meningitis

This affects one in every 4000 babies. It is a very serious illness and is usually due to Gram negative bacilli or group B haemolytic streptococci. It has a high mortality and a majority of survivors have some neurological sequelae. Therapy must be directed towards the ventriculitis which is often associated. Systemic treatment must be with drugs like chloramphenicol or cefotaxime which are known to produce good concentrations in ventricular CSF.

Viral meningitis

Viral meningitis is commoner than it is realised. It may be accompanied by a macular rash or preceded by upper respiratory tract or gastrointestinal complaints. The symptoms of viral meningitis are usually less abrupt and milder than with acute purulent meningitis. Cerebrospinal fluid examination and culture is obviously essential to make the dis-

Cerebrospinal fluid findings in meningitis

	Normal*	Acute purulent meningitis	Aseptic (viral) meningitis	Tuberculous meningitis
Appearance	clear	cloudy	usually clear	opalescent
Cells/mm^3	0–5 lymphocytes	10–100 000 polymorphs	15–2000 lymphocyes	250–500 lymphocytes
glucose (mmol/l)	2.8–4.4 (CSF > 60% blood)	low (CSF < 60% blood)	normal (CSF > 60% blood)	very low (CSF < 60% blood)
Protein (g/l)	0.15–0.35	0.5–5.0	0.2–1.25	0.45–5.00

* in the postnatal period normal CSF contains a higher cell and protein content.

tinction. Serial viral titres, nasopharyngeal and rectal swabs may identify the virus.

Tuberculous meningitis

Tuberculous meningitis must be considered in every case of aseptic meningitis or encephalitis. It follows the rupture of a tubercle (Rich focus) into the cerebrospinal fluid and evolves as the resulting inflammatory reaction and arteritis develops. The cerebrospinal fluid examination is not always diagnostic in early cases. A tuberculin skin test is positive in 75 per cent and a chest X-ray shows a suggestive lesion in 80 per cent. Treatment is dealt with in the section dealing with tuberculosis and may have to be started when the diagnosis is just suspected as any delay can be critical.

Brain abscess

This is a relatively rare condition, there is usually a predisposing cause. Although it is essential to consider lumbar puncture in every child at risk of having intracranial infection, this procedure should be deferred if there are features of raised intra-cranial pressure and a CT scan obtained.

Brain abscess: aetiology, clinical features and treatment

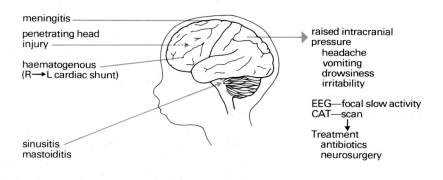

meningitis
penetrating head injury
haematogenous (R→L cardiac shunt)
sinusitis
mastoiditis

raised intracranial pressure
headache
vomiting
drowsiness
irritability

EEG—focal slow activity
CAT—scan
↓
Treatment
antibiotics
neurosurgery

Encephalitis

Causes of viral meningitis

Infectious	Post-infectious
Enterovirus	
coxsackie	
poliomyelitis	
echo	
Myxovirus	
mumps	Measles
rabies	Rubella
Herpes virus	
H. simplex	Varicella
H. zoster	
Arthropod-borne	
yellow fever	
dengue fever	
Other viruses	
lymphocytic	Pox virus
chorio-	
meningitis	
psittacosis	Vaccinia

Encephalitis produces fever, disturbed consciousness, convulsions and focal neurological signs. The majority of cases are viral and there may also be features of meningitis or spinal cord involvement (meningo-encephalitis and encephalomyelitis). Viral invasion of nervous tissue may result in immediate inflammation and destruction, mainly of grey matter, or may provoke a delayed immunologically mediated demyelination of white matter (post-infectious encephalomyelitis).

An encephalitis-like illness without fever or aseptic meningitis raises the possibility of a 'toxic' or metabolic encephalopathy. Lead poisoning and drug ingestion must always be considered.

Herpes simplex encephalitis. This is the most common sporadic severe encephalitis. Only 10 to 15 per cent have associated herpetic gingivo-stomatitis or skin lesions. Focal seizures and neurological signs are frequent and may suggest a temporal lobe space occupying lesion. The untreated mortality rate is 70 per cent and neurological sequelae are frequent in the survivors. The cerebrospinal fluid contains a variably elevated white cell count and may be blood stained. Electroencephalography and computerised axial tomography help to distinguish this encephalitis from a cerebral abscess or tumour. The development of potentially successful anti-viral therapy, acyclovir, has emphasised the need for prompt treatment whenever the disease is suspected. Retrospective diagnosis can be made later by showing increasing antibody titres to H. simplex in blood and CSF.

The more common varieties of post-infectious encephalitis are measles 1 in 1000; varicella 1 in 1000; rubella 1 in 5000; vaccinia 1 in 100 000.

Measles encephalitis. This commences with irritability, drowsiness and multiple seizures 2 to 4 days after the appearance of the rash. The EEG shows a severe diffuse abnormality. The course varies from complete recovery in a few days to death in status epilepticus or grossly impaired recovery. There is no specific treatment.

Subacute sclerosing panencephalitis (SSPE). SSPE is a prototype of human slow virus infection which is now recognised as a late complication of measles. The disease may progress over a period of years or death can occur as soon as 6 weeks after onset. The persistence of virus in the brain may be due to a defective immune response when measles is acquired at an early age. It enters the differential diagnosis of degenerative brain disorders.

Varicella. This causes a relatively benign encephalitis, often an acute self-limiting cerebellar ataxia, although occasionally it can be more serious.

Reye syndrome. This refers to the association of acute encephalopathy with brain swelling and diffuse fatty infiltration of the liver. Viral infections, particularly influenzae B and varicella, have been linked in some cases. Salicylate therapy has also been causally implicated so that these drugs are now no longer given to children. Vomiting or symptoms of an upper respiratory infection often precede the onset of lethargy and seizures and hyperventilation frequently accompany the increasing coma. A CT scan shows cerebral oedema and the CSF cells and protein are normal. Clinical jaundice does not occur but a prolonged prothrombin time and elevated aminotransferases and ammonia in the blood give evidence of liver involvement. Blood and CSF glucose levels are sometimes reduced. The treatment of Reye syndrome is aimed at reducing the raised intracranial pressure by hyperventilation, hypothermia and osmotherapy. Mortality is 40 per cent but the majority of survivors are neurologically intact.

EPILEPSY AND CONVULSIONS

The differential diagnosis of convulsions

Non-epileptic convulsions
Febrile
Metabolic
  hypoglycaemia
  hypocalcaemia
  hypomagnesaemia
  hypo/hypernatraemia
Toxins, poisons
Trauma, inflammation

Epilepsy
Idiopathic
Secondary
  cerebral malformation
  cerebral tumour
  cerebral degeneration
  cerebral damage
Differential diagnosis
  faints or syncopies
  breath holding
  benign paroxysmal vertigo
  migraine
  nightmares
  tics

The definition of terms is important when discussing epilepsy and other causes of transient loss of consciousness in children. The diagnosis of epilepsy has major medical and social implications. Unfortunately it is common for the diagnosis to be made in error and for inappropriate drug regimens to be initiated.

Epilepsy implies a disorder of the brain producing recurrent paroxysmal discharges which result in epileptic attacks. It can only be diagnosed if there has been more than one epileptic attack. A child who has only had one convulsion cannot be said to have epilepsy because he may never have another. The prevalence of epilepsy amongst schoolchildren is in the order of 8 per 1000.

A convulsion is a non-specific term and refers to all tonic–clonic attacks both epileptic and non-epileptic. The terms fit and seizure are also used in this context.

International classification of seizures (older terms in parenthesis)	
Primary generalised seizures	Simple absences ('petit mal') Complex absences Myoclonic Tonic–clonic ('grand-mal')
Partial seizures	Simple partial Complex partial ('temporal lobe') Partial with secondary generalisation

Types of epileptic seizures

Simple absence seizures. The attacks consist of impaired consciousness without falling or involuntary movements. The child stops whatever he is doing and looks vacant for 5–20 seconds and then continues with what he was doing as though nothing had happened. Attacks can be brought on by having the child over-breathe for a minute or two. The

EEG characteristically shows bursts of generalised three per second spike and wave discharges. This form of epilepsy is invariably idiopathic and usually carries a good prognosis.

Complex absence seizures. These tend to be rather a mixed bag. Unlike simple absence seizures the episodes of impaired consciousness may last longer and be associated with involuntary movements such as chewing, myoclonic jerks, loss of postural tone, semi-purposeful movements, or peculiar sensations. Attacks may be difficult to differentiate from partial complex seizures on clinical grounds. The EEG will be helpful in this differential diagnosis as it will show generalised bursts of irregular fast or slow spike and wave activity. The prognosis is not as good as with simple absences.

Myoclonic seizures. Myoclonic seizures take the form of sudden shock-like jerks affecting one part or the whole of the body, the latter are usually bilateral and symmetrical. They may be predominantly flexor or extensor. Mild attacks take the form of sudden head drops but more severe attacks may cause a child to be thrown suddenly forwards or backwards, perhaps injuring his face or back of his head. They may be idiopathic and occur in children without evidence of any other neurological disorder, but more commonly they represent a type of symptomatic epilepsy and are associated with mental handicap or abnormal neurological findings. Myoclonic seizures are common in some rare cerebral degenerative disorders.

Infantile spasms are a kind of myoclonic epilepsy but are usually considered separately because of their particularly bad prognosis for future development. This is a relatively rare but serious type of epilepsy seen only in young children and usually commencing between 3 and 8 months of age. The majority of infants show typical flexion ('jacknife' or 'salaam') spasms which may occur several hundred times a day at their most frequent. The spasm involves sudden flexion of the neck and limbs and lasts 1–3 seconds only but they usually occur in clusters lasting 15–30 minutes. Approximately half the children who develop infantile spasms will be found to have evidence of some underlying neurological disorder by history, examination or investigation. The prognosis for future development in such a child is almost always poor. The other infants have what are called idiopathic infantile spasms and have usually shown quite normal development until the spasms commence at which time they appear to regress developmentally. Sometimes the diagnosis is delayed because the spasms are thought to represent infantile colic or just fretfulness. Infantile spasms are an age-related type of epilepsy and usually cease spontaneously at 2–3 years of age although they may be replaced by tonic–clonic or other types of epileptic attacks. Idiopathic infantile spasms also have a poor prognosis but, after treatment with ACTH and a benzodiazepine, a minority (about 20 per cent) subsequently make satisfactory developmental progress and turn out to be mentally normal.

Tonic–clonic seizures. The attacks start with sudden loss of consciousness, falling and often an initial tonic phase in which the limbs are extended and the back arched. This soon gives way to the clonic phase associated with generalised jerking during which micturition and salivation (foaming at the mouth) may occur. Respiration ceases during the tonic phase but recommences in an irregular fashion during the clonic phase. Commonly the clonic phase settles after a few minutes but if it continues beyond 30 minutes the term status epilepticus is used. When the clonic phase ceases the child gradually regains consciousness but usually remains sleepy for an hour or so afterwards.

Simple partial seizures. Simple partial seizures usually consist of twitching or jerking of one side of the face, one arm or one leg. Consciousness is usually retained or only slightly impaired and the child does not usually fall. Sometimes the jerking can be seen to start in one corner of the mouth and spread across one side of the face or start in one hand and spread up the arm; this is called a 'Jacksonian march'. A simple partial seizure may proceed to a generalised tonic–clonic seizure with loss of consciousness, falling and generalised convulsive movements. Temporary weakness of the affected side of the body is common after a simple partial seizure and is known as a Todd's palsy.

The so-called adversive attack is a rare kind of simple partial seizure which takes the form of turning of the head and eyes to one side and is usually associated with a discharging cortical focus in the opposite frontal cortex. Rarely simple partial seizures with sensory symptoms can occur in which the child complains of tingling or numbness starting in one hand or side of the face and spreading to affect the whole of that side of the body.

Complex partial seizures. Attacks consist of altered or impaired consciousness, usually without falling and associated with strange sensations or complex semi-purposeful movements. The strange sensations may be visual (objects may look too big, too small or distorted, or there may be visual hallucinations), auditory (sounds or voices may appear too loud or too quiet, sensations of vertigo may be experienced or there may be auditory hallucinations), gustatory or olfactory (peculiar tastes or smell) or emotional (sensations of loss of reality, fear, sadness or excessive familiarity). The child may talk during the attack and his words may be just nonsense. Commonly there are chewing, sucking or swallowing movements during the attack and these movements may accompany hallucinations of taste. The child may perform complicated manoeuvres during the attack, such as getting up and walking about. If a sensation of fear accompanies an attack the child may rush to the nearest person and clutch him looking wide eyed and terrified. The attacks commonly last a few minutes and the child on coming round has little recollection of what has happened. A diagnosis of complex partial seizures is very dependant on a careful description of the attacks but the EEG may be helpful if it shows clear discharges arising from one temporal lobe.

Partial seizures with secondary generalisation. Any seizure discharge which starts from a cortical focus may spread across to the other hemisphere through the corpus callosum down to the deep subcortical grey matter regions, from which spread may then occur to both hemispheres simultaneously producing a generalised tonic–clonic seizure. Sometimes it is clear that the tonic–clonic seizure is preceded by a partial seizure (sometimes referred to as an aura) but other times the initial partial seizure is so brief as to pass unnoticed. The EEG is helpful in distinguishing between tonic–clonic seizures which are primary and those which are secondary. In primary generalised tonic–clonic seizures the EEG shows generalised bursts of regular or irregular spike or polyspike and wave activity whereas in secondary generalised tonic–clonic seizures the EEG shows evidence of a cortical focus.

Assessment

All children with suspected epilepsy should be fully assessed. A careful and detailed history from someone who has witnessed the attacks is of the utmost importance. General examination with special emphasis on developmental and neurological aspects is also required. Fasting blood sugar and calcium estimations are sometimes indicated.

An EEG may help to decide if doubtful attacks are epileptic or not, and may give some help in deciding the kind of epilepsy present. Caution is necessary as a normal EEG is seen in a number of children with epilepsy, and conversely abnormal discharges may occasionally be seen in EEGs from children who have never had an attack of any kind. A child with infantile spasms usually has a very severe EEG abnormality termed hypsarrhythmia. Some children have photosensitive epilepsy induced for example by a flickering television screen, and this may be confirmed by the EEG. Partial seizures are associated with cortical spike foci. Bilateral symmetrical discharges of spike and waves are seen in the EEGs of children with primary generalised seizures.

A CT head scan may be required if there are clinical grounds to suspect a structural lesion of the brain or if the EEG shows a persistent slow wave focus.

Management

Children with epilepsy usually require regular drug therapy in an attempt to prevent further seizures. Experience has shown that certain categories of epilepsy respond best to particular groups of anticonvulsants.

Optimal drug dosage and susceptibility to side-effects vary from individual to individual, and serum anticonvulsant levels may be helpful in assessing therapy. The regimen should be kept as simple as possible and it is seldom necessary to use more than two drugs.

A diagnosis of epilepsy raises considerable fears not only in the family but among school teachers and social contacts. Children with epilepsy do not require much limitation of their activities. For obvious reasons they are advised not to cycle in traffic but they may swim provided there is a responsible adult in attendance. Learning difficulties are more common than in other children but the majority of children with epilepsy attend ordinary schools and are average scholars. More

Drug therapy in epilepsy

Type of epilepsy	Drug of first choice	Other drugs
Simple absences	Ethosuximide	Valproate
Complex absences	Valproate	Clonazepam
Myoclonic	Clonazepam	Valproate
Infantile spasms	ACTH	Clonazepam
Primary generalised tonic–clonic	Valproate	Carbamazepine
Simple partial	Carbamazepine	Phenytoin
Complex partial	Carbamazepine	Phenytoin
Secondary generalised tonic–clonic	Carbamazepine	Phenytoin
Status epilepticus	IV or rectal diazepam	Rectal paraldehyde

than 60 per cent of children diagnosed as having epilepsy seem to 'grow out' of their seizure tendency during childhood and anticonvulsant therapy can be discontinued if they have been free of attacks for 2 to 3 years. A very small minority of children continue to have frequent epileptic attacks despite anticonvulsant therapy. Nevertheless the overall prognosis for childhood epilepsy is good with modern management.

Anticonvulsants: dosage and side-effects

Drug	Side-effects Common	Rare
Phenytoin 4–8 mg/kg/day	Cerebellar ataxia** gum hyperplasia hirsutism, rashes	rickets toxic encephalopathy facial coarsening
Carbamazepine 10–20 mg/kg/day	rash* fatigue* dizzyness*	bone marrow depression hepatic toxicity
Sodium valproate 20–40 mg/kg/day	drowsiness* nausea*	thrombocytopenia (high dosage) hair loss*; hepatic toxicity, pancreatitis
Ethosuximide 20–40 mg/kg/day	nausea* rashes	bone marrow depression
Clonazepam 0.05–0.2 mg/kg/day	drowniness** salivation**	

* Transient if drug continued
** May settle with slight dose reduction

Treatment of status epilepticus. It is unfortunate that many children await arrival at a casualty department before any attempt is made to stop status epilepticus. Every family doctor should be prepared to terminate these attacks as promptly as possible. The child should first be placed in a position which assures patency of the airway. Diazepam given rectally 0.5 mg/kg, is the drug of choice as it acts almost immediately. Parents of children who are prone to have prolonged seizures can be instructed in its use and keep a supply at home. Diazepam may be given IV in a lower dose of 0.25 mg/kg but carries a slight risk of causing apnoea so that it should not be used in the absence of facilities for resuscitation. Rectal paraldehyde 0.3 ml/kg mixed with an equal volume of arachis oil is a suitable alternative to rectal diazepam.

Febrile convulsions

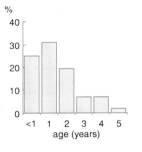

Age at time of first febrile convulsion

Febrile convulsions are very common and affect some 4 per cent of children, most often in the second year of life. They are strongly age-related and hardly ever occur before 6 months or after 6 years of age. The usual history is that the child is noticed to be unwell and hot and then has a major seizure lasting a few minutes. There is often a family history of febrile convulsions. On examination the child has a high temperature, and frequently evidence of upper respiratory tract infection. More serious conditions such as meningitis or urinary tract infections must always be excluded. The attacks are considered to be benign if they last less than 10 minutes and there are no persisting neurological signs. The prognosis for benign febrile convulsions is good, although recurrences are common. The risk of recurrence may be minimised by advising the parents to use cool washes and antipyretics whenever the child becomes febrile. Diazepam suppositories 0.5 mg/kg given at the time of fever further reduce the risk of recurrence and may be indicated. Regular prophylaxis with sodium valproate 20–40 mg/kg/day will also reduce the risk of recurrence but is rarely prescribed for what is usually a very benign condition. The risk of developing epilepsy after one or more febrile convulsion of any kind is only 2 per cent, but this is increased to 4 per cent if any of the febrile convulsions are prolonged or atypical, and to 6 per cent if there was pre-existing neurological abnormality.

Other causes of transient episodes

Breath holding attacks. These are common in toddlers and are usually precipitated by 'not getting his own way'. The child cries, holds his breath and goes blue. The attack usually stops at this point but loss of consciousness sometimes occurs. Drug treatment is not necessary and the attacks cease spontaneously.

Reflex anoxic seizures. These occur in infants who have very sensitive vagal cardiac reflexes. Attacks are usually brought on by pain especially unexpected bangs to the head. This causes reflex cardiac asystole with immediate loss of posture, deathly pallor and floppiness. The heart recommences beating itself and the child then recovers.

Syncope or fainting. This is not uncommon among older children. Careful history reveals likely predisposing factors such as immobility or fear, and recovery without any post-ictal phase.

Benign paroxysmal vertigo. This may present as sudden attacks of falling, swaying or dizziness but consciousness is not lost. Impaired vestibular function is revealed by caloric tests. No treatment is indicated as these attacks are brief and disappear spontaneously.

Migraine, day dreams, night terrors, hysteria and masturbation. These also enter the differential diagnosis.

Tics or habit spasms. These are irregular contractions of muscle groups for example blinking and jerking or facial grimacing. They can be controlled voluntarily but feelings of tension increase until the movement has to be repeated. They are often a reflection of underlying emotional disturbance and should not be confused with focal epilepsy.

NEUROMUSCULAR DISORDERS

Muscle and lower motor neurone disorders present as floppiness, delayed motor milestones, abnormal gait, clumsiness or progressive muscle weakness.

Neuromuscular disorders

Anterior horn cell: genetic—spinal muscular atrophy
infection—poliomyelitis

Nerve fibre: genetic—chronic hereditary polyneuropathy
infectious polyneuritis

Neuromuscular junction: autoimmune—myasthenia gravis

Muscle fibre: genetic—muscular dystrophies
congenital myopathies
metabolic myopathies
autoimmune—dermatomyositis

Muscle disorders

The muscular dystrophies are characterised by progressive degeneration of certain groups of skeletal muscles and are hereditary. A number of different forms have been distinguished on clinical and genetic grounds. Muscular dystrophy is the commonest cause of muscle disease in childhood.

Duchenne muscular dystrophy. This is the commonest and most serious type of muscular dystrophy with 30 per 100 000 live born males affected. A gene deletion at the 21 site on the short arm of the X chromosome (Xp21) can be demonstrated with DNA studies in about 70 per cent of boys with Duchenne dystrophy. This site is known as the dystrophin gene as it codes for the protein dystrophin which is present in all normal muscle cells. Dystrophin is absent in the muscle cells of boys with Duchenne dystrophy. Inheritance is as a sex-linked recessive but mutations are frequent and said to be responsible for 30 per cent of isolated cases. The female carriers are usually asymptomatic.

Symptoms appear in the first 5 years of life and consist of delayed walking, frequent falls, a lordotic waddling gait and difficulty climbing stairs. Prominence of the calf muscles is an early feature and is called 'pseudo-hypertrophy' because the muscles although enlarged are weak.

Gower sign

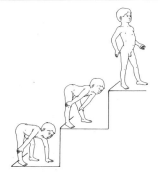

Due to weakness of the gluteal muscles, boys with this condition climb up their legs when they rise from the lying position (Gower sign).

The diagnosis of Duchenne dystrophy is made by finding a serum creatine kinase 10 to 200 times higher than normal, myopathic changes on electromyography and characteristic muscle biopsy features. It is important to consider Duchenne dystrophy in any boy with unexplained generalised developmental delay or delayed walking past 18 months. The serum creatine kinase is always very elevated before muscular weakness becomes clinically evident and is a useful screening test in such cases.

Most of these boys are unable to walk by the age of 8 to 11 years and are confined to a wheelchair. They often develop scoliosis and an equinus deformity of the feet due to muscular weakness and imbalance. The pseudo-hypertrophy is replaced by muscle wasting. Respiratory infections precipitate death by age 15 to 25. Intellectual development is usually normal but there is a slightly increased frequency of mental handicap.

Example of progressive disability in Duchenne muscular dystrophy

age (yrs) 4   5   6   7   8   9   10   11   12   13   14

Site of muscle biopsy

- unable to climb stairs
- unable to stand up from chair
- needs wheelchair
- unable to get from wheelchair to bed
- unable to sit independently
- unable to use wheelchair

Genetic counselling is important in Duchenne dystrophy, and female carriers may be detected by finding a moderately raised serum creatine kinase. When a woman is thought to be a carrier, prenatal diagnosis may be possible by amniocentesis or chorionic villus biopsy. This is particularly true if the index case shows an Xp21 deletion.

Becker muscular dystrophy. This is a milder form of sex-linked recessive muscular dystrophy with a later onset of clinical muscle weakness. Becker dystrophy is now known to be allelic with the gene for Duchenne dystrophy. Muscle dystrophin is present in Becker dystrophy but reduced in amount.

Facioscapulohumeral muscular dystrophy. This has an autosomal dominant pattern of inheritance and presents in late childhood or early adolescence. There may be a marked variation in the severity of the disease within affected families. Shoulder girdle weakness is an early feature followed by facial involvement and inability to close the eyes tightly. Winging of the scapulae is another feature. This condition has a very slow progression and may be compatible with a normal life span.

Limb girdle dystrophy. This type of progressive muscular dystrophy is inherited as an autosomal recessive so that girls are affected as well as boys. The pelvic girdle muscles are more affected than the shoulder girdle muscles. It may mimic Duchenne dystrophy in a boy but muscle dystrophin is normal.

Myotonic dystrophy. This was previously considered to be a disease of adult life but it is now realised that onset in childhood is not uncommon. It differs from the other muscular dystrophies, not only in the presence of myotonia, but also because of the widespread involvement of other tissues. Both males and females are affected and the inheritance is of an autosomal dominant. The muscle weakness characteristically involves the facial and neck muscles producing a myopathic facies, ptosis, an open mouth and a sagging jaw. Myotonia is seen as delayed opening of the eyes after closure or difficulty in relaxing the grasp. Distal limb weakness may also be present. Other features include cardiac involvement, cataracts, testicular atrophy and adrenal dysfunction.

In the congenital form infants have feeding and respiratory difficulties. Many die in the newborn period but those who survive show considerable recovery. The majority are, however, educationally subnormal. It is interesting that in every congenital case the mother is the affected parent.

Congenital myopathies. These are a complex group of disorders which can only be characterised after detailed examination of muscle obtained at biopsy, for example central core disease and nemaline myopathy.

Metabolic myopathies. Type II glycogen storage disease, acid maltase deficiency, is an autosomal recessive condition in which muscle weakness is a major feature. In the infantile form (Pompe disease) infants present with cardiac failure, hepatomegaly and gross hypotonia. The majority die before 18 months.

Acquired muscle disease

Dermatomyositis. Dermatomyositis, an inflammatory disorder of muscle, is rare in childhood. It is characterised by generalised proximal muscle weakness and a violaceous discolouration of the skin, especially over the butterfly area of the face, eyelids, elbows, knees and knuckles. The child is usually miserable and may be febrile. Blood creatine kinase is elevated and the ESR is sometimes raised. EMG show myopathic changes and an inflammatory cell infiltrate is seen in muscle obtained at biopsy. Treatment with corticosteroids often produces a permanent remission.

Neuromuscular junction disorders

Myasthenia gravis. This is now recognised as being an autoimmune disorder and is associated with circulating antibodies to acetylcholine receptors. It is more common in girls. The onset is usually gradual with ptosis, strabismus, difficulty in chewing, loss of facial expression and arm weakness. The weakness may be very variable and is characteristically induced by fatigue. The diagnosis is confirmed by showing prompt improvement after an intravenous injection of edrophonium. The treatment of myasthenia involves the use of long-acting anticholinesterase drugs such as neostigmine or pyridostigmine. Thymectomy may have a place. Infants born to mothers with myasthenia gravis are susceptible to a transient form of the illness due to transplacental antibody transfer.

Nerve fibre disorders

Infectious polyneuritis (Guillain–Barré syndrome). This presents as a rapidly evolving symmetrical flaccid paralysis of the legs but trunk and arms are usually also involved. Respiratory and facial muscles may be affected. The weakness is commonly preceded by symptoms suggestive of viral infection. The cerebrospinal fluid often shows a considerable elevation of protein but no cellular response. The weakness progresses over a matter of days and then remains stationary for some weeks before entering a slow recovery phase. Severe cases may be treated with plasmapherasis which has been shown to improve the rate of recovery. A period of ventilation is required for respiratory paralysis in 10 per cent of cases. Most children make a full recovery but this can take up to a year. It is essential to distinguish spinal cord problems, which may need surgical treatment, from acute infectious polyneuritis.

Anterior horn cell disorders

Werdnig-Hoffman disease (acute spinal muscular atrophy). The early infantile form has autosomal recessive inheritance, and an incidence of 1 in 20 000 births. Mothers may notice a lack of fetal movements and the infants can be floppy and weak at birth. Symptoms are always present within the first few months of life. In spite of the extreme muscle weakness, the infants are alert and watchful. Muscle fasciculation, especially in the tongue, is a feature. The diagnosis is made by electromyography and muscle biopsy. The condition is progressive and usually leads to death from respiratory failure before 18 months of age.

Werdnig-Hoffman disease: clinical features and muscle biopsy appearance

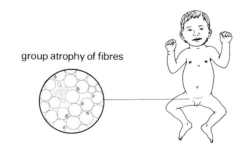

group atrophy of fibres

alert facial expression
fasciculation of tongue

deformed chest
see-saw respiration

frog position
absent reflexes

There are milder forms of spinal muscular atrophy with later onset, for example the Kugelberg–Welander syndrome (chronic spinal muscular atrophy).

Floppy infant syndrome

The term floppy infant describes babies who have marked hypotonia. A useful test is to hold the baby in ventral suspension. A floppy baby will drape over the hands like a rag doll whereas a normal baby will show postural tone appropriate to his age. Severe muscle weakness in addition to hypotonia suggests a neuromuscular disorder. Hypotonia in the absence of obvious muscle weakness suggests a non-paralytic cause for floppiness.

Hypotonia

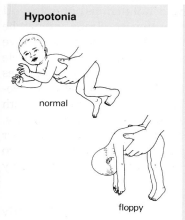

normal

floppy

Paralytic and non-paralytic causes of floppiness in infants

Paralytic	Non-paralytic

Neuromuscular disorders
Spinal cord lesions
  e.g. birth trauma
	Brain disorders
	  e.g. cerebral palsy
	        degenerative CNS disease
	        Prader-Willi syndrome
	Chromosomal disorders
	  e.g. Down syndrome
	Systemic disorders
	  e.g. malnutrition
	        congenital heart disease
	        hypothyroidism
	Connective tissue disorders
	  e.g. osteogenesis imperfecta
	Benign hypotonia

HEADACHE

Headache is a relatively common complaint among older children. Mild, self-limiting headaches are frequent in febrile illness but a severe headache of acute onset raises the possibility of intra-cranial inflammation, subarachnoid haemorrhage, leukaemic infiltration or an intra-cranial tumour (see chapter on Malignancy for cerebral tumours).

Intermittent headaches are usually either tension or migraine headaches but other causes such as dental caries, sinusitis, brain tumour, raised intracranial pressure, hypertension and ocular refractive error should be considered.

Migraine

Migraine affects about 5 per cent of all children at some time. A family history and the characteristic symptoms of throbbing headache, visual disturbance, photophobia and nausea make the diagnosis relatively straightforward in the older child. There may be problems in the recognition of migraine in the preschool child and it may be manifest by acute periods of distress, pallor and nausea. Attacks resulting in ophthalmoplegia or hemiparesis may occur. An underlying vascular malformation is rare association. Treatment is initially with simple analgesics such as paracetamol. More severe cases may benefit from non-ergotamine anti-migraine preparations. Recently there has been renewed interest in the relationship between food allergy and migraine. Some children benefit from the exclusion of cheese, chocolate or citrus fruits from their diets. More severe exclusion diets (oligo-allergenic diets) have been tried with success in some children with difficult migraine.

Ocular headaches

Ocular headaches result from constant muscular activity attempting to correct a latent squint or refractive error, usually long sightedness or astigmatism.

Benign intra-cranial hypertension

This term is used for an illness with raised intra-cranial pressure of unknown cause. It usually presents with vomiting, headache and papilloedema. CT scan shows small or normal sized ventricles and no space occupying lesion. It may be a complication of otitis media or occur after a non-specific viral illness; rarely it develops from too rapid reduction in corticosteroid therapy. Treatment is directed towards reducing the intra-cranial pressure in order to avoid secondary optic atrophy. A course of corticosteroids is usually successful but rarely may have to be complemented by repeated lumbar punctures or a theco-peritoneal shunt.

ATAXIA

Ataxia refers to a disorder of movement manifest by incoordination, clumsiness and poor balance. In the young child, hypotonia and delayed motor development may be the only obvious signs.

Ataxic cerebral palsy is caused by malformation or damage of the cerebellum or its connections. The commonest cause is cerebellar hypoplasia which may be inherited as an autosomal recessive. Dandy-Walker syndrome refers to congenital absence of the foramina of Majendie and Luschka with resulting cystic dilation of the IV ventricle. Affected children have a characteristic prominence of the occipital region and are often ataxic.

Acute ataxia in older children may be due to intoxication with drugs, for example solvent abuse, phenytoin or alcohol. If the history does not reveal a cause, the rapid recovery certainly suggests it. Cerebellar ataxia may also be a manifestation of viral encephalitis, especially that caused by varicella. The differential diagnosis includes an acute presentation of a cerebellar tumour such as medulloblastoma, but CT scanning rapidly resolves this concern.

Friedreich ataxia is the most common of the hereditary ataxias, and is an autosomal recessive condition initially characterised by pes cavus and a progressively clumsy gait. Examination reveals ataxia, loss of postural and vibratory sensation, and impaired leg tendon reflexes. There may, in addition, be optic atrophy and cardiomyopathy. The patients become increasingly handicapped and may be wheelchair-bound by early adult life.

Ataxia telangiectasia is inherited as an autosomal recessive. In addition to slowly increasing cerebellar ataxia, there are characteristic telangiectasia obvious over the bulbar conjunctiva and face. There is an associated impairment of cellular immunity which increases susceptibility to infection and predisposes to neoplasia especially leukaemia and lymphoma.

There are rare metabolic disorders which result in ataxia; Hartnup disease in which there is a derangement of tryptophan metabolism, and Refsum disease in which phytanic acid accumulates.

CEREBRAL PALSY

Cerebral palsy is the leading cause of crippling handicap in children (2 per 1000). The label cerebral palsy implies that the underlying lesion is permanent and non-progressive. However in a developing child the resulting clinical picture will not be static. The lesion is localised in the brain and, as it arises in early life, it interferes with normal motor development. The main handicap is one of disordered movement and posture, but it is often complicated by other neurological and mental problems.

Cerebral palsy is due to brain malformation or damage affecting those areas involved in motor functions. Congenital malformations of the brain include congenital cysts, fusion defects, failure of normal migration of grey matter, and aplasias. Brain damage may occur during fetal life from infection or hypoxia–ischaemia. Birth related cerebral trauma or hypoxia–ischaemia is now considered an uncommon cause of cerebral palsy (perhaps 10 per cent). Postnatal causes include non-accidental injury, road traffic accidents, meningitis, encephalitis, neonatal respiratory distress syndrome, near drowning and cardiopulmonary arrest.

Causes of cerebral palsy

Cerebral malformation
Trauma
  birth
  postnatal
Hypoxia
Kernicterus
Hypoglycaemia
Infection
Cerebrovascular accident
Poisoning
Toxins

Classification

Spastic cerebral palsy. Spastic cerebral palsy, which accounts for 70 per cent of cerebral palsy cases, involves damage to the cerebral motor cortex or its connections, producing clasp-knife hypertonia, abnormally

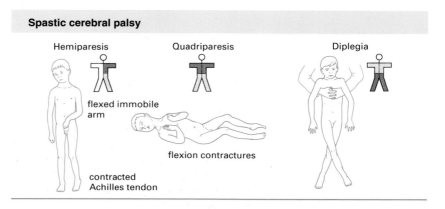

Spastic cerebral palsy

Hemiparesis — flexed immobile arm, contracted Achilles tendon   Quadriparesis — flexion contractures   Diplegia

brisk tendon jerks, ankle clonus and extensor plantar responses. Hemiparesis affects just one side of the body and the arm is usually involved more than the leg. Quadriparesis affects both sides of the body, the arms being affected as much or more than the legs. In spastic diplegia both legs are spastic and the arms are less affected or not affected at all.

Dystonic (Athetoid) cerebral palsy. Ten per cent of cases are characterised by irregular and involuntary movements of some or all muscle groups. These may be continuous or occur only on voluntary active movement. Athetosis is the commonest form with slow purposeless muscle movements and extensor spasms.

Ataxic cerebral palsy. This is associated with hypotonia, weakness, uncoordinated movements and intentional tremor and accounts for 10 per cent of cerebral palsy.

Mixed cerebral palsy. These form the remaining 10 per cent of cases.

Clinical features

Primitive reflexes

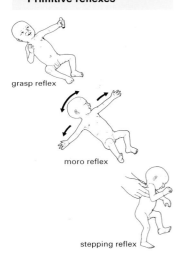

grasp reflex

moro reflex

stepping reflex

Infants who show poor sucking ability, increased or decreased muscle tone, abnormal reflexes, irritability, convulsions or drowsiness in the newborn period are at risk of having cerebral palsy. However, many such infants do develop normally and great care must be exercised in anticipating future development. Usually cerebral palsy is not diagnosed until several months have passed, and when it becomes obvious that motor development is abnormal or delayed. For example, the infant may be brought to the doctor because at 3 months of age he is not showing real head control or at 10 months of age he is not yet sitting alone. His mother may say that he seems stiff on handling. An infant with a spastic hemiplegia will be noted to have developed hand preference before 1 year which is much earlier than normal. The persistence of primitive reflexes, such as the asymmetric tonic neck reflex, beyond the time they usually disappear is suspicious. The characteristic involuntary movements of dystonic cerebral palsy are not usually obvious until near the end of the first year of life or even later. Affected children are usually very floppy and show delayed motor development in infancy. Children with ataxic cerebral palsy are also hypotonic and delayed in motor development but subsequently show an intention tremor.

Management

The child with cerebral palsy requires a multi-disciplinary assessment initially to define the problem, and then to develop a structured treatment programme. Physiotherapy aims to encourage normal motor development, to inhibit abnormal motor development and to prevent contractures. The parents are taught to perform the exercises at home.

Some degree of mental handicap is seen in about 60 per cent of children with cerebral palsy. However, it should not be forgotten that children with severe cerebral palsy may have normal intelligence; this applies particularly to the dystonic group. Epilepsy occurs in approximately 30 per cent and is symptomatic rather than idiopathic. Visual impairment due to errors of refraction, disuse amblyopia, optic atrophy or visual

How to hold a floppy child

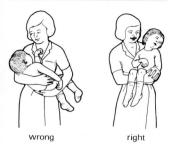

wrong   right

How to hold a spastic child

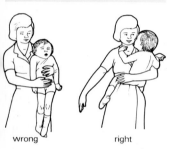

wrong   right

cortical damage occurs in 20 per cent. Squint due to external ocular muscle imbalance or paralysis is present in 30 per cent. Twenty per cent have a degree of hearing loss which is often of the sensorineural type. Children with dystonic cerebral palsy are particularly liable to have associated deafness. Speech disorders are common and are due to a variety of causes including hearing loss, perceptual defects, mental handicap and incoordination of tongue, palate, and lip muscles.

Children with cerebral palsy often do less well in school than would be expected by their estimated abilities. One reason for this is the high frequency of perceptual defects. Behaviour disorders may be due to the frustrations of being handicapped, to strained family life brought about by the presence of a handicapped child, and to the hyperactivity which may be associated with brain damage.

Even with adequate physiotherapy, long-standing muscle weakness or spasticity may produce orthopaedic deformities. These are more common in spastic cerebral palsy where the involved muscles develop fibrotic contractures. Spasticity in the adductors of the thigh may lead to dislocation of the hips and operation may be necessary to correct this. Spasticity and contracture in the calf muscles may produce a fixed equinus deformity of the ankle which requires a tendo-achilles lengthening operation to allow the heel to be used for walking and weight bearing. Neglect of these deformities may lead to painful osteoarthritis.

Drugs have a limited role in the management of cerebral palsy, apart from the treatment of epilepsy. Schools for the physically handicapped provide physiotherapy and speech therapy, and have specially trained staff and equipment. There is, however, a deficiency of opportunity for the handicapped school leaver. The overlap between cerebral palsy and mental handicap is such that some children in schools for children with severe learning disorders also have cerebral palsy.

If a child with a physical handicap comes under your care enquire about his or her 'activities of living' from the child and the carers

---

What is their usual daily schedule?
What can they say?
How do they indicate - Yes, No, Want, Drink, Sleep, Toilet, Pain, Cuddly, Mummy, Daddy etc?
How do they get about? Do they use a special chair or supports?
At meal times do they use special spoons and cups?
Do they wear glasses?
Do they wear hearing aids and when?

BIBLIOGRAPHY

Brett E 1991 Paediatric neurology, 2nd edn. Churchill Livingstone, Edinburgh
Dubowitz V 1978 Muscle disorders in childhood. W B Saunders, Philadelphia
Levene M I, Bennet M J, Punt J (eds) 1988 Fetal and neonatal neurology and neurosurgery. Churchill Livingstone, Edinburgh
O'Donohoe N V 1985 Epilepsies of childhood, 2nd edn. Butterworths, London
Scrutton D (ed) 1984 Management of motor disorders of children with cerebral palsy. Spastics International Medical Publications, London

19 Vision, Hearing, Speech

VISION

Vision is the most highly evolved of man's special senses. Binocular stereoscopic perception and interpretation requires not only an exact optic mechanism but also complex neural interconnections. The retina and eye are relatively mature at birth, and 75 per cent of postnatal ocular growth occurs in the first 3 years of life. Myelination of the optic pathways is, however, still incomplete at term, and experimental work has recently confirmed the clinical impression that normal development of the optic radiation and visual cortex is dependent on undistorted light reception. It is therefore essential to act promptly when, for example, a severe ptosis or a cataract threatens the visual development of a new-born infant.

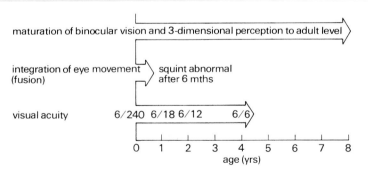

The development of vision

maturation of binocular vision and 3-dimensional perception to adult level

integration of eye movement (fusion) — squint abnormal after 6 mths

visual acuity   6/240 6/18 6/12   6/6

age (yrs)   0 1 2 3 4 5 6 7 8

Assessment of vision

Before the age of 6 months, vision may be assessed by the response to a moving face, a slowly moving ball and by attention to hand-eye skills. Vision must always be considered in the context of general development. Quantification of visual acuity is possible in infancy using a preferential looking test in which the baby is presented a striped and a uniformly grey target simultaneously. Targets with narrower stripes are presented until the baby no longer gives them preferential attention compared with the uniformly grey target. After 3 years single letter

Stycar letter matching cards and after 5 years Stycar letter charts can be used. The Stycar letters have been specially selected as those which cause young children least confusion. Adult type Snellen charts can be used after 7 years.

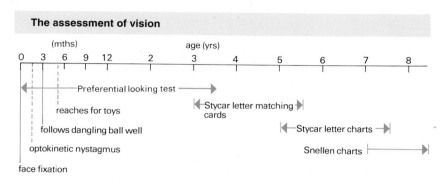

The assessment of vision

Squints

Squints are common in early childhood. All fixed squints and any squint which persists to age 5 or 6 months require careful evaluation. Having detected a squint, expert assessment involves full examination of the eyes to exclude, for example corneal opacities, cataracts, and refractive errors. The usual cause of infantile strabismus is an ill-understood failure to develop binocular fusion at the normal time. Other important causes include refractive errors, particularly hypermetropia and astigmatism, neurological disorders which interfere with the normal function of the extraocular muscles, and eye diseases such as cataracts or retinoblastoma. Whatever the cause, the image of the squinting eye is suppressed, thereby avoiding diplopia and, if neglected, this may lead to an irreversible failure of development of the visual pathways from the squinting eye (amblyopia).

Testing for a squint

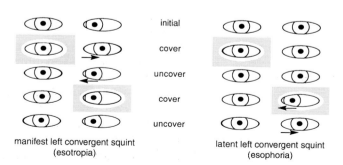

The blind child

For educational purposes a child is defined as blind if he requires education by methods which do not involve sight, for example Braille, and as partially sighted if he requires special educational consideration but can use methods which depend on sight, e.g. large print books. In practice, most blind children have some vision even if it is only recognition of light and dark, or perception of shapes.

In the UK about 500 children each year are newly registered blind or partially sighted, an incidence of approximately 1 in 2500 children but the true incidence may be higher because of incomplete registration. As many as 50 per cent of blind children have additional handicaps, e.g. physical disability, low intelligence, hearing and language difficulties. In their survey of visual handicap, Schappert-Kimmijser et al (1975) reported that the main causes of visual handicap in childhood were optic atrophy (18 per cent), congenital cataracts (16 per cent), and choroidoretinal degenerations (15 per cent). Overall the conditions causing visual handicap were genetically determined in 45 per cent of children and due to some perinatal disturbance in 33 per cent. The incidence of retinopathy of prematurity dramatically decreased in the early 1960s, possibly due to greater care when giving oxygen therapy in the newborn period.

Causes of childhood visual handicap

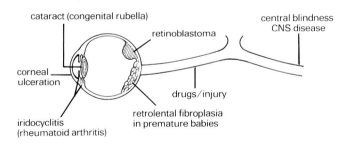

Blindness must be suspected where there is a pendular nystagmus or roving, purposeless eye movements. Normal children cease to show random, uncoordinated eye movements after 6 weeks of age. Some blind infants poke their eyes in a characteristic fashion, probably to produce pleasurable visual hallucinations of retinal origin.

With the exception of cataracts, most causes of blindness in children are not amenable to medical treatment. Recent advances in cataract surgery allow early removal of a congenital cataract and the immediate provision of a lens implant or contact lens thereby avoiding stimulus deprivation amblyopia.

Parents of a blind child need expert, sympathetic advice from a very early stage. Peripatetic preschool teachers from the Royal National Institute for the Blind or local education authority fulfil this role in the UK.

The parents must be taught to stimulate their infant using non-visual means, touch and speech. The home should be adapted so that the child can explore his environment safely. Residential school is often necessary for the blind child who needs to learn Braille. The child with partial sight may cope in an ordinary school with the help of special equipment.

HEARING

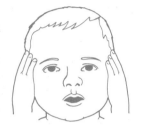

Hearing refers to the reception of sounds, their transduction to nerve impulses and transmission to the relevant areas of the cerebral cortex. Listening implies an attention to the sounds and their interpretation and is a prerequisite for language development. The fetus is sensitive to noise and from the moment of birth there is an important sound inter-play between mother and infant. Hearing provides for emotional contact, language development, identity with the environment and assists in the awareness of posture and body orientation. All children should be screened for deafness by tests which are appropriate to their stage of development and it is usual for these tests to be performed at six to nine months of age, and again at the preschool examination.

The assessment of hearing

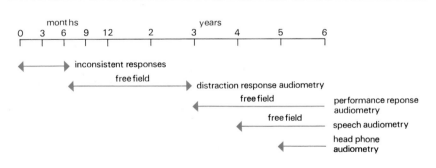

Assessment of hearing

Babies up to about 7 months show inconsistent responses to noises and reliable testing can only be done with sophisticated apparatus such as brainstem evoked response audiometry. From 7 months infants will turn their head and eyes towards the source of a quiet sound (distraction responses). It is essential to have a contented child in a quiet room. The examiner stands one to three feet to the side of the child and just outside his range of vision. The sound stimulus should be given at ear level. Sound makers employed are a high pitched rattle, spoon in cup, tissue paper, hand bell and selected speech sounds, for example 'oo' and 'ss'. A free field pure tone audiometer may be used to generate the sound stimuli. From 3 years, a child will play a game of putting a toy in a box whenever he hears the sound (performance responses). From

4 years, picture cards or toys can be used. The child is asked in a quiet voice to show the examiner a certain picture or toy from an array in front of him (speech audiometry). Most children of 5 years and over will tolerate wearing headphones and give reliable pure tone audiograms showing both air and bone conduction thresholds. The final proof of adequate hearing is the comprehension and imitation of normal speech. Although pure tone audiometry has a place in defining the hearing of children, it cannot replace clinical speech tests.

Causes of childhood deafness

Conductive deafness (4% of school children)	Sensorineural deafness (0.3% of school children)	
Glue ear following otitis media (almost all cases)	Genetic – various types 50%	
	Intrauterine (8%)	congenital infection, e.g. rubella maternal drugs, e.g. streptomycin
	Perinatal (12%)	birth asphyxia severe hyperbilirubinaemia
	Postnatal (30%)	meningitis encephalitis head injury

Types of deafness

Whereas hearing loss of less than 20 dB normally has no effect on the child's development, a loss of over 40 dB creates problems in the development of ordinary speech. Testing over a range of frequencies may show a widespread loss or a loss purely in the high frequency zone. Deafness is classified into two categories, sensorineural and conductive. In sensorineural deafness there is damage to the cochlea or auditory nerve whereas in the conductive type there is middle ear dysfunction. Most severe deafness in children is sensorineural in type and is present from birth. The two types of deafness can be distinguished in older

Audiograms: three patterns of hearing loss

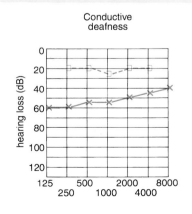

Conductive deafness

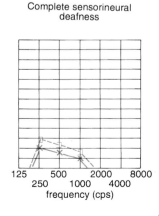

Complete sensorineural deafness

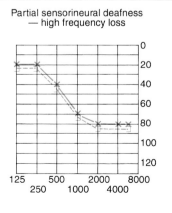

Partial sensorineural deafness — high frequency loss

air conduction ×   bone conduction ▢

children by pure tone headphone audiometry. In the sensorineural type, there is equal impairment of bone and air conduction of sound; in the conductive type, there is an air–bone gap with bone conduction hearing better than air conduction.

Forty per 1000 schoolchildren have mild deafness, usually a conductive middle ear deafness due to glue ear. Two per 1000 children have moderate deafness sufficient to require them to use a hearing aid, and one per 1000 children is severely deaf and requires special education.

Treatment of deafness

More careful management and follow-up of children susceptible to otitis media may reduce the incidence of glue ear. In established cases of glue ear the deafness is usually reversed by aeration of the middle-ear by means of a grommet inserted in the tympanic membrane, and removal of hypertrophied adenoids which often block the Eustachian tubes.

There is no specific therapy for sensorineural deafness apart from cochlear implant surgery which is only suitable for a minority of such children. If there is some residual hearing, a hearing aid is useful. This is simply a device for amplifying sounds within the frequency range of the spoken voice. There are problems in that the receiver is not selective and is liable to cause distressing exaggeration of environmental and background noises, for example rustling clothes. Careful instruction in its use is required as well as attention to such items as the ear moulds. It must be emphasised that the provision of an aid is only part of a more general process of rehabilitation and education. Parents of the young deaf child need expert guidance on how to encourage him to talk and develop language. Such help is given by the peripatetic teacher of the deaf. Many moderately deaf children can attend a normal school, but the more severely affected require specialist education, either at a school for the deaf or in a partially hearing unit attached to a normal school. As genetic causes are present in 50 per cent of children with sensorineural deafness, genetic counselling is often indicated to try to prevent further cases occurring in the family.

SPEECH AND LANGUAGE

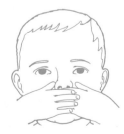

Language is essential to our culture as it provides the symbolic code for communication and for our thought process. The early development of vocalisation (exploratory sounds) and verbalisation (meaningful sounds) is closely linked to the mechanisms of hearing and listening.

There is a wide age range among normal children for the development of vocabulary. Some children with slow speech development may be excellent at non-verbal communication and clearly have a well developed inner language. In others, the physiological basis of speech development is intact but is hindered by detrimental family relationships, social factors or psychiatric disturbances. It is also recognised that children in institutional care have delayed speech development and this is probably due to less intense interpersonal relationships.

Assessment of speech

Speech development must be considered in the context of the wide range of normal development. The parents of the 2-year-old boy with obviously normal development but a vocabulary of only 10 to 20 words may be comparing him with the little girl of similar age down the road with a vocabulary of 200 words. Both are within the normal range. Assessment must consider general development as well as environmental factors. Comprehension and free conversation during play are useful guides before embarking on more specific diagnostic exercises. An experienced speech therapist plays a valuable role in assessing and treating these children, and will be able to make a distinction between comprehension and expressive language delay. It is essential to make sure hearing is normal in any child who is showing delayed speech development.

Causes of speech delay

dysphasia	specific brain lesion generalised brain disorders
deprivation	
	developmental — mental handicap developmental speech disorder
deafness	
	local — structural and functional disorders of larynx

The developmental speech disorder syndrome

About 6 per cent of 3 to 4-year-old children show significant delay in speech development. In half of these children the cause is mental handicap, cerebral palsy or deafness. The remainder have a developmental speech disorder syndrome. It is more common in boys and there is often a family history. With speech therapy help the majority eventually catch up with speech and language development but some of these show later difficulties with reading and spelling (dyslexia). Only a minority, perhaps 1 in 1000 of all children, continue to have major problems with speech and language in later childhood, and the term developmental dysphasia is sometimes used for them. Such children require specialised teaching and may benefit from learning a non-verbal form of communication such as the Bliss or Paget-Gorman systems.

Dysrhythmia (stammering)

It is common for children between 3 and 4 years of age to have a so-called physiological stammer. This corrects itself spontaneously and must not be made a focus of attention. A more persistent stammering or stuttering has a familial predisposition. In younger children, therapy is largely directed towards diverting attention away from the speech difficulty with the expectation of spontaneous improvement. In older children, more formal exercises such as syllable timed speech may be necessary for the most disruptive cases

BIBLIOGRAPHY

Haggard M P, Evans E F 1987 Hearing. British Medical Bulletin 43(4)
Yule W, Rutter M 1987 Language development and disorders. Mac Keith Press and
    Blackwell Scientific Publications, Oxford.

20 Mental handicap

The level of medical care provided within a community may be assessed by the prevalence, identification and care of those who are severely mentally handicapped. Better services result both in fewer people being affected, and in the early recognition of those who are affected due to the effects of deleterious genetic, environmental and social factors. The care offered must also be as supportive and humane as the community can afford.

The words used to describe the mentally handicapped have changed with the years for they quickly become terms of abuse (e.g. moron, idiot, cretin, mongol); and currently the term 'mentally retarded' is being abandoned. As a group, however, these children may be defined as having learning problems. The severely handicapped have difficulty in learning to walk, dress and communicate. The more mildly affected have difficulty acquiring skills to look after themselves and earn a living.

Aspects of mental ability or intelligence can be measured by a variety of tests. They measure what an individual has achieved at the time of the assessment and, although they may be a guide to what he might achieve, they do not necessarily measure his potential. The results of the tests are expressed as a quotient, the child's 'mental' age over chronological age. The distribution of intelligence follows a Gaussian or normal distribution with a distortion in the lower range due to the effects of deleterious environmental and social factors. Fetal and early infant death counteracts some of this distortion.

It is helpful to divide those with low intelligence and who require special education into two groups, mild and severe. The mildly handicapped are composed largely of those in the lower range of the normal distribution, with IQs in the 50 to 70 range. They often come from families of low intelligence and poor social background. The severely handicapped with IQs below 50 usually have some organic disorder: a recognised inherited disorder, a brain deformity or suffered a severe injury which has permanently damaged the brain. Obviously there is some overlap between the two groups.

The following list emphasises the extensive list of disorders which may contribute to mental handicap; each chapter in this book contains problems which may produce this end result. The diseases discussed in the second half of this chapter warrant a separate section, not because of their frequency, but because they do not fit easily into other categories.

The population distribution of intelligence

frequency

SD –3 –2 –1 mean +1 +2 +3 intelligence quotient (IQ)
55 70 85 100 115 130 145

WHO classification
0 profound 20 severe 50 moderate 70

Educational classification
ESN(s) ——————— ESN(m) →

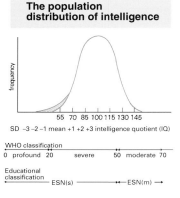

Learning difficulties and social class

IQ < 50, rate per 1000 children

I-IIIa IIIb IIIc IV V

IQ 50-75, rate per 1000 children

I-IIIa IIIb IIIc IV V

social class

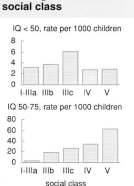

A classification of the recognised causes of mental handicap

Causes of mental handicap	Examples
A Genetic	
• Chromosomal disorder	Trisomy, e.g. Down syndrome
	Deletion, e.g. cri du chat syndrome
	Sex chromosome anomaly, e.g. fragile X syndrome
• Metabolic disorder	Amino acid, e.g. phenylketonuria
	Carbohydrate, e.g. galactosaemia
	Organic acid, e.g. isovaleric acidaemia
• Cerebral degenerative disorder	Gangliosidoses
	Lipidoses
	Complex carbohydrates
	Mucopolysaccharidoses
	Leucodystrophies
• Structural disorders	Tuberose sclerosis
	Familial hydrocephalus
B Intrauterine	
• Congenital infection	Cytomegalovirus
	Rubella
	Toxoplasmosis
• Drugs	Phenytoin, alcohol
• Cerebral malformations	Hydranencephaly, porencephaly
C Perinatal	
• Problems during pregnancy	Pre-eclamptic toxaemia
	Antepartum haemorrhage
	Premature onset of labour
• Problems during labour and delivery	Prolonged labour
	Fetal distress
	Trauma
	Asphyxia
• Neonatal problems	Intraventricular haemorrhage
	Hypoglycaemia
	Meningitis
	Jaundice
D Postnatal	
• Trauma	Accidental or non-accidental injury
• Infection	Encephalitis, meningitis
• Anoxia	Asphyxia, status epilepticus
• Metabolic and endocrine	Hypoglycaemia, hypernatraemia, hypothyroidism
• Poisoning	Lead
• Psychological	Infantile psychosis/autism

THE IDENTIFICATION AND TREATMENT OF MENTALLY HANDICAPPED CHILDREN

Routine developmental checks should be available for all infants, and for those where suspicion arises there must be ready access to the skills of a multidisciplinary assessment team. It is important that prompt, confident reassurance is given to the parents of children who demonstrate innocent variation of development, and that sensitive explanation is provided where abnormality is likely.

Following careful assessment, the cause of severe mental handicap will be found in roughly 80 per cent of cases. The history, examination and investigations may all contribute to the diagnosis. Cerebral palsy although strictly not a cause of mental handicap is an associated finding in 25 per cent of severely mentally handicapped children. A number of conspicuous malformation syndromes are associated with handicap. It is also important to document minor anomalies for these may also provide clues to underlying major disorders. A single minor anomaly is relatively common and occurs in 14 per cent of newborn infants, but the presence of three or four minor anomalies carries a 90 per cent risk of an associated major defect. Particular attention should be paid to eyes, ears, palate, hair pattern, hands and feet. There are invaluable reference atlases which link malformations with defined syndromes.

Features on history, examination and investigations which may identify the cause of mental handicap

Historical items
- Family history of affected males — Fragile X syndrome
- Maternal alcoholism — Fetal alcohol syndrome
- Light-for-dates — Placental dysfunction, congenital infections, fetal alcohol syndrome
- Pica — Lead poisoning
- Deterioration — Cerebral degenerative disorder

Clinical findings
- Floppy infant — Prader-Willi syndrome, congenital myotonic dystrophy, Down syndrome
- Obesity — Pseudohypoparathyroidism, Prader-Willi syndrome
- Funny smell — Organic acidurias, maple syrup urine disease
- Cerebral palsy — Perinatal asphyxia
- Hepatosplenomegaly — Niemann-Pick disease, Gaucher disease, Hurler syndrome
- Cardiac abnormalities — Down syndrome, congenital rubella, infantile hypercalcaemia
- Coarse facies — Hypothyroidism, mucopolysaccharidoses
- Deafness — Congenital rubella, mucopolysaccharidoses
- Large head — Soto syndrome, hydrocephalus, neurofibromatosis, mucopolysaccharidoses
- Microcephaly — Congenital infections, maternal phenylketonuria, fetal alcohol syndrome, Smith-Lemli-Opitz syndrome, perinatal asphyxia, genetic microcephaly
- Large fontanelles — Pseudohypoparathyroidism
- Hypertelorism — Agenesis of the corpus collosum, cri du chat syndrome
- Hypotelorism — Holoprosencephaly
- Slanted palpebral fissures — Down syndrome
- Synophrys (eyebrows meeting) — DeLange syndrome
- Congenital ptosis — Smith-Lemli-Opitz syndrome
- Cataracts — Congenital rubella, galactosaemia
- Corneal opacities — Mucopolysaccharide disorder
- Lens dislocation — Homocystinuria
- Retinal pigmentation — Laurence-Moon-Biedl syndrome, congenital rubella, Leber amaurosis
- Hypopigmented macules — Tuberous sclerosis
- Café au lait patches — Neurofibromatosis
- Port wine stains on face — Sturge-Weber syndrome
- Pigment whorls — Incontinentia pigmenti
- Hirsutism — DeLange syndrome, mucopolysaccharidoses
- Polydactyly — Laurence-Moon-Biedl syndrome
- Small hands and feet — Prader-Willi syndrome
- Large hands and feet — Soto syndrome
- Broad thumbs — Rubenstein-Taybi syndrome
- Simian creases — Down syndrome, DeLange syndrome, Smith-Lemli-Opitz syndrome
- Joint contractures — Mucopolysaccharidoses, sex chromosome disorder
- Cryptorchidism — Smith-Lemli-Opitz syndrome, Prader-Willi syndrome
- Hypospadias — Smith-Lemli-Opitz syndrome

Investigations

Thyroid function tests	Hypothyroidism
Serum and urine amino acids	Aminoacidurias
Blood lead level	Lead poisoning
Blood calcium	Pseudohypoparathyroidism
Blood acid–base balance	Organic acidurias
Urine mucopolysaccharide screen	Mucopolysaccharidoses
Urine organic acids	Organic acidurias
Chromosome studies	Chromosomal abnormalities
Skull X-ray	Intracranial calcification
CT scan	Cerebral malformation, hydrocephalus, leucodystrophy
White blood cell enzymes	Cerebral degenerative disorders

Congenital hypothyroidism and phenylketonuria should not nowadays cause mental handicap as they should be diagnosed by routine neonatal screening tests and treated before they cause permanent damage. Progressive deterioration in performance emphasises the need to look for metabolic, storage or neuro-degenerative disorders. Modern techniques and the identification of specific enzyme deficiencies have improved the yield of such investigations. There is almost no place for brain biopsy.

METABOLIC AND OTHER CEREBRAL DEGENERATIVE DISORDERS

Phenylketonuria

Phenylketonuria causes severe mental deficiency, microcephaly and seizures. It results from a block in the hepatic conversion of phenylalanine to tyrosine. Infants with classical PKU have less than 1 per cent of normal phenylalanine hydroxylase activity. Less severe variants have milder deficiency, 1 to 5 per cent. A rare subgroup lack an essential cofactor, tetrahydrobiopterin (BH4), and have a severe progressive disease refractory to the usual dietary measures but possibly amenable to neurotransmitter replacement.

PKU is a relatively rare, autosomal recessive disorder, 10 cases per 100 000 births, but the effectiveness of prompt therapy justifies routine neonatal screening of blood phenylalanine levels. This is conveniently performed on capillary blood using the Guthrie bacterial inhibition technique in which a specific strain of B. subtilis can multiply only in the presence of phenylalanine. To be valid the infant has to be established on milk, and the test is conventionally performed on samples collected at the end of the first week of life.

Dietary phenylalanine restriction must be established promptly and has to be carefully monitored to meet the twin aims of brain protection while allowing sufficient quantities of this essential amino acid for growth. The overall results of careful treatment are good with 75 per cent of the UK 1974–78 cohort attending normal schools albeit with a higher incidence of behavioural and learning problems. Debate surrounds the issue of when and how to withdraw dietary restriction. Beyond the age of 6 to 8 years the nervous system is less vulnerable to elevated phenylalanine levels, and compliance certainly falls.

Maternal phenylketonuria is now increasing as a problem, and has devastating effects on the fetus, causing microcephaly, severe handicap and other structural anomalies. This emphasises the long-term responsibilities of the health-care team who must maintain patient contact, attempt guidance for planned conception and reintroduce dietary restriction.

Gangliosidoses

Tay-Sachs disease. Tay-Sachs disease is the most frequent of these rare disorders. It is due to the abnormal accumulation of ganglioside GM2 in the grey matter. The developmental regression is usually obvious by 6 to 9 months of age with increasing motor weakness. An exaggerated startle response to sound, hyperacusis, is an early sign. Visual inattention and social unresponsiveness are part of the deteriorating course which includes convulsions and difficulties in swallowing, and ends in death by 3 to 5 years. A cherry red spot at the macula is characteristic of this degenerative disorder. The diagnosis may be confirmed by measuring serum hexosaminidase activity. Prenatal detection is possible, but as 80 per cent of cases mark the first appearance of the condition in families, it is far more valuable to identify at-risk couples before they reproduce. The high frequency of the heterozygote in Ashkenazi Jewish populations has been a stimulus to successful voluntary detection programmes.

Other gangliosidoses include a generalised form with hepatosplenomegaly and skeletal deformities, generalised gangliosidosis, and a variety with later onset neural presentation, juvenile Tay-Sachs disease. The measurement of specific enzyme activity enables precise identification.

The biochemical basis of Tay-Sachs, Gaucher and Nieman-Pick disease

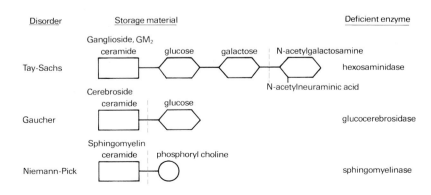

Neural lipidoses

Gaucher disease. Gaucher disease may be classified into neuronopathic and non-neuronopathic or visceral varieties. The former presents in infancy with feeding problems, stridor, and spasticity. There is prominent hepatosplenomegaly and Gaucher cells can be identified in marrow or liver biopsy. Death occurs within months. The non-neuronopathic form presents later in childhood or early adult life with hepatosplenomegaly, pancytopenia and bone involvement. It is compatible with a reasonable life span.

Niemann-Pick disease. Niemann-Pick disease also causes abnormal storage in the reticuloendothelial system and two of the four recognised varieties are neuronopathic. It may resemble Tay-Sachs disease and have a cherry red macular spot. It can also present in the differential diagnosis of neonatal hepatitis. Typical foam cells can be found in marrow and liver biopsy.

Mucopolysaccharidoses

Hurler syndrome

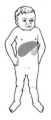

grossly retarded development

coarse facies
hazy corneas
enlarged tongue

cardiac abnormalities

hepatosplenomegaly
umbilical hernia
claw hand
joint deformities

These complex carbohydrate storage disorders typically cause abnormal accumulation in fibroblasts and chondrocytes resulting in coarsened skin, corneal clouding, skeletal dysplasia and hepatosplenomegaly. The manifestations vary and not all have neural involvement. There are currently seven or eight varieties which can be distinguished by the enzyme defect and the major storage substance, dermatan, heparin or keratan sulphate and its excretion in the urine.

Hurler syndrome. This is the best recognised form and results from the deficiency of L-iduronidase.

The mucolipidoses. The mucolipidoses resemble the mucopolysaccharidoses but lack the urine products. Sophisticated biochemical studies are required for their precise identification.

White matter degenerative disorders

These present with progressive motor deterioration and spasticity. There is associated intellectual loss, progressive blindness due to optic atrophy, and convulsions.

Metachromatic leucodystrophy. This is the most commonly recognised variety and usually becomes obvious in the second year. Sulphatides accumulate in nervous and other tissues due to deficiency of the enzyme, aryl sulphatase. The diagnosis is made by demonstrating metachromatic material in urinary sediment or tissue biopsy, and establishing deficient aryl sulphatase activity in white cells or cultured fibroblasts.

SPECIFIC TREATMENT AND GENERAL MANAGEMENT

Treatment. Dietary manipulation assists a small but important group of children with inherited disorders of carbohydrate, amino acid or

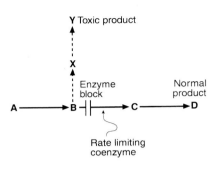

Inborn errors of metabolism: possible therapy

Y Toxic product

X

A ——→ B ┤├ ——→ C ——→ D

Enzyme block

Normal product

Rate limiting coenzyme

1. **Reduce intake of A to a minimum**
   e.g. phenylketonuria
   galactosaemia

2. **Provide high doses of vitamin precursor**
   e.g. pyridoxine-sensitive varieties of homocystinuria
   B_{12} sensitive varieties of methylmalonic aciduria

3. **Provide physiological requirements of C or D**
   e.g. inherited block of thyroxine synthesis

4. **Tissue replacement**
   e.g. bone marrow transplant in mucopolysaccharidoses

organic acid metabolism. We have not yet devised a satisfactory means of replacing deficient enzymes within the tissues, and the blood–brain barrier may prove to be an impenetrable obstacle. Prevention through accurate diagnosis of index cases and genetic counselling provides the only successful method of control in the majority of these disorders.

General management. Mentally handicapped children and their families require the resources of a multidisciplinary approach. In addition to general assessment, the child's social, motor, language, hearing and visual abilities must all be considered. A therapeutic programme must begin as early as possible with parents playing an active role together with physiotherapists, speech therapists, and play counsellors. Health visitors and social workers assist the parents in coming to terms with their problems and advise on financial and equipment help. Seizure disorders and behavioural problems may require specific drug therapy.

The Education Act of 1970 legislated for special schools to be available for all handicapped children. More recently the 1981 Education Act established the basis for a more enlightened framework, evolving away from traditional categories of handicap and promoting integration with normal schoolchildren. Although schools are classified as dealing with moderate learning disordered (MLD) children or severe learning disordered (SLD) children, the system has to be flexible to accommodate coexisting physical problems. Children in the IQ range 50 to 70 often achieve some independence and benefit from the high staff: pupil ratio available in MLD schools. Eighty per cent are capable of an open occupation and the remainder are provided with employment in sheltered workshops, adult occupation centres. Children with IQ below 50 are rarely independent and often need to be dressed and fed. They may not be able to speak and require constant attention. Education at SLD schools is essentially aimed at training the children to do simple social tasks. As these children become older the parents find it increasingly difficult to look after them. Up to the age of 20 only a minority are in residential care but after this age the proportion increases rapidly. Residential facilities vary considerably but there is a tendency towards smaller units which attempt to retain the family structure and links with the surrounding community. Those remaining at home usually attend a day centre run by the local social services department. Community based mental handicap teams play a major role in the provision of services for mentally handicapped adults and their carers.

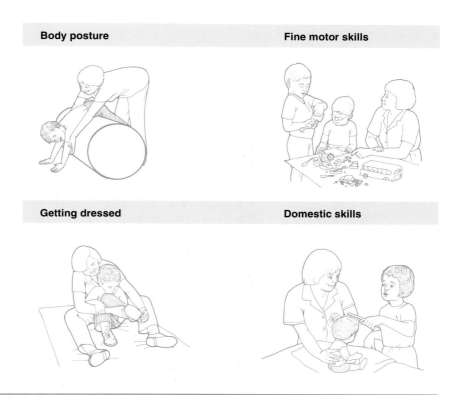

Body posture

Fine motor skills

Getting dressed

Domestic skills

BIBLIOGRAPHY

Craft M Tredgold's mental retardation, 12th edn. Balliere Tindall, London
Heaton-Ward W A, Wiley Y 1984 Mental handicap. Wright, Bristol
Russell O 1985 Mental handicap. Churchill Livingstone, Edinburgh

21

Emotions and Behaviour

People and places

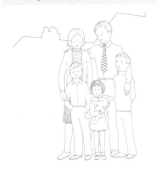

Until recent years, doctors treating children tended to ignore unusual emotions or deviant behaviours, believing them to be the responsibility of the parents or, if the problem was particularly troublesome, the child psychiatrist, social worker, teacher, or the welfare services. However, it is a mistake for a family or hospital doctor caring for children not to have studied the behavioural and emotional disturbances, for on the one hand many childhood illnesses are associated with some disturbance in behaviour, indeed some organic diseases may present with a behaviour problem, and on the other hand children in emotional conflict with themselves or their family or their surroundings may present with symptoms which mimic organic diseases.

Problems with childhood behaviour, or emotions that are severe or prolonged enough to interfere with every day life are classified as psychiatric disorders. The socio-cultural context, and the child's stage of development, are taken into account when deciding whether or not a symptom is abnormal. In different parts of the world, epidemiological surveys using this definition, have reported 1 year prevalence rates of about 1 in 10. Surveys of paediatric patients have shown that about 1 in 4 suffer from a significant psychiatric disorder.

Virtually all the symptoms of psychiatric disturbance in children are non-specific. For example temper tantrums may be a symptom of a mood disorder, such as anxiety or depression. They may also be a sign of disturbed relationships, developmental immaturity, or a reaction to a recent stressful event. Of course temper tantrums can also be normal.

Classification of the recognised causes of mental illness

- Diseases which interfere with vital supplies to the brain:
- Perceptive disorders
- Brain pathologies:
    epilepsy
    mental retardation

- Developmental delays

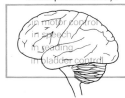

in motor control
in speech
in reading
in bladder control

- Psychiatric syndromes

tics
hyperkinetic syndrome
'minimal brain damage'
autism

In view of the nonspecificity of symptoms when they are considered in isolation, it is important to look at the total picture. A child who is miserable and seems depressed, but has no other associated symptoms, is unlikely to suffer from a depressive disorder; but a child who is occasionally tearful and at the same time has disturbed sleep and appetite, tends to be irritable and expresses feelings of hopelessness and worthlessness, is very likely to be suffering from a serious depressive disorder.

The context in which a symptom occurs is also important. Stealing, for example, may be quite normal if it occurs in the context of a family where criminal behaviour is considered acceptable, and where the child may have actually been taught how to steal. On the other hand, a

Child factors that make emotional and behavioural problems more likely to occur

Boys: more likely to develop behavioural problems when younger
Girls: more likely to develop emotional problems when older
Physical illness: especially temporal lobe epilepsy
Difficult temperament
Developmental delay and learning difficulties
Communication problems: deafness or language disorder
Poor self image: low self esteem, feeling of failure
School failure
Poor peer relationships

Family factors that make behavioural and emotional problems more likely to occur

Marital difficulties, separation and divorce
Death: close relative, friend or pet
Poor discipline: inconsistent, unclear or hostile
Rejecting attitudes
Abuse: emotional, physical or sexual
Poverty: poor housing, unemployment
Four or more children in family
Psychiatric illness in the mother
Criminal behaviour in the father

Social and cultural factors that make emotional and behavioural problems more likely to occur

Bullying
Antisocial influences from other children
Disorganisation within the school
Social/cultural expectations
Social policy

Protective factors that make emotional and behavioural problems less likely to occur

Consistent loving relationships
Age appropriate care
Above average ability
Regular adequate income
Stable family relationships
Support for mother outside the family
3 or more years between children

4-year old who takes something valuable without asking, can hardly be said to have stolen it, because their sense of moral value is still developing; therefore, in the context of the child's developmental stage the stealing does not signify disturbed behaviour.

The different factors that work together to cause a child to develop a disturbance of behaviour or emotions, may interact with each other in such a way that the whole is more than the sum of the parts. For example, a child who is physically ill and has missed school may have no problems, but if the child who is ill has missed particular lessons where crucial bits of information were given and as a result academic failure results, then the disappointment may interact with the child's feeling of ill health and produce a low self-esteem and a feeling of hopelessness, ultimately leading to a depressive disorder. In this instance the depression was not caused by the physical illness, or by missing some time from school; it was the way in which these two factors interacted with each other that caused the problem. In reality, these interactions are usually much more complicated, especially where family factors are involved. In order to understand what is happening to a child it is, therefore, important to consider not only the different factors that might be causing the child's disturbance, but also the way in which they interact. An understanding of this interactive process can be helpful in working out where to target treatment to have the maximum effect. So in the example given, additional teaching help for the child, may be more effective than treatment of the depression.

BRAIN DISORDERS

Diseases affecting the brain It is obvious that any illness which affects the brain might alter a child's emotional stage and affect his behaviour. The list of diseases, metabolic, traumatic, infective, neoplastic which may affect the brain and its function is endless; all may have associated behaviour problems, some of which are easily recognised and understood, but others, for example the odd behaviour of a child with a cerebral tumour, may be overlooked for some time. Their precise relationship to the physical illness is not always clear. There are three ways in which diseases of the brain can affect a child's psychological stage.

Specific effects. Direct damage to the brain can lead to loss of cognitive skills, for example difficulties with language and communication, or with mathematical calculation or problem solving. These problems may combine with short or long term memory loss to present a typical picture of dementia. Hallucinations, particularly if they are either visual or tactile, are characteristic of cerebral dysfunction. Unusual repetitive behaviour and perseveration of spoken language that is abnormal for the child's stage of development, are both commonly associated with abnormal brain function. Finally, clouding of consciousness and dis-orientation in time, place and person, are perhaps the most obvious signs that there is abnormal brain function.

Non-specific effects. Brain dysfunction can result in both emotional and behavioural abnormalities that are not specific to a damaged brain and could occur as a result of a number of different causes. For example, disinhibited behaviour can be the result of brain damage, but it can also lead to lack of social awareness, or inadequate social training. Similarly, emotional lability is commonly associated with an abnormally function-ing brain, but is also typical of immature personality development. Likewise, bizarre behaviour may result from a number of different causes but it is also commonly associated with an abnormally functioning brain.

Secondary causes. Any disease process that interferes with brain func-tion to a sufficient extent to cause the emotional, behavioural and cogni-tive difficulties, is likely to lead to difficulties that are secondary to these symptoms. For example, memory loss and difficulties with cog-nitive skills can lead to academic failure; emotional lability to relation-ship problems and clouding of consciousness and hallucinations to secondary delusional ideas.

It is not unusual for brain dysfunction to be associated with per-ceptual problems. Deafness and blindness are obvious, but often the perceptual difficulties are much more subtle, such as spacial orien-tation, perception of the self and an awareness of social relationships.

Epilepsy is due to an involuntary, uncontrollable activity from the brain which produces a seizure. The usual forms of seizures include grand mal, focal epilepsy, and petit mal seizures and have been discussed elsewhere. Temporal lobe seizures may occur with clouding of aware-ness, confusional states, automatic motor behaviour patterns and angry or terrified outbursts. Epilepsy of whatever form is associated with an increased incidence of behaviour disturbance. This might be related to the brain dysfunction or to the drugs used to control the fits or to the social handicap epilepsy brings to the child in his relationships. Temporal lobe epilepsy is particularly associated with psychiatric disorder with a prevalence rate of 70 per cent.

Mental handicap

Mental handicap whether due to obvious brain injury or to an uncertain mix of genetic and early environmental factors may present primarily with behaviour difficulties. These disturbances may be more of a bur-den to the child, his parents and his teachers, than his basic learning problem. Whether, for example, aggressiveness, negativism, self-destruction or repetitive behaviour in retarded children is due to their abnormal brain function or a consequence of how they are handled in early life is an important question to be considered if appropriate management programmes are to be devised.

There is no doubt that parents of a mentally retarded child tend to have strong feelings of guilt and distress about the child. These strong feelings are unusually channelled towards either rejection or over-protection, and it is not unusual for parents to have a very low expectation of what their child can do. However, up until the point when the handicap is accepted, parents often have very high expectations that are quite unrealistic. These parental expectations that are either too high or too low in relation to the child's natural ability can easily lead to tension in the parent/child relationship, and subsequent emotional behavioural problems.

The prevalence of psychiatric disorder increases as the level of ability decreases. Children with an IQ below 50 are five times more likely to have an emotional or behavioural disorder than a child whose ability falls within the average range. Unlike most other psychiatric disorders in children, boys and girls are equally affected, suggesting that there is an aetiological factor that overrides the more usual childhood factors that make boys more vulnerable. Cerebral dysfunction is the most likely explanation for this.

There is no type of psychiatric disorder that is specifically associated with mental handicap. All disorders of emotion and behaviour are more frequent, but psychosis, hyperactivity, self-injury and stereotypes occur relatively more frequently than would be expected. When assessing a mentally retarded child, it is particularly important to bear in mind the developmental stage that the child has reached before deciding whether or not a psychiatric disorder is present. For example, it would be quite reasonable for a 12-year-old child who is developed mentally at a 2-year-old stage to have temper tantrums of the type that would be quite normal in a toddler.

Specific developmental delay

Children with mental handicap have a generalised delay in development and usually end up with reduced abilities in all areas, so-called global retardation. However the delay may be in one area only and with time, the child may learn to overcome the difficulty or to bypass it. Thus the child may have a functional delay in motor control, language, bladder and bowel control. As we all develop in different ways and at different rates, and end up with different levels of ability, each identified group contains children in the extremes of the normal range, children held back for a variety of reasons, as well as specific functional disorders.

All specific developmental delays occur three or four times more commonly in boys than in girls. They tend to occur in families and follow a normal developmental course, although more slowly than normal. The prognosis is therefore generally good, although it is likely that there will remain a disparity between the specific area of developmental delay and other fields. The relatively slow progress of the specifically delayed area of development can be speeded up using training techniques. So, for example, bladder training exercises will help enuresis and motor control exercises will help clumsy children.

Specific delays in development can lead to emotional and behavioural problems if a sense of failure is allowed to develop as a result of the special area of difficulty the child has. On the whole, young children are remarkably resilient and quickly bounce back from failure, but as self-concept develops, between the ages of 7 to 9 years, children become increasingly vulnerable to the experience of repeated failures which may then lead to the development of poor self-image, and its associated psychological problems.

Clumsiness or motor dyspraxia

Clumsiness in its severe form may result in a child being so uncoordinated that he has problems at home, at school and at play. Fine motor coordination problems result in untidy writing. Children with gross motor incoordination are delayed in learning to dress themselves and have difficulty with sports, particularly ball games, and they continually knock things over and frequently fall over themselves. The academic and social difficulties which follow can cause the child considerable unhappiness and lead to behavioural problems if they are not recognised and dealt with sympathetically. Specific training programmes to improve coordination may help.

Specific reading retardation

Reading is a complex activity which requires a great number of skills, and therefore reading difficulties might be due to a variety of factors. For example children with a general learning problem are slow to read, as are children who are understimulated or badly taught, and children who have a perceptual problem. But apart from those in whom a reading delay might be anticipated, there are many otherwise normal children who have specific reading retardation. Some experts consider that up to 8 per cent of school children have such a problem. As with other specific delays in development, boys are more often affected than girls and there is often a family history. Usually the children are a little slow to develop speech and characteristically they have even more difficulty with spelling than with reading so that, for them, dictation is a nightmare. They may also be delayed in developing handedness. There is an argument for screening all children at 7 years for specific reading retardation not only so that their reading exercises can be approached with insight and sympathy but also to ensure that their general education is not hampered by their limited reading ability. Dyslexia, specific learning difficulty and 'word blindness' have been names given to the most overt form of this problem.

Specific speech and language delay

Hearing, intellectual, or psychosocial impairment are more common factors leading to speech delay than a specific developmental disorder. Nevertheless there are a small group of children, around 2 per cent, of those with speech delay, who have normal intelligence and hearing and come from a happy, stimulating environment but who are unable to speak clearly. Speech difficulty, which is mostly due to motor co-ordination problems of the tongue and structural abnormalities of the mouth and palette, are distinguished from language difficulties. Children with specific language difficulties have the ability to pronounce words correctly, but they make the same mistakes of grammar and syntax that would be typical of a much younger child. It is possible to distinguish between receptive and expressive language disorders but they both present as delay in the acquisition of language. The most extreme form of specific language disorder is infantile autism. It is therefore not surprising that milder forms of specific language delay are associated with autistic like symptoms, such as habits and mannerisms, social difficulties and difficulty coping with change.

Sometimes children with specific language delay present later on in childhood with bizarre behaviour and abnormal social relationships and with a history of being delayed in learning to talk. It is only when their language is carefully analysed that abnormalities of sentence construction, and the use of words, can be identified. These children require a personal education programme aimed at increasing language and social skills.

Nocturnal enuresis

Involuntary emptying of the bladder during sleep is a common and troublesome problem. In round terms the majority of children are dry at night by 3 years of age, some 10 per cent plus regularly wet the bed at 5 years of age, and somewhat less than 5 per cent still do so at 10 years of age. One or two in every hundred will have an organic problem, either a congenital abnormality of the urinary tract, a urinary infection, polyuria or neurogenic bladder. A careful history, thorough examination and urine examination for glucose, infection and specific gravity should exclude these possibilities. Only rarely on the history of nocturnal enuresis alone is radiological investigation of the renal system justified. In another small percentage nocturnal enuresis will be the presenting symptom of a child emotionally upset. Gentle probing enquiry should bring this to light and point the interview in the appropriate direction.

In the majority, clinical enquiry gives no indication of the aetiology. Often there is a family history and there will be relatively more children from poor and unhappy homes than might be expected. It might be hard to refute the parents' suggestion that their child's bladder capacity is too small or that they pass excess amounts of urine during the night, and sleep more deeply than other children. However, there is no evidence to support these ideas. The most likely explanation is that enuresis is due to immature neuromuscular coordination of the bladder muscles and sphincters.

Many children improve, some surprisingly quickly, with whatever method of management is used, whether it be habit training with star charts, lifting at night, drugs or a pad and bell. Suggestion and encouragement are perhaps the most helpful. A distinction is sometimes made between primary and secondary enuresis where primary enuresis is lifelong, and secondary enuresis starts after a period of being dry. Unfortunately this distinction is not a very helpful one since both types of enuresis share the same characteristics and respond in the same way to treatment. The notion that enuresis is a sign of emotional distress is also inaccurate. Treatments for emotional disturbance are remarkably ineffective with enuresis. There is some evidence that enuresis causes an increasing amount of emotional distress as children become older. In this situation the symptomatic treatment of enuresis results in a remarkable improvement in the child's mental state. There is some evidence, however, that children who have experienced social adversity during the first 5 years of life are more likely to suffer from enuresis. The most likely explanation for this is that normal toilet training has been interrupted.

Although the majority of children will eventually become dry, the spontaneous remission rate becomes progressively less as children grow older. At the same time, the secondary, emotional and social consequences of enuresis become more serious. Children who continue to wet over the age of eight years old are at risk of developing a sense of failure and low self esteem. At the same time, they are likely to remain rather immature because it is difficult to feel grown up while at the same time wetting the bed, or the pants. The greatest claim has been made for the bell alarm which is placed in the child's bed so that the alarm rings when the child wets. It is said to help over two-thirds of those who can be brought to use them. Drugs have limited use for enuresis. They may be useful for symptom relief in the short term for example when staying overnight with a friend. Desmopressin has an 80 per cent success rate, but the relapse rate is quite high.

Faecal soiling

Most children are clean by 2 years of age and soiling may be viewed as abnormal after 4 years of age and certainly by the time the child goes to school. Whatever the reason for soiling, as with enuresis, most forms of soiling are more common in boys, and can be seen as a developmental immaturity. Inadequate or disruptive training, or irregular bowel habit, are predisposing factors, as is constipation. One of the main problems with soiling is that it elicits strong negative reactions from those around the child, especially at school, and it doesn't take long for children who soil to become emotionally distressed, purely as a result of the soiling and its consequences. At the same time children who are emotionally stressed are more likely to have difficulties with bowel control, and it is easy to see how a vicious circle soon develops.

The term 'encopresis' is used to describe the passage of formed faeces in unacceptable places. This may be in the pants, but it can also be behind the settee, in a drawer, or indeed anywhere except in the toilet. Occasionally this behaviour is directly linked to a stressful event, and it is clearly meant to be a provocative act. This type of severe encopresis may be difficult to resolve, and expert psychiatric advice is required.

Children who are chronically constipated may develop overflow incontinence and they soil continuously without passing a formed stool. Dealing with the constipation always leads to resolution of the soiling.

The secondary repercussions of soiling are so serious for a child that it is important to deal with the problem actively, rather than waiting and hoping that the child will eventually grow out of it. There are three aspects of treatment:

Toilet training. This involves regular toileting at intervals that are frequent enough to keep the child clean. On each occasion the child is expected to sit on the toilet for about 3 minutes. If a motion is passed, great pleasure and appreciation is shown to the child. It is helpful to keep a record of the child's progress, and it may also be helpful to use a star chart, or some other reward system, for success.

An appropriate diet with adequate amounts of high fibre foods and other foodstuffs that promote bowel action.

The bowel should be kept as empty as possible. Most children who soil, only partially evacuate the contents of the bowel. If regular toileting has not been effective, then regular laxatives, and in more severe cases enemas, may be necessary. It is important to continue an active treatment regime for 3 to 6 months after the child has become clean, otherwise a relapse is likely.

If a child fails to respond to the above regime, the most likely explanation is that it has not been carried out to the letter. However, in a minority of cases, the lack of response to treatment may be because the child is seriously emotionally disturbed, and the causes for this should be sought and dealt with. In the majority of children, once the soiling has stopped, they start to flourish and mature rapidly.

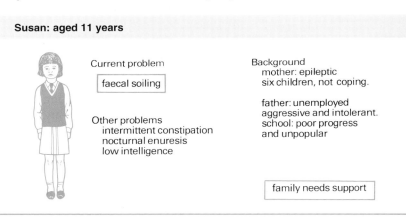

Susan: aged 11 years

Current problem

faecal soiling

Other problems
intermittent constipation
nocturnal enuresis
low intelligence

Background
mother: epileptic
six children, not coping.

father: unemployed
aggressive and intolerant.
school: poor progress
and unpopular

family needs support

Tics

Tics are sudden repetitive coordinated movements of no apparent purpose. They can effect any muscle groups but commonly take the form of blinking, facial grimacing, twisting the head, or shrugging the shoulders. The average age of onset is 2 years and it has been reported that as many as 4 per cent of children develop marked tics at some time and an even larger number develop mild tics especially between the ages of 5 and 8. Tourette described a bizarre syndrome where vocal tics, often rude words, accompany gestures which might be equally embarrassing and may require treatment with a SHT antagonist. In 25 per cent of children with tics there is a family history. In some there is evidence of brain damage or other features of delayed maturation. Tics are more common in boys and are associated with hyperactivity. Usually the tics disappear spontaneously, sometimes in weeks or months, often in late adolescence, and rarely do they persist into adult life. Tics are made worse by stress and they are also worse when a child is excited or relaxed. Anything that draws attention to the tics will make them worse.

Hyperkinetic syndrome

In children with the hyperkinetic syndrome there may be a family history, evidence of a developmental delay or a history which suggests that the child might have had 'minimal brain dysfunction'. In some there is little evidence to suggest any of these alternatives and it is clear that the overactive child has never been given limits for their behaviour or taught to have self control.

Hyperactive children are restless and distractable, they are destructive, impulsive and excitable. It is when they first go to school that they appear to be at their most difficult and it may be then that their problem first comes to light. Pre-school children are naturally active with a short attention span and parents may mistake this normal stage of development for hyperactivity.

In adolescence, though the hyperactivity is less, their learning difficulties with socially disruptive behaviour may lead to further problems and the link between hyperactivity and conduct disorder is a close one. As adults they are more likely to have trouble with the law or need psychiatric help.

Management starts with a careful evaluation of the child's problems and continues by full discussions with parents, teachers and anyone else concerned. Each programme is individual and involves teaching self control and having a regular routine to daily life. Brain stimulants, methylphenidate and other amphetamine related drugs may benefit some affected children, especially where there is evidence of brain dysfunction. Hyperactivity is sometimes reduced by excluding certain foods from the diet but carries a risk of nutritional deficiencies.

Autism and childhood psychosis

Schizophrenia can begin in late childhood, the symptoms are similar to those found in adults. Adults who develop schizophrenia have often shown unusual behaviour when they were youngsters, but the pattern is not characteristic and so prediction and maybe prevention is not yet possible. Bizarre or psychotic behaviour is also seen in encephalopathies and in the severely retarded. About half the children with psychosis have a cluster of clinical features which suggest a specific disorder, infantile autism.

Characteristically, autistic children fail to develop social relationships, they are slow to speak and have little non-verbal communication. They also follow ritualistic behaviour patterns and endlessly perform repetitive movements. Parents seek advice because they wonder if the child is deaf and again later because of delay or absence of speech development. Often the infant's behaviour has been unusual from birth and only occasionally is the child's development for the first year or so apparently normal. There is a strong genetic component to autism, and the organic nature of the disorder is highlighted by the fact that some 40 per cent of autistic children develop epilepsy during adolescence.

Autism is more common in boys, and it seems likely that it is at the extreme end of a continuum of specific language disorders that include Asperger syndrome and developmental dysphasia. Most autistic children are mentally retarded. Those with an IQ below 70 have the worst prognosis. Even those with average intelligence have great difficulty coping when they grow up. Only a few manage to be gainfully employed and they rarely marry.

The essential abnormality in autism is a severe deficit in language ability that effects all aspects of communication and imagination. To be an autistic child is rather like living in a foreign country where not only is the language difficult to understand but gestures and sign language are incomprehensible as well. Management involves intensive training of communication skills, and providing as much routine and regularity in every day life as possible. One of the most difficult problems autistic children have to face is that they look normal, and as they grow older they may achieve reasonable language competence, but they are rarely able to master abstract concepts and the subtleties of relationships. This makes them unusually vulnerable and frequently misunderstood.

Autism is rare: in a population of one million some 20 to 40 children might be identified. They need to be under the care of experts in special schools but because of its rarity it is difficult to provide this for all children whilst maintaining strong home links. Drugs currently play only a small part in management; they may help if there is an associated sleep problem.

THE INTERACTION BETWEEN THE CHILD AND HIS WORLD

A child may develop symptoms of physical disorder or behaviour problems or educational difficulties due to conflicts and confusion within himself, or with his family, with his peers, with school or with society at large. If a schoolgirl gets stomach-ache because she hates her ballet lessons or dislikes her new step-father, then eliciting that information may be just as important for that child as testing the urine in another suspected of having urinary infection. This section merely points to some of the more obvious factors which might lead to problems.

The child

Acute organic disease. Acute organic disease frightens children possibly more than adults, and they show it in different ways according to their maturity. It can be difficult to distinguish the symptoms and signs due to this reaction from those due to the underlying pathology. A terrified 2-year-old with croup may improve dramatically in the arms of a friendly, confident, capable nurse or become even worse if placed on a strange bed surrounded by flashing lights and stainless steel.

Chronic organic disease. Chronic organic disease makes extra demands on the child. The majority of children cope marvellously well but in others the continuing difficulties are just too much and secondary symptoms or behaviour problems add to their difficulties. The burden of the disease for some children can be very heavy; what, for example, can be said to an adolescent with muscular dystrophy or cystic fibrosis when he learns by one means or another of the prognosis of his condition? Sometimes it is the parents who cannot accept or have difficulty managing the child's condition. It is always sad when a child with asthma exaggerates his bronchospasm, or a child with diabetes deliberately breaks diet to precipitate hyperglycaemia, in order to gain admission to hospital where they feel more secure, and where the pressures of coping either with the family or the outside world are avoided.

Deformity and disability. Deformity and disability present at birth may lead to problems if one or both parents have difficulty accepting their own abnormal child; they feel ashamed about him when they should be showing him off. Later as the child grows up he may have trouble at school, for children go through a period of wanting to be the same and of mocking those who are different. Just being different can lead to problems.

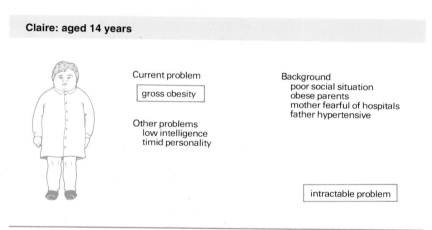

Claire: aged 14 years

Current problem

gross obesity

Other problems
low intelligence
timid personality

Background
poor social situation
obese parents
mother fearful of hospitals
father hypertensive

intractable problem

Intelligence. Intelligence is determined by a mixture of genetic and environmental factors. Happily, in the main, parents have children of similar abilities but misfits occasionally occur, a slow child in an academic family, an awkward child in an athletic family, a gifted child in an average family, a swan amongst ducks. All may lead to conflict and result in bodily symptoms, behaviour disturbances and underachieving. In general, there is an inverse relationship between intelligence and psychiatric disorder. Children with severe learning difficulties have 4–5 times the risk of developing emotional or behavioural problems.

Temperament. Temperament likewise appears to be genetically and environmentally determined. A child's temperament is not only a factor in the risk of disorders developing but may also determine the mode of expression. An outgoing, extrovert child is more likely to develop behaviour problems, while a sensitive, timid child is more likely to internalise conflicts and have disorders of bodily function. The success of any management programme depends on those concerned knowing the child for whom they are making plans. Children with a difficult temperament can be recognised at birth and the combination of strong negative moods, irregular functioning and poor adaptability is associated with an increased risk of behaviour disorder.

The family

A great deal has been written recently about the qualities required of parents. A child needs not only food, warmth and physical protection but also to be loved, to feel important, to be stimulated and encouraged to make the most of his abilities, and to be controlled and guided in the ways of his society. It is the privilege and responsibility of parents to meet these needs and most parents delight in the task. Many factors, some beyond anyone's control, can interfere with the relationship between parents and child. Of course the child is constantly changing and developing and a special task for parents is to modify their management as the child matures.

Maternal deprivation. The bond between *the mother and her child* starts as soon as she knows that she is pregnant. Important stages in the attachment process occur when she first feels the child move and then later at the moment of birth, and the first few weeks after that. The 'bonding' of a *child to the mother* is also a gradual process. Although a child is able to distinguish between some characteristics of his or her own mother and those of other mothers, clear evidence of bonding only becomes apparent when a child is around 5 to 8 months. It is at this stage that stranger anxiety and separation anxiety are first seen; they are part of normal development. The bonding of the child to the mother continues to strengthen over the next few years, and is generally secure by the age of 5 or 6 years. Children who are separated from their mother before the age of 5 to 8 months usually show symptoms that are much less marked than later on, and they adapt remarkably well to alternative parenting. Fathers also become attached to their children, but not only is this a more gradual process, it is also very variable and depends upon the degree of involvement that the father has with the child. Young children who are separated from their

Some reactions a toddler might show on admission to hospital

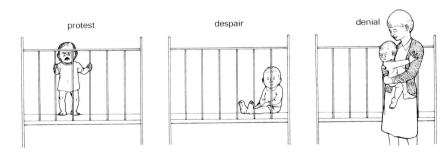

protest   despair   denial

parents, characteristically show three stages of reaction. These are:

1. Protest, screaming and extreme distress
2. Restless searching and frequent crying
3. Withdrawal and despair

For most families brief periods of separation are not as harmful in the long term as was originally thought but in the context of hostile and rejecting family relationships they can be. If either the mother or her dependent infant needs hospital care, they should be admitted together if it is at all possible. One is often important in the other's recovery.

Family breakdown. Unhappily for children in western societies divorce rates are increasing. At least 1 in 5 children will experience the separation of their parents before they reach 16 years of age. Couples seeking divorce are tending to be younger and the duration of their marriages is shorter. Illegitimacy rates are also increasing, and good alternatives for child care have not become available at the same rate as the increase in working mothers. Such situations add to the child's problems and may limit the care he receives. In the year following family breakdown about 80 per cent of children show some significant disturbance and it continues to be higher than normal over the next few years. Boys are more likely to become disturbed than girls.

Parental abilities and attitudes. If a parent is sick, what of the child? If a child has stomach ache it is well to ask about the family symptoms. Children are quick to note how adults gain sympathy and avoid the unpleasant, and they assume that there is no reason why they should not use the same tactics. A parent with a chronic illness may add to the child's anxieties and responsibilities and push the child beyond his limit. A parent with a psychiatric disorder, for example, depression, may have a devastating effect on the child. Sometimes it is the child's illness which draws attention to the mother's need. The effect that the

John: aged 8 years

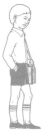

Current problem

stole money from school
and home to buy sweets

Other problems
  high IQ
  reading retardation

Background
  unmarried mother who
  despised and did not
  mention his father.
  Catholic school taught
  the sanctity of marriage

he wanted to be told about his father

death of a parent has on a child varies with his maturity. It is not until 6–8 years old that children develop a reasonably clear concept of death. A disturbed child may be considerably helped by having the opportunity to talk frankly about it with a sympathetic but uninvolved adult. Unclear limit setting and unpredictability are especially linked with an increased risk of disturbed behaviour.

Even when both parents are well and able to provide a comfortable home, their attitudes and expectations of their children can still lead to difficulties. In the extremes they may over-protect them or over-discipline them or ignore and reject them or they may wish to dominate them, even when they are capable of being independent. On the other hand, they may have unrealistic expectations of their abilities; for example, a mother who expected a 6-month-old infant to use a pot, a father who expected his children to move at the blow of a whistle, a professional woman who thought her 7-year-old should realise when she wished to be left alone.

Adoption. The situation of a couple longing for children that they cannot have and adopting into their family an unwanted child has its own peculiar problems. Inevitably the child has those characteristics, appearance, abilities and personality, determined by his genetic make-up from his parents but also he is influenced by the environment provided by his new home. Since adoptive parents are usually specially selected as being capable, adopted children usually do better than they would have done in their natural family. The rate of emotional–behavioural problems in adopted children differs very little from the general population.

Children in care. It has been said that bad parents are better than no parents. This is not true. However, in the absence of a larger family to embrace a child who loses both parents, the best efforts of the social services often fall well short of the child's needs. It is easy to be pessimistic about the long-term prognosis of such children. However, many children build happy and successful lives out of appalling childhoods. One important factor to determine outcome is a continuing stable and caring relationship.

Environment

Deprivation. Ineffectual parents tend to be poor and to live in bad housing in deprived sections of the towns or country. It is difficult to be sure of the extent that a child's problems are due to his make-up, the care and attitudes of his parents or to his physical surroundings. But there is no doubt that poverty, overcrowding and poor housing, are associated not only with increased rates of illness and death in infancy and childhood but also behaviour problems and school failure. It is so difficult for children from such backgrounds to become good parents themselves. The poor are at a threefold disadvantage; they are more likely to fall ill, they have less family reserves to meet new problems and they are less able to make use of the support the state provides. Even in the UK with a National Health Service, the deprived are still at a disadvantage in comparison with the middle classes and almost a million children are being brought up in poverty.

Neighbourhood. Wealth is relative, and poverty as defined in western societies need not bring misery. It has been shown that the prevalence of health and social problems varies considerably from one community to another with apparently similar levels of wealth, housing, and services. In some communities there is stability and mutual responsibility, in others there is aggression, cruelty and conflict. Race, culture, religion, industrial troubles can all lead to a family being rejected by the neighbourhood. Families continually on the move may create problems of insecurity for their children.

School. School is where children go to work, where they make friends and enemies, where they test out their personality against others, where they find out how other families think and behave. So problems at school may be far more than difficulties with learning. A child who has difficulty with his school such that special education is considered necessary, should have a thorough and expert medical assessment so that the handicap due to a medical condition is reduced to a minimum.

Schools vary quite significantly in the rate of behaviour problems shown by their pupils over and above that which can be explained by social factors. In other words, some schools have a positive effect on children, whereas others make it more likely that children will be disruptive and difficult. Schools with high staff morale, low teacher turnover, good organisation, clear methods of discipline, and a detailed knowledge of children as individuals, tend to have a low rate of antisocial behaviour.

BEHAVIOURAL PROBLEMS

From what has been said so far it can be appreciated that many factors may contribute to the genesis of any particular problem which brings a child to the doctor's attention. The physician is particularly concerned with symptoms which suggest physical disease but have their origins in a psychological disturbance, and with behavioural problems which are a consequence of a physical disorder, either as a direct effect of brain disturbance or indirectly due to the difficulty the child has coping with his illness or handicap.

The preschool child

Feeding problems. Interaction between an uncertain or insecure mother with a healthy baby, or a happy mother with a determined or difficult baby may lead to the baby vomiting, refusing food or failing to gain weight satisfactorily. Sometimes the problem is resolved by patience and counselling either from the health visitor, relative or friendly neighbour but it is not uncommon for a child to have to be admitted to hospital to exclude an organic cause and to reassure both mother and her baby. Battles over food are always best avoided. Anxiety reduction for all concerned is the most effective approach, relying on the child's natural thirst and hunger drive to take enough food.

Sleep problems. Adults used to a regular biological rhythm differ in their tolerance of the baby's desire for a feed in the middle of the night. Occasionally infants appear to scream and cry through most of the night and this may be tolerated when the baby is young and weak but a playful demanding toddler in the middle of the night can stretch the patience of most parents. A regular pattern of sleep/waking is usually established by 7 months. But if not, the temptation for the parents is to take the child in their bed or for one or other parent to sleep with the child to comfort him but this is really no solution and can lead to further problems. Adults without sleep perform poorly in their work and this adds to the strain. In this situation there is an argument for establishing a regular bedtime routine and not responding to a child's crying. This approach is usually rapidly effective, but can only be carried out if the child is obviously well and not in pain, and the parents are sure that their child is safe in the bedroom or in the cot. Night sedation is best avoided, it should only be used as a last resort.

Breath-holding attacks. Infants and toddlers quickly find that they can control their parents by refusing to do what they are asked. For example, they may refuse to eat or to go the toilet, but perhaps their most dramatic card to play is to refuse to breathe. Breath holding attacks to the point of going unconscious, when they may or may not provoke a fit, are not uncommon. They certainly terrify the parents and may reduce them to quivering slaves. From the medical point of view it is important to distinguish the episodes from convulsions due to other causes and to reassure parents about the nature of the attacks. In the vast majority of cases the children come to no harm and parents should be encouraged to take no action during the episode. These determined, often stubborn youngsters need to be handled firmly and consistently.

Jason: aged 1 year 6 months

Current problem
head-banging

Other problems
febrile convulsions
advanced development

Background
cried a lot as baby
mother very tense
parents not married
—both divorced!

an extreme of normal behaviour

Rhythmic behaviour. Head rocking, head banging, thumb sucking, self stimulation, baby behaviour, and many other variants may all occur during normal development. They are more likely to appear when the child is bored, anxious or tired. In the very disturbed, autistic or retarded child they can become bad habits and strategies need to be devised to avoid or suppress them by diverting, disrupting or preventing the behaviour.

Delayed development and regression. Understimulation with or without undernutrition may limit a child's development and growth. It is not surprising perhaps that a child left alone for hours with no toys in a high rise flat is quite withdrawn, apathetic, and has little muscle tone or strength, and delayed motor, social and mental development. Physical illness or emotional stress frequently causes regression with the loss of the more recently acquired skills and a return to a more immature stage of development.

Bowel and bladder control. Again inappropriate training or anxiety and conflict will interfere with the development of bodily control and appropriate social habits. Nocturnal enuresis which in the main is probably due to a disorder in maturation and encopresis has been discussed in the first part of this chapter.

School children

Recurrent abdominal pain. One of the common symptoms which bring children to clinic is recurrent pains usually in the abdomen or head, occasionally in the limbs. A few will have organic disease and so all require a careful clinical evaluation. In others it may be a cry for help, the child having a psychiatric disorder or a terrible domestic situation. But for the majority, the clinical investigations will be negative and there will be no major psychosocial problems. There may have been mild or moderate disturbances in the child's life, and the symptoms become a way of communicating distress. Finding words to express emotional problems is difficult for children and most parents respond more quickly to physical symptoms than to emotional reactions in their children.

Jane: aged 8 years

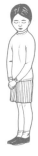

Current problem

| recurrent abdominal pain |

Other problems
none

Background
quiet, sensitive shy child
mother had migraine
father travelling salesman
away from home.
brother—big and extrovert

| sibling rivalry |

A thorough examination and reassurance with explanations will help many. However in those referred to hospital, a good percentage continue to have recurrent pains into adolescence and adult life. Headaches rather than abdominal pains tend to persist, especially if there is a positive family history.

Periodic syndrome. This describes a condition when attacks of abdominal pain are associated with severe vomiting. The vomiting can sometimes result in dehydration to a degree that requires correction by intravenous therapy. In this situation it is difficult to believe that the child has not got an organic disease but so far no pathology has been identified. However in its milder form it merges with the clinical entity of 'recurrent abdominal pain'.

School refusal and truancy. Illness is the commonest reason for school absence. Sometimes children are kept away from school by their parents to help in the home. It is important to distinguish these two categories from those children who refuse to go to school because they are anxious, frightened or depressed, and from those children who play truant from school because they dislike the atmosphere in which they appear to fail and are subject to ridicule and as they see it, to unfair discipline.

The distinction between school refusal on the one hand, and truancy on the other, is characteristic of the contrast between neurotic disorders and conduct disorders.

School refusal is a neurotic/emotional disorder and is associated with:	Truancy is a conduct/antisocial disorder and is associated with:
School phobia, depression and separation anxiety	Disruptive and aggressive behaviour
Equal frequency in boys and girls	Higher frequency in boys
Stable family background	Disrupted family background
Good progress at school	Academic failure
Close, overinvolved family	Lack of supervision at home
Emotional distress in the family	Social deprivation

The main distinction between school refusal and truancy is that in the former, everyone knows where the child is, but in the latter the child disappears during school hours but may turn up at home after school as if it were just another ordinary school day. It can sometimes be helpful to distinguish between school phobia and separation anxiety. In separation anxiety there is characteristically a long history of separation problems, the problems of going to school are at their worst on leaving home. On the other hand, school phobia is often triggered by a distressing event at school and the symptoms become progressively worse as the child approaches the school.

Truancy is rare in primary school and if it does occur it usually has a very poor prognosis. However, truancy becomes increasingly frequent in secondary school and reaches a peak in the last year of schooling. The majority of children truant at one time or another.

Conduct disorders. Often parents are concerned because their young children are unacceptably aggressive, destructive, cruel or antisocial. Again individual tolerance will depend on the family and the community. In some lively teenagers, outbursts of aggressive, destructive, foolish or antisocial behaviour may be dismissed as high spirits but in others living in inner city areas with mixed cultures and limited outlets it results in delinquency.

It is now clear that as children grow older, persistent aggressive or antisocial behaviour has an increasingly poor prognosis. In fact the continuity of aggression after the age of 5 is almost as strong as it is for intelligence. Aggressive children are significantly more likely to grow up into adults who have a poor employment record, are convicted criminals and form unsatisfactory relationships. It is therefore unwise to expect persistently aggressive and antisocial children to grow out of it.

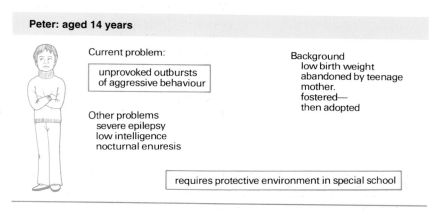

Peter: aged 14 years

Current problem:

> unprovoked outbursts
> of aggressive behaviour

Other problems
  severe epilepsy
  low intelligence
  nocturnal enuresis

Background
  low birth weight
  abandoned by teenage
  mother.
  fostered—
  then adopted

> requires protective environment in special school

EMOTIONAL DISORDERS

Children, like adults can get unduly anxious; they may suffer from unreasonable fears and they can have outbursts of hysterical behaviour. By nature, children are optimistic and confident about the future, but occasionally even without obvious cause they can become severely depressed and seriously attempt suicide. These children should have the counsel of a child psychiatrist.

Anxiety states

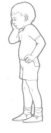

Children frequently experience worries and fears in much the same way that adults do, and there is a similar variation in the way that some are much more reactive and sensitive to fearful situations than others. Normal fears do not interfere with the child's everyday life, and usually fade away after a few weeks. On the other hand, pathological anxiety is disruptive to the child's life to the point where family functioning may also be affected. It is often helpful to see anxiety as being 'infectious', in that it is very easy to pick it up from other people. It is therefore helpful to consider 'where does the anxiety come from, who does it belong to'. The source of the problem has to be dealt with.

Fears at different ages

Strangers	0.5 – 3 years
Animals	2 – 4 years
Darkness, storms, imaginary monsters	4 – 6 years
Mysterious happenings	6 –12 years
Social embarrassment, academic failure, death and wars	12 –18 years

Anorexia nervosa

In this odd condition, young people either just before or during puberty, deliberately avoid food so that they lose weight, and they often go on losing weight till they become tragically thin. It is thought that they have an irrational fear of growing up, of becoming sexually and physically mature. Usually they are able youngsters if somewhat obsessional and precise. Rarely are there major psychological problems which need attention.

As they can starve themselves to death, some management must be attempted but as no pathology or avoidable environmental factors are usually identified, it has to be symptomatic. It sounds somewhat crude, but the most effective approach appears to be to remove all the child's privileges and return them one by one as she begins to eat more and more. Antidepressive drugs may help.

Alison: aged 12 years

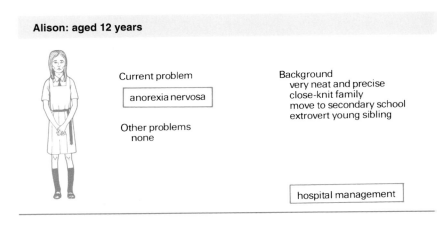

Current problem

anorexia nervosa

Other problems
none

Background
very neat and precise
close-knit family
move to secondary school
extrovert young sibling

hospital management

Depression

Babies cry a great deal, but this does not mean that they are depressed. Indeed, crying in very young children can have a wide range of meanings, including ' I am hungry', 'I am in pain', 'my nappy needs changing' and 'I am just bored and fed up'. The term 'depression' can be used as a general description for everyday distress and unhappiness. When it is used in the technical sense, there is in addition to feelings of misery, thoughts of hopelessness about the future and feelings of worthlessness about oneself. Thus, in order to be depressed, a child must have developed to the stage where there is a clear concept of time in order to understand hopelessness for the future, and a clear concept of the self in order to feel worthless. Both of these abilities become reasonably well established between the ages of 7 to 9, and it is not until this stage that children are developmentally able to experience a depressive disorder. Even then, it is rare and requires a high level of stress. Additional symptoms of depression include poor concentration, deterioration of school work and some or all of the symptoms of emotional distress, such as alterations to appetite and sleep patterns, psychosomatic aches and pains and other symptoms of physiological disturbance.

The development of a depressive disorder during childhood has a very serious significance. This is partly because a child must be subjected to high levels of stress, but also because relationships and progress at school are often adversely affected. The child becomes stuck in a vicious circle. Recent research indicates that the long term prognosis for depressed children is very poor.

Phobias and obsessions

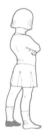

The link between phobias and obsessions is quite a strong one. For example, obsessional cleanliness could be described as dirt phobia, or dog phobia could be described as an obsessional avoidance of dogs. Both conditions are classified as neurotic disorders and occur with equal frequency in boys and girls.

Phobias. A phobia is an overwhelming but unrealistic fear which is accompanied by avoidance behaviour. Mild phobic reactions occur quite commonly in young children, reaching a peak between 5 and 7 years of age. The prognosis for single phobias is good, but if they are multiple or complex, the phobic reactions tend to continue, with one being replaced by another.

Obsessions. An obsession is an irresistible urge to repeat a thought or action. The term 'compulsion' is used to describe an obsessional behaviour or ritual. Overall the condition is known as 'obsessional compulsive disorder' (OCD). It is classified as a neurotic condition and occurs with equal frequency in boys and girls. Children between the ages of 4 and 7 commonly go through a phase of ritualistic behaviour, where they insist that something is done in exactly the same way on each occasion. Where obsessions are complex, they have a tendency to persist, even into adult life.

MANAGEMENT

The above paragraphs merely list some of the symptoms and problems which children under medical care may have. Management includes recognising them for what they are, identifying the contributing factors and conferring with the other people concerned. The latter may include the family doctor and other members of the primary care team, the health visitor, the school teacher, school health services and school welfare officers, the educational psychologist and social service workers. When, after review, a programme of care has been agreed, it is essential that a person is identified to be responsible for counselling the child and parents, and ensuring that all concerned are properly informed. Being thorough at the outset can avoid many problems later. With the more intractable emotional and conduct disorders a child psychiatrist will be the key person, but the majority will fall within the responsibility of the health visitor or the family doctor or the paediatrician.

Perhaps the most important factor in determining a successful outcome in the management of children with emotional–behavioural problems, is to achieve an agreed understanding and approach to the problem. It is particularly important to gain cooperation and agreement between all adults who have direct care of a child. This will usually involve a considerable amount of time spent in delicate negotiations. However, agreement and understanding are not sufficient in themselves. One of the most common reasons for treatment plans being ineffective is that they are not carried through. The role of the key person should be to make frequent checks to ensure that the agreed treatment approach is in fact being carried out, and to arrange further discussion with those involved if no progress has been made. The detailed treatment programmes

---

Guidelines for management

* A child's emotional–behavioural problems may be the symptom of disturbance elsewhere, for example in the family or in the school, in which case treatment needs to be directed, not at the child, but at the source of the problem.

* The younger the child the more likely it is that the source of the problem is outside the child. Treatment approaches for young children should therefore be directed at changing a child's family and environment.

* As children approach adolescence it is important to consider individual treatment needs and the child's inner world.

* Behaviour problems respond best to clear limit setting, high levels of supervision, and training in appropriate behaviour.

* Developmental problems, such as soiling, wetting and specific language problems, require intensive training programmes aimed at increasing competence and confidence in the skill that is delayed.

* Anxieties and phobias are best tackled by finding ways in which the child can be helped to face up to them. This can either be done very gradually, or by going in at the deep end. This latter approach is often rapidly effective, but it is important to have the agreement of all those concerned if this approach is going to be used.

* Miserable and depressed children are unlikely to respond to treatment unless the cause has been identified and dealt with.

* Medication has a very limited role to play in the treatment of childhood behaviour and emotional problems, and should only be prescribed by those who have specialised knowledge of this area.

* Children easily become stuck in a vicious circle that maintains the psychiatric disorder. Treatment can be directed at any part of this circle and still be effective, even if it is not directed at the problem itself. For example, a child with academic failure, leading to school phobia, may be helped merely by treatment directed at boosting self image.

* It is never acceptable to wait for a child to grow out of a problem, even though behavioural and emotional problems eventually resolve spontaneously. Children easily become stuck in particular patterns of behaviour and develop characteristic emotional reactions. If these are maladaptive, a range of adverse consequences quickly follows, such as rejection, scapegoating and hostility, which will leave the child psychologically damaged, even though the problem may have been resolved.

that are currently available are beyond the scope of this book, but there are some general guidelines which should be considered in each case.

THE MALTREATMENT OF CHILDREN

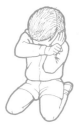

Deviant behaviour by adults may take the form of injuring their children. Child murder, child cruelty, child neglect, child abuse, child molesting and the use of children for pornography all fall into this category. The obvious examples are easily recognised, but defining the limits of child abuse or child neglect is difficult. It might be considered that it is the right of every child to be allowed to develop to his full potential. Child abuse could then be defined as any action or omission by an adult responsible for that child which either temporarily or permanently interferes with that development. In a real world we must settle for something less. What we are able to achieve is a good measure of our success as a society. In this section we will not be concerned with mental or social abuse or educational ineptitude, not because these are unimportant, but because they are not primarily medical problems. Similarly child cruelty and murder will not be considered further.

Child physical abuse

Clinical features. Non-accidental injuries (NAI) and other forms of child abuse occur when parents, at their wits end, strike out at their helpless but demanding infant. It also happens when ignorant, inept, cruel, selfish, irresponsible or mentally sick parents do not exert reasonable self-control. Gripping and shaking the baby may produce finger tip bruising on his chest and arms. Forcing his mouth open to give food may cause similar bruises on the cheeks. The frenulum may be torn or the palate

Gripping injuries

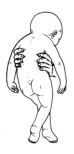 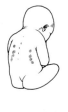 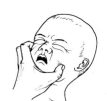

scratched by objects pushed in the mouth. Slapping and hitting the infant may also cause black eyes or characteristic strap marks. The skin of the attacked infant may also show scratches, bite marks, cigarette burns of scalds. Rough handling may fracture long bones, ribs or skull. Swinging the baby by the legs or arms can cause epiphyseal separation at the end of the long bones. Squeezing the limbs with rotation can separate the periosteum and cause periosteal haematomas. Repeated injuries of the same bone leads to large callus formation. Banging the head not only produces fractures of the skull but haemorrhages in the eyes and occasionally blindness.

Other non-accidental injuries

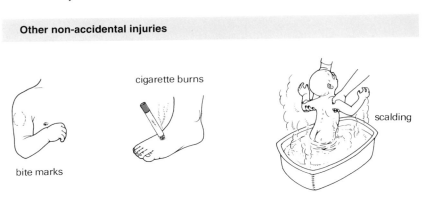

Shaking the head can tear superficial veins over the brain and cause subdural haematomas. The child may weather the initial injury, but the blood clot may then draw in fluid; the infant then develops the clinical features of a space occupying lesion of slow onset. He may present with vomiting or fits or changes in the level of responsiveness and activity. The fontanelle is full and there may be papilloedema and retinal bleeds. This injury may kill the child; if it does not, it often leaves him mentally retarded, hemiplegic or blind.

Bony injuries

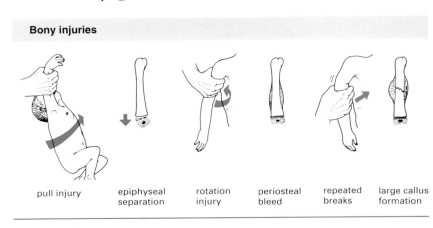

All the baby's injuries must be noted in detail and photographed if possible.

A careful enquiry is essential. The parents often delay in bringing the child for medical attention. Their story does not accord with the injuries. Their explanation for the injuries may change if they are pressed. Their concern for the child may be inappropriate, they may show too much concern or anger or they may be off-hand and indifferent. Often they are relieved when hospital admission is advised. Sometimes they will talk at length about their own anxieties and problems and say how difficult and demanding the baby has been. It is very important to record precisely the history as it is given, with an evaluation of the parents' attitudes.

The injury that can kill or leave a child with brain damage

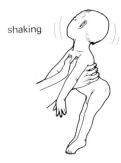

shaking

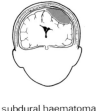

subdural haematoma

Slow onset

enlarging head

full fontanelle

vomiting

drowsiness

fits

Child abuse occurs in families from all walks of life but it is more common in the under-privileged and in families where actions speak louder than words. As Professor Kempe has suggested, the setting in which child abuse might occur includes a number of elements:

1. The parents have usually had troubled childhoods themselves; they may be from broken homes or have suffered deprivation or abuse themselves when children.

2. There are problems with the marriage; for example the marriage may be between two young people from disturbed homes who married for the wrong reasons, perhaps because they wanted to leave home or were in need of affection. Some people mistakenly believe that a pregnancy will help to reverse a breaking relationship.

3. The child may be difficult to rear, he may have been premature or have a blemish or handicap. More often than not the child's problems are imaginary, the baby's first cry is seen as rejection, he fails to respond as his mother feels he should to her and this is felt to be his fault. An unloved child may be difficult, a difficult child may be unloved.

4. Against this background there may be added stresses, for example the father in trouble with the law or there may be financial or housing problems.

5. Finally, there are no life lines available, no close friends to whom the parents can turn for advice, support and relief.

Management. If a health visitor, social worker or casualty doctor suspects non-accidental injury the child must be admitted to a place of safety until a fuller enquiry has been made. This might be a police station, a social service institution or a hospital. If his parents are deliberately injuring him, society has a responsibility to protect him. If the parents are unwilling to release their child then he may have to be taken from them on the grounds laid down to obtain the necessary care order.

Whilst providing temporary protection, the primary medical responsibility is to identify and treat the injuries, attend to the child's general well being, and to exclude possible contributing factors and alternative diagnoses. It is equally important for others to evaluate the parents and the family situation and provide support and guidance if this is appropriate.

The distribution of the bruises is usually diagnostic. Babies when they begin to walk frequently fall and bruise their foreheads and shins but do not bruise their upper arms and chests. Nevertheless bleeding diseases should be excluded. Brittle-bone disease is a rare condition where bruising as well as bone fractures occur with the slightest injury but the fractures are in the shaft and not at the end of the long bones. Although some bony injuries are obvious, others are not, so a full skeletal survey by radiography is essential.

The social work team will usually take the lead in planning the strategy for management, but they depend on the full cooperation of medical and nursing personnel involved and the police. Initial policy is usually worked out at a case conference held as soon as possible after the diagnosis is firm. Subsequent management will depend on the background and on the attitudes of the parents. When investigations have been completed a full case conference with representatives from all agencies concerned in attendance is held to decide what legal action is required, what social work activity is to be attempted and what medical surveillance is desirable.

Many children may be allowed home, initially under supervision and although they may not live happily ever after they do appear to thrive and to be content. Occasionally it is necessary to take the child away from his parents and put him into care of others. The decisions are very difficult and even those with most knowledge and experience can get it wrong. Unhappy experiences in this area can harden the hearts of the wisest and kindest of men and produce vicious reaction in others.

Child neglect

A child may also be harmed by omission. This might be due to unavoidable circumstances, or ignorance or ineptness on the part of his guardians as well as deliberate attempts to hurt or punish him. The children are generally undernourished and undersized, the skin and hair are often in poor condition and they may be dirty and infested. Nasty rashes may be present in those places where the most dirt collects, the skin creases and nappy area.

Sexual misuse or abuse

Sexual abuse, that is a child being involved by an adult in sexual activities that he or she is not old enough to understand, or to give informed consent to, and which breaks the community taboos and expectations, appears to be on the increase. Although there is a notion that such activities happen at the hands of strangers, in fact it is three times more likely to occur within the family or within a circle of trusted friends. The first step is to recognize the problem for what it is, for both the adult and the child involved need expert counselling.

Emotional abuse

It is important to remember that emotional abuse may occur on its own in the form of open hostility, rejection or scapegoating, in which case it is obvious, or it may occur in less obvious ways, for example by not recognising the child's emotional need for affection, security and consistent care. All forms of child abuse and neglect involve emotional abuse. It is always necessary to attend to the emotional needs of abused children.

Deprivation

A child in a repressive atmosphere may appear to be well nourished and clean, but still fail to thrive, his hands and feet may be cold and small, and his growth suppressed. These more subtle forms of negligence or abuse are more difficult to recognise and define. The management as with most of the problems in this chapter includes a thorough clinical evaluation, a detailed enquiry about him, his family life and his neighbourhood, and a programme of care which is realistic and accepted by all concerned.

Munchausen syndrome by proxy

This is a bizarre form of child abuse in which one of those who cares for a child, usually the mother, persistently fabricates symptoms and signs such that the child becomes ill or is in danger of, or is subject to, unnecessary investigations and treatment. The diagnosis should be considered in any child whose illness is unexplained and prolonged or extraordinary in some way; when the child's signs and symptoms seem particularly inappropriate or incongruous, or only occur when the parent is present. It should also be suspected when treatments are surprisingly ineffective or not well tolerated. As in other instances of child abuse the parent may be inappropriately concerned, or alternatively not concerned about the severity of the child's supposed problems, or they may in some way benefit from the child's illness by way of support, attention or money.

Making a firm diagnosis can be difficult. There is no alternative to taking a clear history, particularly noting the time and place of the events described, and then making enquiries from others for supporting evidence. This means seeking information from other members of the family and other health professionals concerned with the child's care. If the diagnosis is suspected, it is important that the child and the parent be observed carefully. Perhaps the easiest way of making the diagnosis is to see if the signs and symptoms disappear when the parents are excluded.

Management can be difficult and it is vital for the child's sake for it to be firm and determined. This will involve case conferences and may mean keeping the child in a place of safety at least in the short term until the situation has been clarified.

BIBLIOGRAPHY

Graham P 1991 Child psychiatry: a developmental approach. Oxford University Press, Oxford
Rutter M, Hersov L 1985 Child and adolescent psychiatry. Blackwell Scientific Publications, Oxford

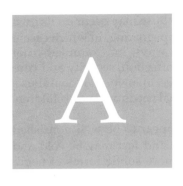

A Essential Paediatric Formulary

The range of drugs regularly prescribed in general paediatric practice is considerably more limited than in adult medicine. This therapeutic caution is well founded. The pattern of many childhood disorders is short-lived and self-limiting, and does not justify drug therapy. Many common disorders are amenable to long established agents with a low incidence of side-effects. Simple measures, such as the use of glucose-electrolyte solution in gastroenteritis, make an enormous contribution to child health. On the other hand, casual use of anti-emetics and anti-diarrhoeal agents is indefensible. The prescribing habits of a doctor not only determine future demand for drug intervention, but also modify parental attitudes to their child's health.

The efficacy of a drug depends on the doctor selecting an appropriate preparation, calculating the correct dosage, and motivating the family to ensure regular administration. Infancy raises problems of immaturity of absorption, transport, enzymatic biotransformation and excretion. Drug dynamics may be profoundly altered in preterm infants reflecting not only immaturity but also altered body fluid compartments. The awareness of altered drug metabolism in young children has resulted in more restricted licensing of newly introduced drugs. The ethical and practical problems of drug trials add to this restraint. Paradoxically these same restraints may delay studies which bring to light side-effects in older established drugs. Fortunately carefully designed multi-centre studies have enabled certain paediatric subspecialities, such as oncology, to move rapidly ahead in the introduction of complex but effective drug regimens.

Selecting an acceptable oral preparation for a miserable child is usually dictated by finding a palatable liquid preparation. The formulary provides a useful range of these; the majority contain a convenient children's dose in a 5 ml spoonful. The British National Formulary (BNF) recommends that smaller doses be diluted so that they also match a 5 ml spoonful. Liquids containing sucrose promote dental caries and should be avoided for long-term use. Colouring agents are also coming under critical review.

Drug dosage in children is a potentially complex topic but, for most drugs, readily available guidance is based on either age or body weight.

Age-related doses are appropriate when prescribing commonly used drugs with high therapeutic indices to average-sized children. Body weight calculations are also convenient but tend to underestimate dosage in infancy, and overestimate dosage in older or obese children. Body surface area measurements are less amenable but have a closer relationship to physiological functions which influence drug effects. Again caution is required in the immature infant with a disproportionately large surface area. The percentage method, derived from surface area, provides a simple scheme for calculating dose as a percentage of an adult dose.

Faced with these contrasting methods the wise doctor will not hesitate to reach for a reliable formulary rather than rely on a fallable memory. He must also be obsessionally careful about providing correct instructions for critically dose-dependent drugs such as digoxin.

This list has been selected from the British National Formulary to reflect drugs most commonly prescribed in our department. It does not encompass drugs used in specialised branches of paediatrics. It aims to provide an easily accessible guide to rational prescribing in childhood but is definitely not an alternative to more comprehensive formularies.

Abbreviations

I	indications
CI	contraindications
SE	side-effects
S/F	sugar-free liquid
S/R	slow release

GASTROINTESTINAL SYSTEM

ANTACIDS

Gaviscon	I		Gastro-oesophageal reflux
	CI		Prematurity, impaired renal function
	SE		Gastric distension
Sachets – Infant			1/2–1 sachet with feed
Liquid – child			5–10 ml after meals

ANTISPASMODICS

Dicyclomine	I		Smooth muscle spasm, e.g. of bowel
	CI		Infants under age 6 months
	SE		Respiratory irregularity, dry mouth, thirst, dizziness
Syrup 10 mg/5 ml		6–24 months	5–10 mg before feeds (max 40 mg/day)
Tabs 10 mg		2–12 years	10 mg 3 times daily

ULCER-HEALING

Cimetidine	I		Peptic ulcer. Gastro-oesophageal reflux
	CI		—
	SE		Rare reversible liver damage
Syrup 200 mg/5 ml			20–40 mg/kg/day in 3–4 doses
Tabs 200 mg			

ANTIDIARRHOEAL

Loperamide	I		Prolonged non-specific diarrhoea
	CI		Infective gastroenteritis
	SE		Occasional rashes
S/F syrup 1 mg/5 ml		2–5 years	1 mg 3 times daily
Capsules 2 mg		6–12 years	2 mg 3 times daily

LAXATIVES
Stimulant
Senna

	I	Chronic constipation
	CI	Undiagnosed abdominal pain
	SE	Mild discomfort

Syrup 7.5 mg/5 ml   5–20 ml once daily

Softener
Dioctyl/sodium sulphosuccinate
Paed syrup   12.5–25 mg 3 times daily
12.5 mg/5 ml

Osmotic
Lactulose

Elixir 3.35 mg/5 ml	Under 1 year	2.5 ml twice daily
	1–5 years	5 ml twice daily
	6–12 years	10 ml twice daily

PANCREATIN REPLACEMENT
Pancreatin

	I	Pancreatic exocrine failure
	CI	–
	SE	Anal irritation

Creon capsules containing
enteric-coated granules   5–15 capsules daily with meals

CARDIOVASCULAR SYSTEM

CARDIAC GLYCOSIDE
Digoxin

	I	Heart failure, supraventricular arrhythmias
	CI	Hypokalaemia
	SE	Vomiting, bradycardia, arrhythmias

Elixir PG 50 μg/ml   5–10 μg/kg/day in 2 doses
Tabs PG 62.5 μg
Tabs 125, 250 μg

DIURETICS
Frusemide

	I	Fluid overload, hypertension
	CI	Liver failure
	SE	Rashes, electrolyte imbalance

S/F liquid 1 mg/ml   1–3 mg/kg/day in 2 doses
Tabs 20, 40 mg

Spironolactone

	I	Fluid overload in liver failure
	CI	Hyperkalaemia
	SE	GIT upset, gynaecomastia

S/F liquid – various
Tabs 25 mg   1–3 mg/kg/day

BETA-ADRENOCEPTOR BLOCKING DRUGS
Propranolol

	I	Hypertension, supraventricular arrhythmias, thyrotoxicosis
	CI	Cardiac failure, asthma
	SE	Cardiac failure

S/F liquid 5 mg/5 ml
Tabs 10, 40 mg   1 mg/kg three times daily

RESPIRATORY SYSTEM

BRONCHODILATORS

Beta₂ adrenoreceptor	I		Reversible asthma
stimulants	CI		—
	SE		Tremor, headaches, tachycardia

Salbutamol

S/F syrup 2 mg/5 ml	2–5 years	1–2 mg 3–4 times daily
S/R tabs 4 mg	3–12 years	4 mg 1–2 times daily
Aerosol 100 µg/puff		1–2 puffs 3–4 times daily max 4 hourly
Rotacaps 200 µg		200 µg 3–4 times daily max 4 hourly
Ventodisks 200 µg		
Nebulised solution 2.5 mg/2.5 ml		2.5–5 mg max 4 hourly

Terbutaline

S/F syrup 1.5 mg/5 ml	3–7 years	0.75–1.5 mg 3 times daily
Aerosol 250 µg/puff		1 puff 3–4 times daily
Powder inhalation		1 puff 3–4 times daily
500 µg/puff		

Xanthine bronchodilators	I		Reversible asthma
	CI		Tachycardia
	SE		Tachycardia, vomiting, irritability, headache (measure plasma levels)

Theophylline

Capsules containing		
S/R granules	2–6 years	60–120 mg 12 hourly
60, 125, 250 mg	7–12 years	125–250 mg 12 hourly

ANTI-ALLERGY

Inhaled corticosteroids	I		Asthma
	CI		—
	SE		Oral candidiasis

Beclomethasone

Inhaler 50 µg/puff	50–100 µg 2–4 times daily
Rotacaps 100 µg	100 µg 2–4 times daily

Budenoside

Inhaler 50 µg/puff	50–200 µg 2 times daily

Prophylactic drugs	I		Asthma
	CI		—
	SE		Upper airway irritation

Sodium cromoglycate

Inhaler 5 mg/puff	5 mg 4 times daily
Spincaps 20 mg	20 mg 4–6 times daily
Nebulizer 20 mg/2 ml	20 mg 4–6 times daily

Antihistamines	I		Hayfever, urticaria, emergency treatment of anaphylaxis
	CI		Caution in epilepsy
	SE		Sedation, dry mouth

Chlorpheniramine

Tabs 4 mg	1–5 years	1–2 mg 3 times daily
Syrup 2 mg/5 ml	6–12 years	2–4 mg 3 times daily

Promethazine HCl

Tabs 10, 25 mg	6–12 months	5–10 mg at night
Syrup 5 mg/5 ml	1–5 years	5–15 mg at night
	6–12 years	10–25 mg at night

Terfanidine

Suspension 30 mg/5 ml	I	Non-sedative
Tabs 60 mg	6–12 years	30 mg twice daily

CENTRAL NERVOUS SYSTEM

HYPNOTICS, SEDATIVES

Chloral	I	Sedation
	CI	Airways obstruction
	SE	GIT upsets, rashes
Elixir paediatric 200 mg/5 ml		30–50 mg/kg at night
Trimeprazine	I	Sleep disturbance with pruritus
	CI	Epilepsy, infants under 6 months
	SE	Paradoxical stimulation
Syrup 7.5 mg/5 ml Syrup forte 30 mg/5 ml		3 mg/kg at night

ANALGESICS/ANTIPYRETICS

Paracetamol	I	Mild to moderate pain, pyrexia
	CI	Hepatic impairment
	SE	Liver damage in overdosage
S/F elixir 120 mg/5 ml	0–1 years	60–120 mg 4–6 hourly
Tabs 500 mg	1–5 years	120–250 mg 4–6 hourly
	6–12 years	250–500 mg 4–6 hourly
Ibuprofen	I	Pain, inflammation, pyrexia
	CI	GIT bleeding
	SE	GIT symptoms, rashes
S/F syrup 100 mg/5 ml Tab 200 mg		10–20 mg/kg/day

ANTIEPILEPTICS

Sodium valproate	I	All epilepsies
	CI	Hepatic impairment
	SE	GIT symptoms, lethargy, weight gain, thrombocytopenia, liver toxicity, pancreatitis
Tabs 100, 200, 500 mg S/F elixir 200 mg/5 ml		20–40 mg/kg/day divided doses
Carbamazepine	I	Partial epilepsies
	CI	Hepatic impairment
	SE	Lethargy, dizziness, transient rash, rare marrow, liver toxicity
Tab 100, 200 mg S/R tab 200, 400 mg S/F syrup 100 mg/5 ml		10–20 mg/kg/day
Phenobarbitone	I	Short-term seizure control, e.g. encephalopathy
	CI	Acute intermittent porphyria
	SE	Lethargy, behaviour disturbance, rashes
Tabs 15, 30, 60, 100 mg S/F elixir 15 mg/5 ml Injection 200 mg/ml		Loading dose i.v. 15–20 mg/kg once Maintenance i.v./oral 5–10 mg/kg/day
Phenytoin	I	All epilepsies except absence seizures
	CI	Hepatic impairment
	SE	Nausea, ataxia, gum hypertrophy, rashes, facial coarsening, haematological effects, rickets
Phenytoin sodium Tabs 25, 50, 100 mg Phenytoin base susp 30 mg/5 ml		4–8 mg/kg day
Ethosuximide	I	Absence seizures
	CI	Hepatic impairment
	SE	Nausea, headaches, rashes, bone marrow depression
Caps 250 mg Syrup 250 mg/5 ml		20–40 mg/kg/day

Clonazepam	I	Myoclonic seizures
	CI	—
	SE	Drowsiness, salivation
Tabs 500 µg, 2 mg		50–200 µg/kg/day. Gradual introduction recommended

DRUGS USED IN STATUS EPILEPTICUS

Diazepam	I	Status epilepticus
	CI	—
	SE	Respiratory depression, venous thrombophlebitis at injection site (minimised by using an emulsion)
Injection 5 mg/ml	Slow i.v.	200–300 µg/kg
Rectal tube 5, 10 mg	1–3 years	5 mg
	Over 3 years	10 mg

Paraldehyde	I	Status epilepticus
	CI	Hepatic impairment
	SE	Sterile abscesses, rashes
Injection 5, 10 ml ampoule	Deep i.m.	0.1 ml/kg to max 5 ml

JOINT DISEASE

ANTI-INFLAMMATORY

Ibuprofen	I	Juvenile chronic polyarthritis
	CI	GIT bleeding
	SE	Mild GIT symptoms, rashes
Syrup 100 mg/5 ml	Child	10–40 mg/kg/day
Tabs 200 mg	Max.	500 mg/day in child under 30 kg

Naproxen	I	Juvenile chronic polyarthritis
	CI	GIT bleeding
	SE	GIT symptoms
Suspension 125 mg/5 ml		
Tabs 250 mg		5 mg/kg twice daily

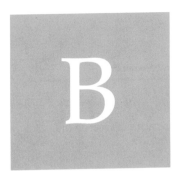

Normal Values

CLINICAL CHEMISTRY

These values are offered as a guide only. Local laboraties may differ. Check normal values with the laboratory you use. For less common tests check with your local laboratory.

Acid–base	pH 7.3–7.45 PCO_2 4.5–6 kPA (32–45 mmHg) PO_2 11–14 kPA (78–105 mmHg) Bicarbonate 18–25 mmol/l Base excess -4 to +3 mmol/l
Alanine amino- transferase (ALT)	Newborn–1 month up to 70 iu/l; infants and children 15–55 iu/l
Albumin	Preterm 25–45 g/l; newborn (term) 25–50 g/l; 1–3 months 30–42 g/l; 3–12 months 27–50 g/l; 1–15 years 32–50 g/l
Alkaline phosphatase	Newborn: 150–600 u/l; 6 months–9 years: 250–800 u/l
Ammonia	Newborn < 80 μmol/l; infants and children < 50 μmol/l
Amylase	70–300 iu/l
Aspartate amino- transferase (AST)	<45 iu/l
Base excess	See acid–base
Bicarbonate	See acid–base
Bilirubin	Full term day 1 < 65 μmol/l; day 2 < 115 μmol/l; 3–5 days < 155 μmol/l; > 1 month < 10 μmol/l
Calcium (ionised)	Adult value is 1.19–1.29 mmol/l
Calcium (total)	Preterm 1.5–2.5 mmol/l; infants 2.25–2.75 mmol/l; > 1 year 2.25–2.6 mmol/l; correction for protein binding—measure Ca^{2+} + (40 - albumin/40 g/l) mmol/l
Calcium (urine)	Children < 0.1 mmol/kg per 24 hours
Chloride	95–105 mmol/l
Creatine kinase	Newborn < 600 iu/l; 1 month < 400 iu/l; 1 year < 300 iu/l; children < 190 iu/l (male), < 130 iu/l (female)
Creatinine	0–2 years 20–50 μmol/l; 2–6 years 25–60 μmol/l; 6–12 years 30–80 μmol/l; >12 years 65–120 μmol/l (male), 50–110 μmol/l (female)
Creatinine clearance	0–3 months 17–50 ml/min/m²; 3–12 months 26–75 ml/min/m²; 12–18 months 36–95 ml/min/m²; 2 years–adult 50–85 ml/min/m²

Creatinine (calculation of GFR from serum level)	GFR = (49.5 × ht (cm))/plasma creatinine (µmol/l)
C-reactive protein	< 20 mg/l
Gammaglutaryl transferase (GGT)	Neonate < 200 iu/l; 1 month–1 year < 150 iu/l; > 1 year < 30 iu/l
Glucose	Newborn—3 days 2–5 mmol/l; > 1 week 2.5–5 mmol/l
Glycosylated haemoglobin	4.5–7.5%
Lactate	0.7–1.8 mmol/l
Liver function	see Bilirubin, AST, GGT and Protein
Magnesium	Newborn 0.7–1.2 mmol/l; child 0.7–1.0 mmol/l
Osmolality	275–295 mmol/kg
Phosphate	Preterm first month 1.4–3.4 mmol/l; full term newborn 1.2–2.9 mmol/l; 1 year 1.2–2.2 mmol/l; 2–10 years 1.0–1.8 mmol/l; > 10 years 0.7–1.6 mmol/l
Potassium	0–2 weeks 3.7–6 mmol/l; 2 weeks–3 months 3.7–5.7 mmol/l; > 3 months 3.5–5 mmol/l
Protein (total)	1 month 50–70 g/l; 1 year 60–80 g/l; 1–9 years 60–81 g/l
Sodium	135–145 mmol/l
Urea	0–1 year 2.5–7.5 mmol/l; 1–7 years 3.3–6.5 mmol/l; 7–16 years 2.6–6.7 mmol/l (male), 2.5–6.0 mmol/l (female)

HAEMATOLOGY

Normal haematological indices for various ages

Age	Hb (g/dl) Mean (range)	MCV (fl) Mean (range)	WBC (× 10⁹/l) Range	Reticulocyte (%) Range
Birth	18.5 (14.5–21.5)	108 (95–116)	5–26	3–7
1 month	14.0 (10.0–16.5)	104 (85–108)	6–15	0–1
6 months	11.0 (8.5–13.5)	88 (80–96)	6–15	0–1
1 year	12.0 (10.5–13.5)	78 (70–86)	6–15	0–1
6 years	12.5 (11.5–14.0)	81 (75–88)	6–15	0–1
12 years	13.5 (11.5–14.5)	86 (77–94)	5–15	0–1

Note: an artefactual high neonatal WBC may be reported because automatic cell counters may wrongly include in the WBC the many normoblasts (red cell precursors) in the neonate.

Blood pressure

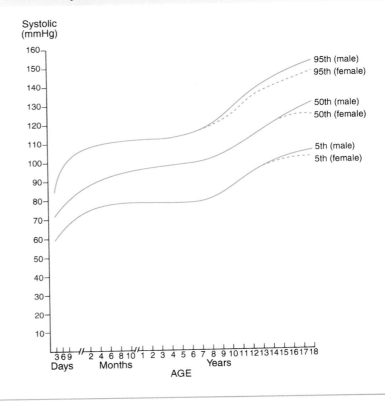

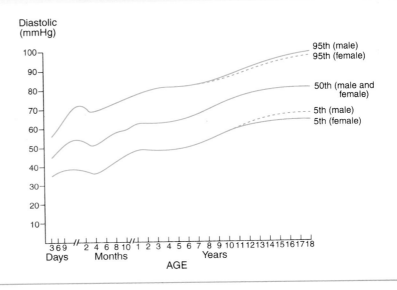

CALCULATING THE BODY SURFACE AREA FROM HEIGHT AND WEIGHT

Nomogram

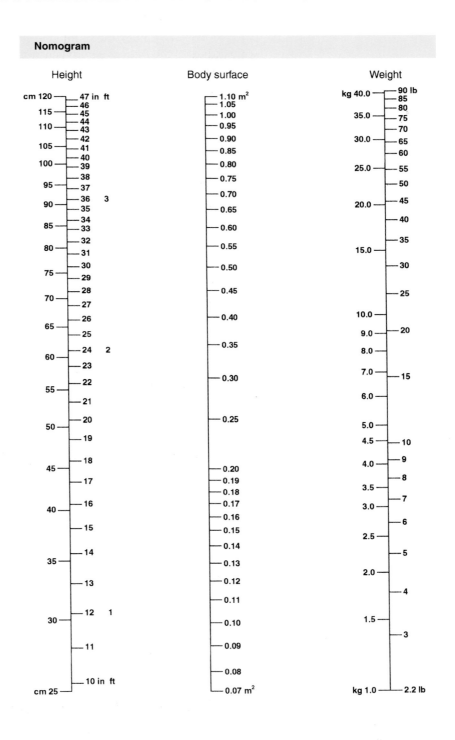

Height	Body surface	Weight

The nomogram may be used to calculate the body surface area from the weight and height of the patient. Note the patient's height on the left-hand scale and weight on the right-hand scale, and put a rule between the two points; the point at which the line intersects the centre scale indicates the patient's body surface area.

Surface area and weight

	Weight (kg)	Surface area (m²)
Newborn	3	0.2
1 year	10	0.5
3 years	15	0.6
5 years	20	0.7
9 years	30	1.0
14 years	50	1.5
Adult	70	1.7

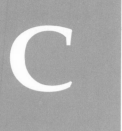

Immunisation Schedule (UK)

National Immunization Schedule (subject to usual contraindications)

INFANT

Birth	BCG for babies in Asian and other immigrant families with high TB rates and those in contact with active respiratory tuberculosis
2 months	Polio + diphtheria/tetanus/pertussis (DTP) + haemophilus influenzae B (HIB)
3 months	Polio + DTP + HIB
4 months	Polio + DTP + HIB
12 – 18 mths	Combined measles, mumps, and rubella (MMR) or measles (preferably at 15 months)
12 – 48 mths	HIB if not given before

PRE-SCHOOL

4 – 5 years	MMR, if not previously given, + polio + diphtheria/tetanus booster

SECONDARY SCHOOL

10 – 14 years	Heaf or Mantoux and, if negative, BCG
10 – 14 years	Rubella (girls only)

SCHOOL LEAVING

15 – 19 years	Polio + tetanus

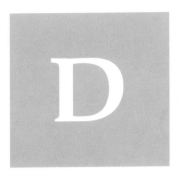

Child Health Surveillence Programme

The following is taken from *Health for All Children* edited by Dr David Hall.

THE CORE PROGRAMME

The core programme of surveillance for all children incorporates those screening procedures (<u>underlined</u>) which can be supported in the light of the available evidence. It consists of a series of checks and reviews which, it is hoped, will strike a balance between the risk of 'missing' children with problems on the one hand, while on the other avoiding an excessive number of examinations. In individual cases, parental concern or professional judgement may dictate that the child is seen on more or different occasions. In a minority of families, more intensive support and guidance may be needed.

No two primary care teams will function in exactly the same way and it would not be appropriate to specify rigid rules regarding the delivery of the Child Health Surveillance programme. Nevertheless, each of the key examinations has a different content and purpose and it seems reasonable to suggest which members of the primary care team might be responsible for them.

The following summary of the recommended programme:
* incorporates details of the specified health checks and immunisations;
* gives examples of topics for health education at different ages;
* stresses the importance of record systems that facilitate communication, clinical audit and epidemiological monitoring.

Consideration should always be given to social and psychological aspects of family life, whatever the nature of the examination or review. Housing and financial problems, parental depression and illness, and difficulties with siblings, are all relevant to the health and development of the individual child.

Neonatal examination

This should usually be the responsibility of suitably trained hospital staff, but should be the responsibility of the primary care team in the case of home deliveries, babies born in GP obstetric units, and very early (<6 hours) discharges.

It consists of:

Elicit and consider any concerns expressed by parents. Review of family history, pregnancy and birth. <u>Full physical examination including weight and head circumference.</u> <u>Check for congenital dislocation of hips (CDH) and testicular descent. Inspect eyes, view red reflex of fundus with ophthalmoscope</u> but do not attempt fundoscopy. If <u>high risk category</u> for hearing defect, consider <u>otoacoustic emissions (OAE) or brainstem evoked response (BSER)</u> test of hearing. <u>PKU and thyroid</u> tests to be done at usual time. Haemoglobinopathy screen if specified in local policy.

Completion of record sheet; preferably in Parent Held Record.

Topics for Health Education could include: Feeding and nutrition; baby care, sibling management; crying and sleep problems; transport in cars.

First 2 weeks

Many GPs consider it good practice to visit all new babies as soon as possible after discharge from hospital. This provides an opportunity to evaluate any concerns raised by the parents, and to cement the relationship with the family. In addition to the immediate benefits, this contact can be the prelude to an effective programme of surveillance and helps the members of the primary care team to estimate the level of support and assistance that each new parent is likely to require. Further physical examination should be undertaken if appropriate. Check <u>hips</u> again (this may be done by either a doctor or a nurse, <u>provided that</u> the person is adequately trained).

Topics for Health Education could include: Nutrition; supine sleeping position and clothing; effects of passive smoking; accident prevention — bathing, scalding by feeds, fires; immunisation; reason for doing PKU and thyroid tests (and haemoglobinopathy if indicated).

6–8 weeks

This examination should be undertaken by the doctor responsible for the child's surveillance. The presence of the health visitor facilitates the sharing and follow-up of any anxieties. The examination may be undertaken at the same visit as the first immunisation and/or the post-natal check for the mother; this is a matter for individual practices to decide.

It consists of:

Check history and ask about parental concerns. <u>Physical examination, weight and head circumference (± length if indicated). Check for CDH.</u> Enquire particularly about concerns regarding vision, squint and hearing. <u>Inspect eyes.</u> Do not attempt hearing test (there is no simple clinical test of hearing suitable for primary care use in this age group). If a high-risk hearing screening service is provided, check again whether baby is in <u>high risk category for hearing loss</u> and refer if necessary. Give parents check list of advice for detection of hearing loss ('Hints for Parents'), or draw parents' attention to relevant information in Parent Held Record.

Discuss immunisation; signed consent is NOT essential, but should be obtained at this visit if thought desirable by individual practitioners.

Complete the record and ensure information is transferred to the agency responsible for monitoring the CHS programme (FHSA/Health Authority/Health Board).

Topics for Health Education could include: Immunisation; nutrition; dangers of fires, falls, overheating and scalds; recognition of illness in babies and what to do.

2, 3 and 4 months

The baby should receive the primary course of immunisations at these ages. No specific checks are required, but the parent should have the opportunity to discuss any concerns with the appropriate member of the primary health care team.

Weighing in the first 6 months: Regular weighing of normal healthy babies is of uncertain value. There is no doubt that parents value this procedure because of the reassurance it gives them that all is well, but health professionals should be aware of both the unnecessary anxiety and the false sense of security it can provide.

Facilities for weighing should be available as part of a Child Health Surveillance service. The parent(s) should be encouraged to weigh the baby themselves, if they so wish.

6–9 months

This examination can be regarded as primarily the health visitor's responsibility, provided that the essential items of physical examination are undertaken (on an opportunistic basis if necessary); or it can be undertaken by the health visitor working together with the doctor.

Enquire about parental concerns regarding health and development. Ask specifically about vision and hearing. Check weight if parents request or if indicated. Measure length if indicated. Look for evidence of <u>CDH</u>. Check for <u>testicular descent</u>. Observe visual behaviour and look for squint. Carry out <u>distraction test of hearing</u>. NB TWO adequately trained staff, and adequate testing conditions, are essential for this test.

Complete the record and ensure information is transferred to the agency responsible for monitoring the CHS programme.

Topics for Health Education could include: Accident prevention: choking, scalds and burns, falls, anticipate increasing mobility, i.e. safety gates, guards, etc; nutrition; dental prophylaxis; reinforce advice about safety in cars and passive smoking; developmental needs; sunburn.

18–24 months

This review does not involve any specific medical screening procedures and is concerned primarily with parental guidance and education. It is often carried out at the family home and it is suggested that the health visitor is the most appropriate person to take responsibility for this examination. The doctor provides support and advice where necessary. In some families however, opportunistic review by the doctor may be desirable, for example where the health visitor experiences difficulty in contacting the family at home.

The amount of time devoted to this review in each case should be decided on the basis of the primary care team's overall knowledge of the child and family.

The content of the review is as follows:

Enquire about parental concerns, particularly regarding behaviour, vision and hearing Confirm that child is <u>walking with normal gait;</u> and that speech production and comprehension are appropriate for age. Do not attempt formal tests of vision, hearing or language development. Arrange detailed assessment if in doubt. Remember high prevalence of iron deficiency anaemia at this age. Carry out <u>Hb estimation</u> if local policy. Measure <u>length or height</u> IF child is sufficiently cooperative for accurate measurement.

Complete the record and ensure information is transferred to the agency responsible for monitoring the CHS programme.

Topics for Health Education could include: Accident prevention: falls from heights including windows, drowning, poisoning, road safety; developmental needs: language and play need to mix with other children — playgroup, etc; avoidance and management of behaviour problems.

Special needs of children and the Education Act 1981 The Education Act of 1981 requires the Health Authority to notify the Local Education Authority if it believes that a child has, or may have, Special Educational Needs, when the child reaches the age of 2 years (or sooner than this if the parents so wish). The primary care team should ensure that the specialist paediatric services are informed if there is ANY anxiety about a child's educational potential, so that the doctor with responsibility for liaison with the Education Authority can arrange the notification. This provision of the Act was designed to ensure that children and parents benefit from the expertise of specialist teachers in the pre-school years, and deserves the support of all professionals.

36–48 months

This can be regarded as a 'school readiness examination'. The aims are to ensure that the child is physically fit and that there are no medical disorders or defects which may interfere with education; that the immunisations are up to date; and to determine whether there are problems with development, language, or behaviour which may have educational implications. The review can be shared between health visitor and doctor, on a single occasion. Alternatively, the health visitor can carry out a general progress review and the doctor can undertake the physical examination on a separate occasion, perhaps in combination with the pre-school booster. (The latter can be given at any time once 2 years have elapsed from the last of the three primary immunisations.) The review consists of:

Enquiry and discussion about vision, squint, hearing, behaviour, language acquisition and development. If any concerns, discuss with the parent whether the child is likely have any special educational problems or needs and arrange further action as appropriate.

Measure <u>height</u> and plot on chart. Check for <u>testicular descent and heart abnormalities</u> (if not checked on any other occasion since 8 months — these checks are often done on an opportunistic basis). If concerned about possible hearing impairment, perform hearing test <u>IF</u> adequately trained and equipped, otherwise refer.

Complete the record and ensure information is transferred to the agency responsible for monitoring the CHS programme.

Topics for Health Education could include: Accidents: fires, roads, drowning; begin to teach road safety; preparation for school; nutrition and dental care.

5 years (school entry — range approximately 54 – 66 months)
The school entrant medical examination is undertaken by the staff of the School Health Service, and a detailed review of this subject is not relevant to primary care teams.

Some authorities believe that ALL school entrants should be offered not only a physical examination but also a full developmental evaluation. However, in many Districts and Boards, the universal 'cohort' examination of all school entrants has been discontinued, because the yield of new abnormalities is small. Only selected children are examined, on the basis of previously inadequate or poorly documented pre-school surveillance, or concerns raised by parents or teachers.

Whichever policy is adopted, it seems likely that a well-conducted pre-school surveillance programme, as outlined above, will progressively reduce the need for, and the yield of, detailed school entrant examinations. For ALL children the following are recommended at school entry:

Enquire about parental and teacher concerns. Review pre-school records, including immunisation status. Measure <u>height</u> and plot on chart. Check <u>vision</u> using Snellen chart. Check hearing by <u>'sweep'</u> test.

Complete the record and ensure information is transferred to the agency responsible for monitoring the CHS programme.

In many schools these checks are combined in a health interview in which the opportunity is taken to provide health education relevant to school health. The school nurse may be solely responsible for this task or may share it with the school doctor.

Index

puberty 234–8
    delayed 228, 237–8
    precocious 236
pulmonary
    haemorrhage 60
    hypertension 139–40
    hypoplasia 65
    stenosis 143–4
    tuberculosis 102–3
    see also lungs
purpura
    Henoch Schönlein 184–5, 262–3
    immune thrombocytopenic 42, 204–5
pyloric stenosis 82
pyruvate kinase deficiency 200

R

radiotherapy 209
    cranial, and disordered puberty 237
rashes 84–5, 252–3
reading retardation 315
Refsum disease 291
regression 327
renal
    agenesis 178
    disease, fetal 34
    dysplasia 178
    failure, acute 187–9
    failure, chronic 189–90
    function tests 176–8
    hypoplasia 178
    tract infection 157
    tubular disorders 187
    tumours 218–19
    see also kidneys
respiratory distress syndrome 52, 59–60
    preterm infants 55
respiratory syncytial virus infection
        120–21
respiratory system
    at birth 49–50
    disorders 117–29
    drugs 341
    examination 6
    problems, neonates 58–61
    respiratory rates, normal 117
resuscitation, neonate 51–2
retinoblastoma 27, 221
retinopathy
    diabetic 249
    of prematurity 56
Reye syndrome 171–2, 278–9
rhabdomyosarcoma 218
rhesus haemolytic disease 36
rhesus incompatibility 62–3
rheumatic fever 150
rhythmic behaviour 327
rickets 85–6

ringworm 255–6
Ritter disease 255
road traffic accidents 108, 109
roseola infantum (exanthum subitum) 98
roundworm 166
rubella (German measles) 38, 92–3
Russell-Silver syndrome 228

S

sacrococcygeal teratoma, congenital 220
sarcomas, soft tissue 218
scabies 256
scalded skin syndrome 255
scalds 111
scarlet fever 101
school 325
    behaviour problems 327–9
scoliosis 266–7
scurvy 85
septic spots 72
sexual abuse 182, 336
sexual differentiation, disorders 238–9
short stature 225–31
sinusitis 119
skin 251–60
    congenital lesions 257–8
    fold thickness 88–9
    infections 254–6
    infestations 256
    tags, accessory 46
skull
    asymmetrical 224
    fractures 109–10
    growth 223–4
sleep problems 326
small bowel obstruction 65
small-for-dates infants 54
smoking
    by children 115
    effect on fetus 37
social factors
    abuse 9
    deprivation 324–5
    growth 228
    infant death 10
    small-for-dates infants 54
soft tissue sarcomas 218
spasms, infantile 280
spasticity 291–2
speech 299–301
    delay 315–16
    disorder syndrome 300
spherocytosis, hereditary 63, 199
spina bifida cystica 67–9
spina bifida occulta 69
spine
    scoliosis 266–7
    tumours 217–18